AF768323

PROGRESS IN CLINICAL AND BIOLOGICAL RESEARCH

Series Editors

Nathan Back, Vincent P. Eijsvoogel, Kurt Hirschhorn, Sidney Udenfriend, George J. Brewer, Robert Grover, Seymour S. Kety, Jonathan W. Uhr

RECENT TITLES

Vol 278: **Advances in Cancer Control: Cancer Control Research and the Emergence of the Oncology Product Line,** Paul F. Engstrom, Paul N. Anderson, Lee E. Mortenson, *Editors*

Vol 279: **Basic and Clinical Perspectives of Colorectal Polyps and Cancer,** Glenn Steele, Jr., Randall W. Burt, Sidney J. Winawer, James P. Karr, *Editors*

Vol 280: **Plant Flavonoids in Biology and Medicine II: Biochemical, Cellular, and Medicinal Properties,** Vivian Cody, Elliott Middleton, Jr., Jeffrey B. Harborne, Alain Beretz, *Editors*

Vol 281: **Transplacental Effects on Fetal Health,** Dante G. Scarpelli, George Migaki, *Editors*

Vol 282: **Biological Membranes: Aberrations in Membrane Structure and Function,** Manfred L. Karnovsky, Alexander Leaf, Liana C. Bolis, *Editors*

Vol 283: **Platelet Membrane Receptors: Molecular Biology, Immunology, Biochemistry, and Pathology,** G.A. Jamieson, *Editor*

Vol 284: **Cellular Factors in Development and Differentiation: Embryos, Teratocarcinomas, and Differentiated Tissues,** Stephen E. Harris, Per-Erik Mansson, *Editors*

Vol 285: **Non-Radiometric Assays: Technology and Application in Polypeptide and Steroid Hormone Detection,** Barry D. Albertson, Florence P. Haseltine, *Editors*

Vol 286: **Molecular and Cellular Mechanisms of Septic Shock,** Bryan L. Roth, Thor B. Nielsen, Adam E. McKee, *Editors*

Vol 287: **Dietary Restriction and Aging,** David L. Snyder, *Editor*

Vol 288: **Immunity to Cancer. II,** Malcolm S. Mitchell, *Editor*

Vol 289: **Computer-Assisted Modeling of Receptor–Ligand Interactions: Theoretical Aspects and Applications to Drug Design,** Robert Rein, Amram Golombek, *Editors*

Vol 290: **Enzymology and Molecular Biology of Carbonyl Metabolism 2: Aldehyde Dehydrogenase, Alcohol Dehydrogenase, and Aldo-Keto Reductase,** Henry Weiner, T. Geoffrey Flynn, *Editors*

Vol 291: **QSAR: Quantitative Structure-Activity Relationships in Drug Design,** J.L. Fauchère, *Editor*

Vol 292: **Biological and Synthetic Membranes,** D. Allan Butterfield, *Editor*

Vol 293: **Advances in Cancer Control: Innovations and Research,** Paul N. Anderson, Paul F. Engstrom, Lee E. Mortenson, *Editors*

Vol 294: **Development of Preimplantation Embryos and Their Environment,** Koji Yoshinaga, Takahide Mori, *Editors*

Vol 295: **Cells and Tissues: A Three-Dimensional Approach by Modern Techniques in Microscopy,** Pietro M. Motta, *Editor*

Vol 296: **Developments in Ultrastructure of Reproduction,** Pietro M. Motta, *Editor*

Vol 297: **Biochemistry of the Acute Allergic Reactions: Fifth International Symposium,** Alfred I. Tauber, Bruce U. Wintroub, Arlene Stolper Simon, *Editors*

Vol 298: **Skin Carcinogenesis: Mechanisms and Human Relevance,** Thomas J. Slaga, Andre J.P. Klein-Szanto, R.K. Boutwell, Donald E. Stevenson, Hugh L. Spitzer, Bob D'Amato, *Editors*

Vol 299: **Perspectives in Shock Research: Metabolism, Immunology, Mediators, and Models,** John C. Passmore, *Editor,* Sherwood M. Reichard, David G. Reynolds, Daniel L. Traber, *Co-Editors*

Vol 300: **Alpha$_1$-Acid Glycoprotein: Genetics, Biochemistry, Physiological Functions, and Pharmacology,** Pierre Baumann, Chin B. Eap, Walter E. Müller, Jean-Paul Tillement, *Editors*

Vol 301: **Prostaglandins in Clinical Research: Cardiovascular System,** Karsten Schrör, Helmut Sinzinger, *Editors*

Vol 302: **Sperm Measures and Reproductive Success: Institute for Health Policy Analysis Forum on Science, Health, and Environmental Risk Assessment,** Edward J. Burger, Jr., Robert G. Tardiff, Anthony R. Scialli, Harold Zenick, *Editors*

Vol 303: **Therapeutic Progress in Urological Cancers,** Gerald P. Murphy, Saad Khoury, *Editors*

Vol 304: **The Maillard Reaction in Aging, Diabetes, and Nutrition,** John W. Baynes, Vincent M. Monnier, *Editors*

Vol 305: **Genetics of Kidney Disorders,** Christos S. Bartsocas, *Editor*

Vol 306: **Genetics of Neuromuscular Disorders,** Christos S. Bartsocas, *Editor*

Vol 307: **Recent Advances in Avian Immunology Research,** Balbir S. Bhogal, Guus Koch, *Editors*

Vol 308: **Second Vienna Shock Forum,** Günther Schlag, Heinz Redl, *Editors*

Vol 309: **Advances and Controversies in Thalassemia Therapy: Bone Marrow Transplantation and Other Approaches,** C. Dean Buckner, Robert Peter Gale, Guido Lucarelli, *Editors*

Vol 310: **EORTC Genitourinary Group Monograph 6: BCG in Superficial Bladder Cancer,** Frans M.J. Debruyne, Louis Denis, Ad P.M. van der Meijden, *Editors*

Vol 311: **Molecular and Cytogenetic Studies of Non-Disjunction,** Terry J. Hassold, Charles J. Epstein, *Editors*

Vol 312: **The Ocular Effects of Prostaglandins and Other Eicosanoids,** Laszlo Z. Bito, Johan Stjernschantz, *Editors*

Vol 313: **Malaria and the Red Cell: 2,** John W. Eaton, Steven R. Meshnick, George J. Brewer, *Editors*

Vol 314: **Inherited and Environmentally Induced Retinal Degenerations,** Matthew M. LaVail, Robert E. Anderson, Joe G. Hollyfield, *Editors*

Vol 315: **Muscle Energetics,** Richard J. Paul, Gijs Elzinga, Kazuhiro Yamada, *Editors*

Vol 316: **Hemoglobin Switching,** George Stamatoyannopoulos, Arthur W. Nienhuis, *Editors*. Published in two volumes: Part A: *Transcriptional Regulation*. Part B: *Cellular and Molecular Mechanisms*.

Vol 317: **Alzheimer's Disease and Related Disorders,** Khalid Iqbal, Henryk M. Wisniewski, Bengt Winblad, *Editors*

Vol 318: **Mechanisms of Chromosome Distribution and Aneuploidy,** Michael A. Resnick, Baldev K. Vig, *Editors*

Vol 319: **The Red Cell: Seventh Ann Arbor Conference,** George J. Brewer, *Editor*

Vol 320: **Menopause: Evaluation, Treatment, and Health Concerns,** Charles B. Hammond, Florence P. Haseltine, Isaac Schiff, *Editors*

Vol 321: **Fatty Acid Oxidation: Clinical, Biochemical, and Molecular Aspects,** Kay Tanaka, Paul M. Coates, *Editors*

Vol 322: **Molecular Endocrinology and Steroid Hormone Action,** Gordon H. Sato, James L. Stevens, *Editors*

Vol 323: **Current Concepts in Endometriosis,** Dev R. Chadha, Veasy C. Buttram, Jr., *Editors*

Vol 324: **Recent Advances in Hemophilia Care,** Carol K. Kaspar, *Editor*

Vol 325: **Alcohol, Immunomodulation, and AIDS,** Daniela Seminara, Ronald Ross Watson, Albert Pawlowski, *Editors*

Vol 326: **Nutrition and Aging,** Derek M. Prinsley, Harold H. Sandstead, *Editors*

Vol 327: **Frontiers in Smooth Muscle Research,** Nicholas Sperelakis, Jackie D. Wood, *Editors*

Vol 328: **The International Narcotics Research Conference (INRC) '89,** Rémi Quirion, Khem Jhamandas, Christina Gianoulakis, *Editors*

Please contact publisher for information about previous titles in this series.

ALCOHOL, IMMUNOMODULATION, AND AIDS

ALCOHOL, IMMUNOMODULATION, AND AIDS

Proceedings of the Alcohol-Immunology AIDS Conference Held in Tucson, Arizona, April 27–29, 1989

Editors

Daniela Seminara
National Institute on Alcohol
Abuse and Alcoholism
Rockville, Maryland

Ronald Ross Watson
University of Arizona
Tucson, Arizona

Albert Pawlowski
National Institute on Alcohol
Abuse and Alcoholism
Rockville, Maryland

ALAN R. LISS, INC. • NEW YORK

Address all Inquiries to the Publisher
Alan R. Liss, Inc., 41 East 11th Street, New York, NY 10003

Copyright © 1990 Alan R. Liss, Inc.

Printed in United States of America

Under the conditions stated below the owner of copyright for this book hereby grants permission to users to make photocopy reproductions of any part or all of its contents for personal or internal organizational use, or for personal or internal use of specific clients. This consent is given on the condition that the copier pay the stated per-copy fee through the Copyright Clearance Center, Incorporated, 27 Congress Street, Salem, MA 01970, as listed in the most current issue of "Permissions to Photocopy" (Publisher's Fee List, distributed by CCC, Inc.), for copying beyond that permitted by sections 107 or 108 of the US Copyright Law. This consent does not extend to other kinds of copying, such as copying for general distribution, for advertising or promotional purposes, for creating new collective works, or for resale.

While the authors, editors, and publisher believe that drug selection and dosage and the specifications and usage of equipment and devices, as set forth in this book, are in accord with current recommendations and practice at the time of publication, they accept no legal responsibility for any errors or omissions, and make no warranty, express or implied, with respect to material contained herein. In view of ongoing research, equipment modifications, changes in governmental regulations and the constant flow of information relating to drug therapy, drug reactions and the use of equipment and devices, the reader is urged to review and evaluate the information provided in the package insert or instructions for each drug, piece of equipment or device for, among other things, any changes in the instructions or indications of dosage or usage and for added warnings and precautions.

The publication of this volume was facilitated by the authors and editors who submitted the text in a form suitable for direct reproduction without subsequent editing or proofreading by the publisher.

Library of Congress Cataloging-in-Publication Data

Alcohol-Immunology AIDS Conference (1st : 1989 : Tucson, Ariz.)
Alcohol, immunomodulation, and AIDS : proceedings of the Alcohol-Immunology AIDS Conference, held in Tucson, Arizona, April 27–29, 1989 / editors, Daniela Seminara, Ronald Ross Watson, Albert Pawlowski.
p. cm.—(Progress in clinical and biological research ; v. 325)
Includes bibliographical references.
ISBN 0-471-56215-7
1. AIDS (Disease)—Risk factors—Congresses. 2. Alcoholism— Immunological aspects—Congresses. 3. Alcohol—Physiological effect—Congresses. 4. Immunosuppression—Congresses.
I. Seminara, Daniela. II. Watson, Ronald R. (Ronald Ross) III. Pawlowski, Albert, 1925– . IV. Title. V. Series.
[DNLM: 1. Acquired Immunodeficiency Syndrome—immunology—congresses. 2. Alcohol, Ethyl-adverse effects—congresses. 3. Alcoholism—complications—congresses. 4. Immune System—drug effects—congresses. 5. Immunity—drug effects—congresses. W1 PR66BE v. 325 / WD 308 A354a 1989]
RC607.A26A369 1989
616.97′92071—dc20
DNLM/DLC
for Library of Congress

89-12166
CIP

Contents

Contributors ... **xi**

Preface
Daniela Seminara and Albert Pawlowski ... **xvii**

Acknowledgments ... **xix**

ALCOHOL ABUSE: EPIDEMIOLOGIC AND BEHAVIORAL CHANGES THAT COULD INFLUENCE AIDS

Methodological Issues Concerning the Sensitive Query in AIDS/Alcohol Research: Sample Size Estimates for Randomized Response Procedures
Amanda L. Golbeck and Craig A. Molgaard ... **1**

Alcohol Use and Sexual Risk-Taking Among Adolescents: Methodological Approaches for Addressing Causal Issues
M. Lynne Cooper, Jeremy B. Skinner, and William H. George ... **11**

Preliminary Results on Sexual Risk-Taking in a General Population Sample
Karen Trocki ... **21**

Drinking Patterns and Drinking Problems in a Community Sample of Gay Men
John L. Martin ... **27**

Alcohol and Unsafe Sex: An Overview of Research and Theory
Barbara Critchlow Leigh ... **35**

ALCOHOL AND HIV: NEUROIMMUNOMODULATION

Neuroimmunotoxic Effects in Offspring of Paternal Alcohol Consumption
Ernest L. Abel, Linda S. Hazlett, Richard S. Berk, and Milton G. Mutchnick ... **47**

Interaction Between Alcohol and HIV in the Central Nervous System Detected by the Auditory Brainstem Response: Methodology
Don L. Jewett ... **57**

ALCOHOL, HIV, AND LIVER DISEASES

Human Immunodeficiency Virus and Hepatitis B Virus Infections in Alcoholics
Jeffrey M. Jacobson, Theresa M. Worner, Henry S. Sacks, and Charles S. Lieber ... **67**

Alcohol and Immune System: Role of Gastric Tissue
Salwa A. Elgebaly, Robert A. Kozol, and Donald L. Kreutzer 75

ALCOHOL, DRUGS OF ABUSE, IMMUNOMODULATION, AND AIDS

Suppression by Morphine and Ethanol of Tumor Cell Cytotoxic Activity Released by Macrophages From Retrovirally Infected Mice Upon In Vitro Stimulation by Beta Carotene
Ronald R. Watson and Tuan H. Nguyen 79

The Search for Cofactors in AIDS, Including an Analysis of the Association of Nitrite Inhalant Abuse and Kaposi's Sarcoma
Harry W. Haverkos 93

Alcohol and Immune Function in HIV-1 Seronegative, HTLV-I/II Seronegative and Positive Men on Methadone
Nancy G. Klimas, Robert Morgan, Nancy T. Blaney, Dale Chitwood, J. Bryan Page, Karen Milles, and Mary Ann Fletcher 103

ALCOHOL AND THE IMMUNE SYSTEM NETWORK

Ethanol Modulation of the Effects of Platelet-Activating Factor on Human Platelets and a Macrophage Cell Line
Rodney C. Baker 113

Evaluation of Interferon System Among Chronic Alcoholics
Kailash C. Chadha, Robert B. Whitney, Michael K. Cummings, Marilyn Norman, Michael Windle, and Istvan Stadler 123

The Effect of Ethanol on Signal Transduction in the Rat Alveolar Macrophage
Raymond J. Dorio 135

In Vitro Effects of Ethanol and Acetaldehyde on Cell-Mediated Cytotoxicity
Amrik S. Walia and E.W. Lamon 145

Effects of Various Alcohols Applied In Vitro on Human Lymphocyte Subtypes and Mitogenesis
Rao H. Prabhala and Ronald R. Watson 155

Effects In Vitro of Ethanol and Acetaldehyde on Natural Killer Activity From Rats
Olcay Yeralan and Joe M. Jones 165

Mechanisms of Ethanol-Induced Immunosuppression
Thomas R. Jerrells, Michael J. Eckardt, and Joanne Weinberg 173

Modulation of Natural Killer Cell Activity by Alcohol Consumption and Nutritional Status
Gary G. Meadows, Sally E. Blank, and Deborah A. Duncan 181

Lymphocyte Populations and Immune Responses in Mice Prenatally Exposed to Ethanol
Sandra J. Ewald and Ching Huang 191

Effects of Chronic Alcohol Intake on Placental Transport of IgG
William P. Jollie and Hamdy M. Aly 201

Alcohol-Induced Suppression of Tumor Necrosis Factor—A Potential Risk Factor for Secondary Infection in the Acquired Immunodeficiency Syndrome
Steve Nelson, Gregory J. Bagby, and Warren R. Summer 211

Immunoregulatory Effects of Alcohol on Lymphocyte Responses to Human Immunodeficiency Virus Proteins
Madhavan P.N. Nair, Stanley A. Schwartz, Ziad A. Kronfol, Edgar P. Heimer, Raveendran Pottathil, and John F. Greden 221

Biochemical Changes in Ethanol-Treated HL-60 Cells
Lester K. Leung, Peter Kinkade, and Joseph M. Wu 231

An Observed Mechanism for Decreasing Blood Alcohol Levels in Rats by Using Sodium Acetate
C.D. Eskelson, L. Meeks, L. Myers, R. MacDonald, P. Thut, and E. Tucker .. 239

Ethanol, Acetaldehyde, and Kupffer Cell Function: Potential Role for Kupffer Cells in Alcohol Induced Liver Injury
David L. Earnest, Winnie W. Sim, Thomas L. Smith, and Cleamond D. Eskelson 255

The Effect of Alcohol on HIV Infection In Vitro
Louis D. Saravolatz, Robert F. Cerra, Donald J. Pohlod, and Susan Smereck .. 267

Suppression of Lymphocyte Activity After Acute Morphine Administration Appears to Be Glucocorticoid Independent
Barbara M. Bayer, Monica Hernandez, and Lauren Irvin 273

Effect of Chronic Ethanol Consumption and Retroviral Infection on Carcinogenesis and Its Possible Inhibition by an Immunostimulant, Canthaxanthin: Definition of a Murine Model
Siraj I. Mufti and Ronald R. Watson 283

Receptor Modulation as a Primary Target of the Immunological Effects of Alcohol and Other Drugs of Abuse
Robert M. Donahoe 305

Ethanol Induced Alteration of Immune Function May Involve Hormones of the Hypothalamic-Pituitary-Adrenal Axis
Eva Redei, William R. Clark, and Robert F. McGivern 313

Cell-Mediated Immunity in Alcoholic Liver Disease
Antonio Chedid, Charles L. Mendenhall, and the Veterans Administration Cooperative Study # 275 321

Immune Response to Acetaldehyde Adducts
Lynell W. Klassen, D.S. Xu, and Dean J. Tuma 333

In Vivo Microscopy of the Liver Following Acute Administration of Ethanol
R.S. McCuskey, P.A. McCuskey, H. Eguchi, E.G. Crichton, R. Urbaschek, and B. Urbaschek **341**

ALCOHOL, HIV, AND INFECTIOUS DISEASE PATHOGENESIS

Effects of Alcohol Ingestion on In Vitro Susceptibility of Peripheral Blood Mononuclear Cells to Infection With HIV-1 and on CD4 and CD8 Lymphocytes
Omar Bagasra, Patricia Whittle, Andre Kajdacsy-Balla, and Harold W. Lischner **351**

An Animal Model of Immune Response Associated With Alcohol-Related Cancers
Siraj I. Mufti **359**

Chronic Alcohol Consumption Prevents the Sepsis-Induced Increases in Gluconeogenesis and Metabolic Clearance Rate
Charles H. Lang, Patricia E. Molina, Gregory J. Bagby, and John J. Spitzer ... **373**

Ethanol and Survival of *Mycobacterium avium* Complex Within Macrophages
Luiz E. Bermudez and Lowell S. Young **383**

Clinical and Immunologic Spectrum of HIV Infection in Infants and Children and Disease Pathogenesis
Savita Pahwa, Narendra Chirmule, and Naoki Oyaizu **393**

EFFECTS OF ETHANOL AND OTHER DRUGS OF ABUSE UPON NUTRITIONAL STATE AND IMMUNE FUNCTION

Malnutrition-Induced Impairment of Resistance Against Experimental Pulmonary Tuberculosis
David N. McMurray, Rebecca A. Bartow, and Carole Mintzer **403**

Effects of Morphine, Cocaine, and Heroin on Nutrition
Ronald Ross Watson and Mary E. Mohs **413**

Vitamin and Trace Metal Disturbances in Alcoholism: Potential Effects on the Immune System
Nancy W. Alcock **419**

Ethanol Induced Malnutrition, a Potential Cause of Immunosuppression During AIDS
Mary E. Mohs and Ronald R. Watson **433**

Index **445**

Contributors

Ernest L. Abel, Department of Obstetrics and Gynecology, Wayne State University, Detroit, MI 48201 **[47]**

Nancy W. Alcock, Department of Preventive Medicine and Community Health, University of Texas Medical Branch, Galveston, TX 77550-5520 **[419]**

Hamdy M. Aly, Department of Anatomy, Medical College of Virginia, Virginia Commonwealth University, Richmond, VA 23298-0709 **[201]**

Omar Bagasra, Department of Microbiology, School of Osteopathic Medicine, University of Medicine and Dentistry of New Jersey, Camden, NJ 08103-1505 **[351]**

Gregory J. Bagby, Department of Physiology, Louisiana State University Medical Center, New Orleans, LA 70112 **[211,373]**

Rodney C. Baker, Department of Pharmacology, University of Colorado Health Sciences Center, Denver, CO 80262 **[113]**

Rebecca A. Bartow, Department of Medical Microbiology and Immunology, College of Medicine, Texas A&M University, College Station, TX 77843 **[403]**

Barbara M. Bayer, Department of Pharmacology, Georgetown University School of Medicine, Washington, DC 20007 **[273]**

Richard S. Berk, Department of Immunology/Microbiology, Wayne State University, Detroit, MI 48201 **[47]**

Luiz E. Bermudez, Department of Infectious Diseases, Kuzell Institute for Arthritis and Infectious Diseases, Medical Research Institute of San Francisco at Pacific Presbyterian Medical Center, San Francisco, CA 94115 **[383]**

Nancy T. Blaney, Department of Psychiatry, University of Miami School of Medicine, Miami, FL 33176 **[103]**

Sally E. Blank, College of Pharmacy, Washington State University, Pullman, WA 99164-6510 **[181]**

Robert F. Cerra, Surgical Research Laboratory, Henry Ford Hospital, Detroit, MI 48202 **[267]**

Kailash C. Chadha, Department of Molecular and Cellular Biology, Roswell Park Memorial Institute, Buffalo, NY 14263 **[123]**

The numbers in brackets are the opening page numbers of the contributors' articles.

Antonio Chedid, Department of Pathology, University of Health Sciences/ The Chicago Medical School at Veterans Administration Medical Center, North Chicago, IL 60064 **[321]**

Narendra Chirmule, Division of Allergy/Immunology, Department of Pediatrics, North Shore University Hospital, Manhasset, NY 11030 **[393]**

Dale Chitwood, Department of Oncology, University of Miami School of Medicine, Miami, FL 33176 **[103]**

William R. Clark, Department of Biology, University of California-Los Angeles, Los Angeles, CA 90024 **[313]**

M. Lynne Cooper, Center for the Study of Behavioral and Social Aspects of Health, and Department of Psychology, State University of New York at Buffalo, Buffalo, NY 14260 **[11]**

E.G. Crichton, Department of Anatomy, University of Arizona College of Medicine, Tucson, AZ 85724 **[341]**

Michael K. Cummings, Roswell Park Memorial Institute, Buffalo, NY 14263 **[123]**

Robert M. Donahoe, Laboratory of Psychoimmunology, Departments of Psychiatry and Pathology, Georgia Mental Health Institute, Emory University, Atlanta, GA 30306 **[305]**

Raymond J. Dorio, Division of Neonatology and Pediatric Pulmonology, Department of Pediatrics, and Department of Pathology and Laboratory Medicine, Childrens Hospital of Los Angeles, University of Southern California, Los Angeles, CA 90027 **[135]**

Deborah A. Duncan, College of Pharmacy, Washington State University, Pullmam, WA 99164-6510 **[181]**

David L. Earnest, Department of Internal Medicine, University of Arizona College of Medicine, Tucson, AZ 85724 **[255]**

Michael J. Eckardt, Laboratory of Clinical Studies, National Institute on Alcohol Abuse and Alcoholism, Bethesda, MD 20892 **[173]**

H. Eguchi, Department of Anatomy, University of Arizona College of Medicine, Tucson, AZ 85724 **[341]**

Salwa A. Elgebaly, Department of Surgery, University of Connecticut Health Center, Farmington, CT 06032 **[75]**

Cleamond D. Eskelson, Department of Surgery, University of Arizona Health Sciences Center, Tucson, AZ 85724, and Veterans Administration Hospital, Tucson, AZ 85723 **[239,255]**

Sandra J. Ewald, Department of Microbiology, Montana State University, Bozeman, MT 59717 **[191]**

Mary Ann Fletcher, Department of Medicine, University of Miami School of Medicine, Miami, FL 33176 **[103]**

William H. George, Center for the Study of Behavioral and Social Aspects of Health, and Department of Psychology, State University of New York at Buffalo, Buffalo, NY 14260 **[11]**

Amanda L. Golbeck, Division of Statistics, Department of Mathematical Sciences, College of Sciences, San Diego State University, San Diego, CA 92182 **[1]**

John F. Greden, Department of Psychiatry and the Alcohol Research Center, The University of Michigan, Ann Arbor, MI 48109-0120 **[221]**

Harry W. Haverkos, Clinical Medicine Branch, Division of Clinical Research, National Institute on Drug Abuse; Alcohol, Drug Abuse, and Mental Health Administration, Rockville, MD 20857 **[93]**

Linda S. Hazlett, Department of Anatomy, Wayne State University, Detroit, MI 48201 **[47]**

Edgar P. Heimer, Roche Diagnostic Systems, Hoffmann-La Roche, Inc., Nutley, NJ 07110 **[221]**

Monica Hernandez, Department of Pharmacology, Georgetown University School of Medicine, Washington, DC 20007 **[273]**

Ching Huang, Department of Microbiology, Montana State University, Bozeman, MT 59717 **[191]**

Lauren Irvin, Department of Pharmacology, Georgetown University School of Medicine, Washington, DC 20007 **[273]**

Jeffrey M. Jacobson, Infectious Diseases Section, Bronx Veterans Administration Medical Center, Bronx, NY 10468, and Department of Medicine, Mount Sinai School of Medicine, New York, NY 10029 **[67]**

Thomas R. Jerrells, Department of Pathology, University of Texas Medical Branch, Galveston, TX 77550 **[173]**

Don L. Jewett, Department of Orthopaedic Surgery, University of California-San Francisco, San Francisco, CA 94143-0728 **[57]**

William P. Jollie, Department of Anatomy, Medical College of Virginia, Virginia Commonwealth University, Richmond, VA 23298-0709 **[201]**

Joe M. Jones, Departments of Pathology and Microbiology/Immunology, University of Arkansas for Medical Sciences, Little Rock, AR 72205 **[165]**

Andre Kajdacsy-Balla, Department of Pathology, University of Oklahoma, Oklahoma City, OK 73190 **[351]**

Peter Kinkade, Department of Biochemistry and Molecular Biology, New York Medical College, Valhalla, NY 10595 **[231]**

Lynell W. Klassen, Department of Internal Medicine, University of Nebraska Medical Center, Omaha, NE 68105 **[333]**

Nancy G. Klimas, Department of Medicine, University of Miami School of Medicine, Miami, FL 33176 **[103]**

Robert A. Kozol, Department of Surgery, University of Connecticut Health Center, Farmington, CT 06032; present address: Veterans Administration Medical Center, Allen Park, MI 48101 **[75]**

Donald L. Kreutzer, Department of Pathology, University of Connecticut Health Center, Farmington, CT 06032 **[75]**

Ziad A. Kronfol, Department of Psychiatry and the Alcohol Research Center, The University of Michigan, Ann Arbor, MI 48109-0120 **[221]**

E.W. Lamon, Veterans Administration Medical Center and Department of Surgery, University of Alabama School of Medicine, Birmingham, AL 35294 **[145]**

Charles H. Lang, Department of Physiology, Louisiana State University Medical Center, New Orleans, LA 70112 **[373]**

Barbara Critchlow Leigh, Alcohol Research Group, Medical Research Institute of San Francisco, Berkeley, CA 94709, and Alcohol and Drug Abuse Institute, University of Washington, Seattle, WA 98103 **[35]**

Lester K. Leung, Department of Biochemistry and Molecular Biology, New York Medical College, Valhalla, NY 10595 **[231]**

Charles S. Lieber, Alcohol Research and Treatment Center, Bronx Veterans Administration Medical Center, Bronx, NY 10468 **[67]**

Harold W. Lischner, Department of Pediatrics and Department of Microbiology and Immunity, Temple University School of Medicine, Philadelphia, PA 19140 **[351]**

R. MacDonald, Veterans Administration Hospital, Tucson, AZ 85723 **[239]**

John L. Martin, Division of Sociomedical Sciences, Columbia University School of Public Health, New York, NY 10032 **[27]**

P.A. McCuskey, Department of Anatomy, University of Arizona College of Medicine, Tucson, AZ 85724 **[341]**

R.S. McCuskey, Department of Anatomy, University of Arizona College of Medicine, Tucson, AZ 85724 **[341]**

Robert F. McGivern, Department of Medicine, UCLA/Harbor Medical Center, Torrance, CA 90502 **[313]**

David N. McMurray, Department of Medical Microbiology and Immunology, College of Medicine, Texas A&M University, College Station, TX 77843 **[403]**

Gary G. Meadows, College of Pharmacy, Washington State University, Pullman, WA 99164-6510 **[181]**

L. Meeks, Veterans Administration Hospital, Tucson, AZ 85723 **[239]**

Charles L. Mendenhall, Department of Medicine, Veterans Administration Medical Center, and University of Cincinnati College of Medicine, Cincinnati, OH 45220 **[321]**

Karen Milles, Department of Pediatrics, University of Miami School of Medicine, Miami, FL 33176 **[103]**

Carole Mintzer, Department of Medical Microbiology and Immunology, College of Medicine, Texas A&M University, College Station, TX 77843 **[403]**

Mary E. Mohs, Department of Family and Community Medicine, University of Arizona, Tucson, AZ 85724 **[413,433]**

Craig A. Molgaard, Division of Epidemiology and Biostatistics, Graduate School of Public Health, College of Health and Human Services, San Diego State University, San Diego, CA 92182 **[1]**

Patricia E. Molina, Department of Physiology, Louisiana State University Medical Center, New Orleans, LA 70112 **[373]**

Robert Morgan, Department of Psychiatry, University of Miami School of Medicine, Miami, FL 33176 **[103]**

Siraj I. Mufti, Department of Pharmacology and Toxicology, University of Arizona Health Sciences Center, Tucson, AZ 85724 **[283,359]**

Milton G. Mutchnick, Department of Gastroenterology, Wayne State University, Detroit, MI 48201 **[47]**

L. Myers, Veterans Administration Hospital, Tucson, AZ 85723 **[239]**

Madhavan P.N. Nair, Departments of Pediatrics, Epidemiology, and Psychiatry, and the Alcohol Research Center, The University of Michigan, Ann Arbor, MI 48109-2029 **[221]**

Steve Nelson, Department of Pulmonary/Critical Care Medicine, Louisiana State University Medical Center, New Orleans, LA 70112 **[211]**

Tuan H. Nguyen, Medical Class of 1992, University of Arizona, Tucson, AZ 85724 **[79]**

Marilyn Norman, Roswell Park Memorial Institute, Buffalo, NY 14263 **[123]**

Naoki Oyaizu, Division of Allergy/ Immunology, Department of Pediatrics, North Shore University Hospital, Manhasset, NY 11030 **[393]**

J. Bryan Page, Department of Psychiatry, University of Miami School of Medicine, Miami, FL 33176 **[103]**

Savita Pahwa, Division of Allergy/ Immunology, Department of Pediatrics, North Shore University Hospital, Manhasset, NY 11030 **[393]**

Albert Pawlowski, National Institute on Alcohol Abuse and Alcoholism, Rockville, MD 20857; present address: Alcohol Beverage Medical Research Foundation, Baltimore, MD 21205 **[xvii]**

Donald J. Pohlod, Infectious Diseases Laboratory, Henry Ford Hospital, Detroit, MI 48202 **[267]**

Raveendran Pottathil, Roche Diagnostic Systems, Hoffmann-La Roche, Inc., Nutley, NJ 07110 **[221]**

Rao H. Prabhala, Department of Family and Community Medicine, University of Arizona Health Sciences Center, Tucson, AZ 85724; present address: Department of Physiology, Dartmouth Medical School, Hanover, NH 03756 **[155]**

Eva Redei, Department of Psychiatry, University of Pennsylvania, Philadelphia, PA 19104 **[313]**

Henry S. Sacks, Departments of Medicine and Biomathematical Science, Mount Sinai School of Medicine, New York, NY 10029 **[67]**

Louis D. Saravolatz, Infectious Diseases Laboratory, Henry Ford Hospital, Detroit, MI 48202 **[267]**

Stanley A. Schwartz, Departments of Pediatrics and Epidemiology, and the Alcohol Research Center, The University of Michigan, Ann Arbor, MI 48109-2029 **[221]**

Daniela Seminara, National Institute on Alcohol Abuse and Alcoholism, Rockville, MD 20857; present address: Office of AIDS Programs, National Institute of Mental Health, Rockville, MD 20857 **[xvii]**

Winnie W. Sim, Department of Internal Medicine, University of Arizona College of Medicine, Tucson, AZ 85724 **[255]**

Jeremy B. Skinner, Center for the Study of Behavioral and Social Aspects of Health, and Department of Psychology, State University of New York at Buffalo, Buffalo, NY 14260 **[11]**

Susan Smereck, Infectious Diseases Laboratory, Henry Ford Hospital, Detroit, MI 48202 **[267]**

Thomas L. Smith, Department of Pharmacology, University of Arizona College of Medicine, Tucson, AZ 85724 **[255]**

John J. Spitzer, Department of Physiology, Louisiana State University Medical Center, New Orleans, LA 70112 **[373]**

Istvan Stadler, Roswell Park Memorial Institute, Buffalo, NY 14263 **[123]**

Warren R. Summer, Department of Pulmonary/Critical Care Medicine, Louisiana State University Medical Center, New Orleans, LA 70112 **[211]**

P. Thut, Department of Pharmacology, University of Arizona Health Sciences Center, Tucson, AZ 85724, and Veterans Administration Hospital, Tucson, AZ 85723 **[239]**

Karen Trocki, Alcohol Research Group, Medical Research Institute of San Francisco, Berkeley, CA 94709 **[21]**

E. Tucker, Veterans Administration Hospital, Tucson, AZ 85723 **[239]**

Dean J. Tuma, Research Service, Omaha Veterans Administration Medical Center, Omaha, NE 68105 **[333]**

B. Urbaschek, Department of Immunology and Serology, Institute for Hygiene and Medical Microbiology, University of Heidelberg, 6800 Mannheim, Federal Republic of Germany **[341]**

R. Urbaschek, Department of Immunology and Serology, Institute for Hygiene and Medical Microbiology, University of Heidelberg, 6800 Mannheim, Federal Republic of Germany **[341]**

Amrik S. Walia, Veterans Administration Medical Center and Department of Surgery, University of Alabama School of Medicine, Birmingham, AL 35294 **[145]**

Ronald Ross Watson, Department of Family and Community Medicine, University of Arizona Health Sciences Center, Tucson, AZ 85724 **[79,155,283,413,433]**

Joanne Weinberg, Department of Anatomy, University of British Columbia, Vancouver, BC, Canada V6T 1W5 **[173]**

Robert B. Whitney, Department of Alcoholism, Erie County Medical Center, Buffalo, NY 14215 **[123]**

Patricia Whittle, Department of Microbiology, School of Osteopathic Medicine, University of Medicine and Dentistry of New Jersey, Camden, NJ 08103-1505 **[351]**

Michael Windle, Research Institute on Alcoholism, Buffalo, NY 14203 **[123]**

Theresa M. Worner, Alcohol Research and Treatment Center, Bronx Veterans Administration Medical Center, Bronx, NY 10468 **[67]**

Joseph M. Wu, Department of Biochemistry and Molecular Biology, New York Medical College, Valhalla, NY 10595 **[231]**

D.S. Xu, Research Service, Omaha Veterans Administration Medical Center, Omaha, NE 68105 **[333]**

Olcay Yeralan, Department of Microbiology/Immunology, University of Arkansas for Medical Sciences, Little Rock, AR 72205 **[165]**

Lowell S. Young, Department of Infectious Diseases, Kuzell Institute for Arthritis and Infectious Diseases, Medical Research Institute of San Francisco at Pacific Presbyterian Medical Center, San Francisco, CA 94115 **[383]**

Preface

In 1989 the National Institute on Alcohol Abuse and Alcoholism, with the collaboration of the Alcohol Research Center on Alcohol and Immunologic Disorders at the University of Arizona, sponsored the First Alcohol and Acquired Immunodeficiency Syndrome (AIDS) Network Conference. This symposium, held on April 27–29 in Tucson, Arizona, was the first national meeting on the relation between alcohol consumption, HIV infection, and AIDS, and it featured presentations by a number of experts in the epidemiological, behavioral, and biomedical research related to this theme.

The occurrence of the HIV epidemics has given a further impulse to this field of research. In 1989 the cumulative number of reported AIDS cases, according to the CDC definition, has reached 87,188. However, it has often been observed that this number represents only a fraction of the number of infected persons, including the large number of undiagnosed cases. The latter are asymptomatic carriers who can remain infected, and infectious, for up to ten years before developing the full-blown syndrome.

On the behavioral side, many behaviors leading to high risk for HIV infection are now well identified. However, not much is known about the factors that may influence or modify these behaviors. On the biomedical side, remarkable advances have been made in the study of the pathogenesis of HIV infection, but there is still quite a bit of uncertainty on the biological factors that could determine susceptibility to HIV infection or influence the development of full-blown AIDS.

Despite its influence as a behavioral modifier, its disturbing effects on the immune system, and its high diffusion in high-risk populations such as drug abusers, homosexuals, blacks, and Hispanics, the possible role of alcohol abuse as a potential risk factor for HIV infection and AIDS development has not been adequately studied in the past.

Research evidence supports the hypothesis that the role of alcohol in the acquisition of HIV infection and the development of AIDS is two-fold. First, alcohol consumption can operate as a disinhibiting factor, leading to unsafe sexual behaviors and therefore unprotected exposure to HIV infection. Second, alcohol consumption has been associated with pronounced abnormalities of immune system function, ranging from immunosuppression to autoimmune phenomena. In addition, several landmark studies have found that there is increased incidence of opportunistic infections, such as tuberculosis and pneumonia, in alcohol populations, and a correlation has been drawn between this phenomena and the immunodysregulation caused by alcohol.

Accordingly, the Alcohol and AIDS Network Conference was divided into two parts. The first addressed the substantive relationship between drinking, high-risk sexual behavior, and AIDS. Epidemiological and behavioral studies performed on homosexual and heterosexual populations, as well as in specific racial and ethnic subgroups, were presented. Specific problems related to alcohol and drug use and AIDS in adolescents were also addressed. The second part covered the full spectrum of the ongoing biomedical research on alcohol and AIDS. Both the direct alcohol effect on cellular and humoral immune response and the interaction between medical complications of alcoholism (such as liver disease, viral infections other than HIV, and central nervous system involvement) and HIV infection, were discussed. Other topics of particular interest were the role of alcohol in affecting immune system development as related to pediatric AIDS, the effect of alcohol on immunoneuroendocrine homeostasis, and the role of nutritional factors in alcoholism and AIDS. Particular interest was elicited by the research presentations on the mechanisms underlying the interactions between alcohol, other drugs of abuse, and the immune system, since polydrug abuse occurs very frequently in individuals at high risk for HIV.

This book is a partial report of the proceedings from the conference and is meant to provide the reader with a comprehensive update of the ongoing AIDS-related alcohol research. We hope that it will elicit the interest of scientists in related disciplines toward this young but rapidly growing field.

A copy of the book of abstracts from the First Alcohol and AIDS Network Conference can be obtained by writing to:

AIDS Coordinator
Room 14C-20
5600 Fishers Lane
Rockville, MD 20857

Daniela Seminara
Albert Pawlowski

Acknowledgments

We appreciate the assistance of the NIAAA-funded Specialized Alcohol Research Center (AA08037) in Tucson, the host of the conference that brought together the speakers whose presentations form the basis of this book. In addition, we thank the National Institute on Alcohol Abuse and Alcoholism for its encouragement and support of the participants' research and for its support of the conference.

We especially appreciate the dedicated work of Cindy L. Wallace, who managed the logistics of the conference and allowed it to be brought about in a short period of time. We also gratefully recognize Sue Theiss and Gayle W. Croft, whose efforts were critical to the preparation of the manuscripts and the travel arrangements of the speakers.

Alcohol, Immunomodulation, and AIDS, pages 1–10
© 1990 Alan R. Liss, Inc.

METHODOLOGICAL ISSUES CONCERNING THE SENSITIVE QUERY IN AIDS/ALCOHOL RESEARCH: SAMPLE SIZE ESTIMATES FOR RANDOMIZED RESPONSE PROCEDURES

Amanda L. Golbeck, Ph.D., and
Craig A. Molgaard, Ph.D., M.P.H.

Division of Statistics, Department of Mathematical Sciences, College of Sciences, (A.L.G.), and Division of Epidemiology and Biostatistics, Graduate School of Public Health, College of Health and Human Services,(C.A.M.), San Diego State University, San Diego, California 92182

INTRODUCTION

It is generally accepted that alcohol consumption during sexual activity is associated with increased risk of Acquired Immunodeficiency Syndrome (AIDS) through the practice of risky sexual behaviors which increase the chance of exposure to HIV (Stall and Wiley, 1988; Loue, et al, 1989). It is also generally accepted that chronic alcohol abuse is associated with immune system modification and impairment (Molgaard, et al, 1988). Yet empirical data driven estimates of the joint distribution of alcohol abuse, homosexual/bisexual practices, and IV drug use are: 1) rare; 2) often contradictory; and 3) usually constructed with conventional methodological effort. In general, the relative impact of alcohol use and abuse on the risk for and clinical manifestation of AIDS is unclear. In this paper, we would like to examine some methodological issues for the epidemiologist concerned with the construction of sensitive queries in AIDS-Alcohol research. We would like to focus on the feasibility of use of the randomized response technique (RRT).

RANDOMIZED RESPONSE TECHNIQUES

The RRT has been used to study abortion (Abernathy, et al, 1970), alcohol use and non-compliance in hypertensives (Volicer and Volicer, 1982), generic drug use (Goodstadt and Gruson, 1975), smoking behavior (Akers, et al, 1983), problem use of alcohol among employed females (Volicer, et al, 1983), prevalence of drinking (Barth and Sandler, 1976), and other sensitive questions. RRT's can be formulated with several types of models. Here we discuss two frequently employed types: the Warner model (Warner, 1965), and the unrelated question model (Greenberg, et al, 1969).

In the Warner model, the subject is presented with two questions, one asking about membership in group A, and one asking about membership in the group defined by the complement of A. One must then instruct the subject to answer only one of the questions. That question is chosen in a probabilistic fashion. For example, the subject might toss two coins, and depending on the outcome, answer question 1 (about membership in A) if the outcome is two heads, and question 2 (about membership in the complement of A) if the outcome is anything else. The researcher records responses without knowing which question is asked. Because the probability with which each question is answered is known, one can estimate π_A, the unknown population proportion of members in group A.

In the unrelated question model, the subject is also presented with two questions. This time, however, one is a sensitive question and one is an innocuous question. The sensitive question asks about membership in A. The innocuous question asks about membership in group Y instead of the complement of A. Memberships in groups Y and A are unrelated, and memberships in groups Y and the complement of Y are innocuous. As in the Warner model, the subject chooses which of the two questions to answer by using a randomization device, and the subject conceals from the interviewer which question he is answering. There are two cases of the unrelated question model according to whether π_y, the population proportion of members in group Y, is known or unknown to the investigator. Below we illustrate the case of known π_y.

In a brief report by Comstock and colleagues (1985), it was noted that RRT's have been rarely applied or reported in the literature by epidemiologists (Rider, et al, 1976). This was despite the frequent need of epidemiologists to ascertain reliable information on sensitive matters from individuals on potentially embarrassing or incriminating topics.

Use of RRT's in alcohol research *per se* has also not been widely reported in the literature. Initial enthusiasm oriented to using the technique to overcome the problem that level of consumption of alcohol reported by survey data is less than that estimated based on sales of alcoholic beverages. A strong underreporting bias was assumed (Goodstadt, et al, 1978). Later work, especially that of Volicer and Volicer (1982), showed that alcohol consumption is not uniformly underreported but instead varies by demographic characteristics such as age and sex.

SAMPLE SIZE AND RANDOMIZED RESPONSE TECHNIQUES

The RRT has been recently criticized by Campbell (1987). In brief, Campbell's critique of using RRT's to estimate the prevalence of high-risk behaviors focused on sample size requirements. The randomization procedure, according to Campbell, greatly increases sampling error, which drives a requirement for larger sample sizes to derive estimates with a set level of reliability than with conventional survey instruments. However, no example or illustration of this effect of the RRT was provided. Also, Campbell did not quantify how much larger this number of cases would be for use of the RRT. Below we perform some quantification to elucidate the sample size differences that can occur between randomized response and direct response surveys.

Following Chaudhuri and Mukerjee (1988), let $\hat{\pi}_{AD}$, $\hat{\pi}_{AW}$, and $\hat{\pi}_{AU1}$ denote the estimators of π_A for the direct question survey, the Warner model randomized response survey, and the unrelated question randomized response survey, respectively. Also, N is the size of the sample, and P is the probability that the subject answers the question relating to membership in A. Then 1-P in the Warner model is the probability that the subject answers the question relating to membership in the complement of A, and 1-P in the unrelated question model is the probability of answering the question relating to membership in Y.

The RRT has the feature, via the existence of the parameter P under the design control of the investigator, that maintenance of confidentiality can be increased at the expense of efficiency. In other words, the investigator can design the specific application of the RRT to increase the possibility of truthful reporting, if he is willing to pay a price in an increase in the variance of his estimates, and hence an increase in sample size. Chaudhuri and Mukerjee (1988) devote an entire chapter of their recent book on RRT methodology to the treatment of optimally efficient estimation in randomized response subject to practical constraints imposed by the requirement of protecting the privacy of a respondent.

The following formulas for the variances of each of the estimators of π_A are well known:

$$\mathrm{Var}(\hat{\pi}_{AD}) = [\pi_A(1-\pi_A)] / N$$

$$\mathrm{Var}(\hat{\pi}_{AW}) = [\pi_A(1-\pi_A) - .25 + \{16(P-.5)^2\}^{-1}] / N$$

$$\text{Var}(\hat{\pi}_{AU1}) = \left[\{P\pi_A + (1-P)\pi_Y\}\{1-P\pi_A - (1-P)\pi_Y\} \right] / [NP^2]$$

These variance formulas can be used together with standard statistical procedures based on normal theory to derive formulas for the size of the sample that would be required for each type of survey under specified degrees of accuracy of the estimates.

Suppose we are concerned with testing the null hypothesis H_0: $\pi_A=\pi_0$ against the one-sided alternative H_1: $\pi_A>\pi_0$. Let π_1 denote the value of π_A for which we desire the power function to have a specified value $1-\beta$. $Z_{1-\alpha}$ and $Z_{1-\beta}$ are the $(1-\alpha)$-th and $(1-\beta)$-th percentile, respectively, of the standard normal distribution. Let N_{AD}, N_{AW}, and N_{AU1} denote the sample sizes for the direct question survey, the Warner model randomized response survey, and the unrelated question randomized response survey, respectively. Then formulas for sample sizes for the three types of surveys can be written as follows:

$$N_{AD} = \left[\; [Z_{1-\alpha}\{\pi_0(1-\pi_0)\}^{1/2} + Z_{1-\beta}\{\pi_1(1-\pi_1)\}^{1/2}] \; / (\pi_0-\pi_1) \right]^2$$

$$N_{AW} = \left[\; [Z_{1-\alpha}\{\pi_0(1-\pi_0) - .25 + \{16(P-.5)^2\}^{-1}\}^{1/2} + Z_{1-\beta}\{\pi_1(1-\pi_1) - .25 + \{16(P-.5)^2\}^{-1}\}^{1/2}] \; / (\pi_0-\pi_1) \right]^2$$

$$N_{AU1} = \Big[\ \big[\ Z_{1-\alpha} \{ [P\pi_0 + (1-P)\pi_Y][1 - P\pi_0 - (1-P)\pi_Y] \}^{1/2}$$

$$+ \ Z_{1-\beta} \{ [P\pi_1 + (1-P)\pi_Y][1 - P\pi_1 - (1-P)\pi_Y] \}^{1/2} \ \big]$$

$$/ \{ (\pi_0 - \pi_1) P \} \ \Big]^2$$

As in Levy (1978), suppose we are concerned with values of π_1 such that $\pi_1 - \pi_0 = .10$, and we specify a level of significance α of .05. Levy shows a table of sample sizes required to achieve a power $1-\beta$ of at least .80 for both the direct question survey and the Warner model randomized response survey under various values of π_0 and P. In Table 1, we show selected sample sizes required to achieve a power of at least .90 for both types of surveys that Levy considered, and also for the unrelated question randomized response survey. In Table 2 we show the ratios of the various RRT sample sizes to the sample sizes that are required for the direct question survey. Tables 1 and 2 illustrate a theorem by Dowling and Schachtman (1975) which proves that the sample size in the unrelated question model will always be less than the sample size in the Warner model whenever $P > .339333\ldots$.

TABLE 1: Sample Sizes for Direct Question Surveys, Warner Model Randomized Response Surveys, and Unrelated Question Randomized Response Surveys

π_0	P	N_{AD}	N_{AW}	$N_{AU1}, \pi_Y=$				
				.05	.25	.45	.65	.85
.05	.15	67	293	2023	6670	9110	9349	7386
.05	.25	67	713	776	2279	3160	3424	3070
.05	.35	67	2237	419	1096	1533	1733	1696
.05	.45	67	21275	267	621	869	1013	1056
.05	.55	67	21275	187	385	535	637	694
.05	.65	67	2237	140	253	344	414	465
.05	.75	67	713	109	171	225	270	307
.05	.85	67	293	88	118	145	170	192
.15	.15	131	355	2523	6974	9220	9264	7107
.15	.25	131	775	1071	2469	3247	3408	2951
.15	.35	131	2298	626	1237	1610	1746	1645
.15	.45	131	21336	425	735	940	1043	1043
.15	.55	131	21336	314	482	603	678	706
.15	.65	131	2298	245	338	410	462	493
.15	.75	131	775	199	248	289	323	348
.15	.85	131	355	166	189	209	227	243
.25	.15	176	399	3005	7261	9312	9162	6811
.25	.25	176	819	1347	2641	3317	3374	2815
.25	.35	176	2342	814	1361	1670	1742	1578
.25	.45	176	21380	564	831	995	1056	1014
.25	.55	176	21380	422	561	654	700	701
.25	.65	176	2342	332	405	459	492	505
.25	.75	176	819	270	307	336	358	372
.25	.85	176	399	224	241	255	267	277
.35	.15	203	426	3469	7530	9388	9044	6498
.35	.25	203	845	1606	2797	3369	3324	2662
.35	.35	203	2369	985	1468	1713	1721	1493
.35	.45	203	21407	686	911	1032	1051	967
.35	.55	203	21407	513	623	688	706	679
.35	.65	203	2369	401	455	490	505	500
.35	.75	203	845	323	348	366	376	379
.35	.85	203	426	265	275	283	289	293

TABLE 2: Ratio of Sample Sizes for Warner Model and Unrelated Question Model Randomized Response Surveys, Each Compared to Direct Question Surveys ($R_{AW}=N_{AW}/N_{AD}$, and $R_{AU1}=N_{AU1}/N_{AD}$)

π_0	P	R_{AW}	$R_{AU1}, \pi_y=$				
			.05	.25	.45	.65	.85
.05	.15	4.37	30.19	99.55	135.97	139.54	110.24
.05	.25	10.64	11.58	34.01	47.16	51.10	45.82
.05	.35	33.39	6.25	16.36	22.88	25.87	25.31
.05	.45	317.54	3.99	9.27	12.97	15.12	15.76
.05	.55	317.54	2.79	5.75	7.99	9.51	10.36
.05	.65	33.39	2.09	3.78	5.13	6.18	6.94
.05	.75	10.64	1.63	2.55	3.36	4.03	4.58
.05	.85	4.37	1.31	1.76	2.16	2.54	2.87
.15	.15	2.71	19.26	53.24	70.38	70.72	54.25
.15	.25	5.92	8.18	18.85	24.79	26.02	22.53
.15	.35	17.54	4.78	9.44	12.29	13.33	12.56
.15	.45	162.87	3.24	5.61	7.18	7.96	7.96
.15	.55	162.87	2.40	3.68	4.60	5.18	5.39
.15	.65	17.54	1.87	2.58	3.13	3.53	3.76
.15	.75	5.92	1.52	1.89	2.21	2.47	2.66
.15	.85	2.71	1.27	1.44	1.60	1.73	1.85
.25	.15	2.27	17.07	41.26	52.91	52.06	38.70
.25	.25	4.65	7.65	15.01	18.85	19.17	15.99
.25	.35	13.31	4.63	7.73	9.49	9.90	8.97
.25	.45	121.48	3.20	4.72	5.65	6.00	5.76
.25	.55	121.48	2.40	3.19	3.72	3.98	3.98
.25	.65	13.31	1.89	2.30	2.61	2.80	2.87
.25	.75	4.65	1.53	1.74	1.91	2.03	2.11
.25	.85	2.27	1.27	1.37	1.45	1.52	1.57
.35	.15	2.10	17.09	37.09	46.25	44.55	32.01
.35	.25	4.16	7.91	13.78	16.60	16.37	13.11
.35	.35	11.67	4.85	7.23	8.44	8.48	7.35
.35	.45	105.45	3.38	4.49	5.08	5.18	4.76
.35	.55	105.45	2.53	3.07	3.39	3.48	3.34
.35	.65	11.67	1.98	2.24	2.41	2.49	2.46
.35	.75	4.16	1.59	1.71	1.80	1.85	1.87
.35	.85	2.10	1.31	1.35	1.39	1.42	1.44

SUMMARY

Quantification of sample size requirements for two common models of the RRT as compared to conventional survey techniques demonstrates that Campbell is fundamentally correct. However, the absolute increase in sample size necessitated by either model of the RRT is not of such a magnitude as to make use of the method always impractical. Where the appropriate sample size exists, it may well be the method of choice for selected issues pertaining to AIDS and alcohol research.

REFERENCES

Abernathy JR, Greenberg BG, Horvitz DG (1970). Estimates of induced abortion in urban North Carolina. Demography 7:19-29.

Akers RL, Massey J, Clarke W, Lauer RM (1983). Are self-reports of adolescent deviance valid? Biochemical measures, randomized response, and the bogus pipeline in smoking behavior. Social Forces 62:234-251.

Barth JT, Sandler HM (1976). Evaluation of the randomized response technique in a drinking survey. J of Studies on Alcohol 37:690-693.

Campbell AA (1987). Randomized response technique. Science 236:1049.

Chaudhuri A, Mukerjee R (1988). Randomized Response, Theory and Techniques. New York: Marcel Dekker.

Comstock GW, Conde JG, Knud JH (1985). A simple randomized response device. Am J of Epidemiology 122:187-190.

Dowling TA, Shachtman R (1975). On the relative efficiency of RR models. J Am Stat Assoc 70:84-87.

Goodstadt MS, Cook G, Gruson V (1978). The validity of reported drug use: the randomized response technique. Int J Addict 13(3):359-367.

Goodstadt MS, Gruson V (1975). The randomized response technique: A test on drug use. J Am Stat Assoc 70:814-818.

Greenberg BG, Abul-Ela A-La, Simmons WR, Horvitz DG (1969). The unrelated question randomized response model: Theoretical framework. J Am Stat Assoc 64:520-539.
Levy KJ (1978). Sample size comparisons involving the randomized response technique. J of Experimental Education 47:21-23.
Loue S, McCutchan JA, Brysk L, Spechko P, Weinrich J, Molgaard C, et al. (1989). Cocaine, marijuana and alcohol as risk factors for HIV infection in homosexual men: A pilot study. Presented at Fifth International Conference on AIDS in Montreal, June 4-9, 1989.
Molgaard CA, Nakamura C, Hovell M, Elder JP (1988). Assessing alcoholism as a risk factor for acquired immunodeficiency syndrome (AIDS). Soc Sci Med 27:1147-1152.
Rider RV, Harper PA, Chow P, Cheng CI (1976). A comparison of four methods for determining prevalence of induced abortion, Taiwan. Am J Epidemiol 103:37-49.
Stall R, Wiley J (1988). A comparison of alcohol and drug use patterns of homosexual and heterosexual men: The San Francisco Men's Health Study. Drug and Alcohol Dependence 22:63-73.
Volicer BJ, Volicer L (1982). Randomized response technique for estimating alcohol use and noncompliance in hypertensives. J of Studies on Alcohol 43:739-750.
Volicer BJ, Cahill MH, Neuburger E, Arntz G (1983). Randomized response estimates of problem use of alcohol among employed females. Alcoholism: Clinical and Experimental Research 7:321-326.
Warner SL (1965). Randomized response: a survey technique for eliminating evasive answer bias. J Am Stat Assoc 60:63-69.

Alcohol, Immunomodulation, and AIDS, pages 11–19
© 1990 Alan R. Liss, Inc.

ALCOHOL USE AND SEXUAL RISK-TAKING AMONG ADOLESCENTS: METHODOLOGICAL APPROACHES FOR ADDRESSING CAUSAL ISSUES

M. Lynne Cooper, Jeremy B. Skinner and William H. George
Center for the Study of Behavioral and Social Aspects of Health and Department of Psychology
State University of New York at Buffalo,
Buffalo, New York, 14260

Costs associated with adolescent sexual activity have risen dramatically in recent years due to the potentially lethal threat posed by acquired immune deficiency syndrome (AIDS). Given that no effective cure or vaccination for AIDS is imminent, prevention of sexual risk-taking among adolescents is recognized as a primary avenue for reducing the incidence of human immunodeficiency virus (HIV) infection (Flora & Thorensen, 1988). However, development of effective prevention programs requires an understanding of the causal mechanisms underlying sexual risk-taking.

Alcohol use has recently been cited as a potential cause of sexual risk-taking among adolescents (Flora & Thorensen, 1988). Indeed, numerous correlational studies document an association between alcohol use and sexual behavior among adolescents. Work by Jessor and others (Bentler & Newcomb, 1986; Donovan & Jessor, 1985; Mott & Haurin, 1988) indicates that alcohol use, drug use, early onset of sexual activity, more frequent sexual activity and degree of sexual involvement are consistently interrelated. Although less well-documented, available evidence also suggests that alcohol use is associated with contraceptive risk-taking behavior among adolescents (e.g., Zucker, Battistich, & Langer, 1981). Despite consistent evidence suggesting covariation among these behaviors, little is known about the underlying causal mechanisms.

The present paper outlines a methodological approach for examining one prominent hypothesis regarding this relationship -- that alcohol use and sexual behavior reflect correlated manifestations of some underlying personality or lifestyle dimension, such as unconventionality or deviance proneness (Donovan & Jessor, 1985). The proposed approach examines covariation between alcohol use and sexual risk-taking on specific occasions while controlling for global measures of alcohol use and sexual risk-taking behaviors. Applied to our own data, this strategy indicates that such a third variable hypothesis cannot adequately account for the relationship between alcohol use and risk-taking on specific occasions. We therefore propose several alternative models to explain this covariation, and suggest general strategies for examining these models.

IMPLICATIONS OF EXPLANATORY HYPOTHESES FOR PREVENTION

To the extent that the link between alcohol use and sexual risk-taking reflects some enduring lifestyle or dispositional characteristic, attempts to decrease risky sexual behavior by altering patterns of alcohol use may prove ineffectual. Indeed, assuming that both behaviors serve a similar underlying need or function, successfully reducing alcohol use may have the untoward effect of "re-channeling" those impulses into increased sexual behaviors (Ensminger, 1987).

Alternately, if the link between alcohol use and sexual risk-taking is more directly causal in nature, reducing alcohol consumption -- and especially alcohol consumption proximal to intercourse -- should constitute an effective intervention strategy for reducing sexual risk-taking among adolescents. Thus, distinguishing between these alternative causal explanations may have important practical implications for the design of effective prevention programs.

A STRATEGY FOR EVALUATING THE THIRD VARIABLE HYPOTHESIS

In our view, a major limitation of most previous research linking alcohol use to sexual risk-taking has been the failure to examine the co-occurence of alcohol use and sexual behavior on a given occasion. Typically, usual alcohol use or the frequency of drinking proximal to intercourse over some specified time period are correlated with similar aggregate reports of sexual risk-taking behaviors. Importantly, however, covariation among aggregate measures would be expected whether it was due to third variable or direct causation.

In contrast, demonstrating covariation of alcohol use and sexual risk behaviors on the same occasion provides more diagnostic information regarding underlying causal mechanisms. If acute alcohol consumption causally promotes sexual risk-taking behavior, then alcohol consumption and risk-taking must be temporally linked. If, on the other hand, alcohol use and sexual risk-taking both stem from some underlying third variable (e.g., a personality or lifestyle dimension), these behaviors <u>may or may not</u> be simultaneously expressed in a particular situation. Thus, establishing a temporal link between alcohol use and sexual risk behaviors may best be regarded as a <u>necessary but not sufficient</u> condition for inferring causality. That is, demonstrating significant covariation between these behaviors on a given occasion does not prove a causal relationship; however, failure to do so substantially weakens a causal interpretation of their relationship. Thus, examining alcohol use and sexual risk-taking in specific situations is an important first step toward understanding the causal significance of their relationship.

We have thus far suggested that confirmation of the situational association between alcohol use and sexual risk-taking constitutes logically inconclusive evidence regarding the proposed direct causal link between alcohol use and sexual risk-taking. The following figure illustrates one way in which this ambiguity may arise. Hypothetically, some underlying third variable gives rise to the behavioral predispositions to drink heavily and to engage in risky behaviors. In turn, individuals who typically drink heavily will be more likely to drink on any given occasion than those who don't drink heavily. Similarly, individuals who characteristically engage in a range of sexual risk-taking behaviors will also be more likely to exhibit sexual risk behaviors on any particular occasion. Thus, these predispositions should predict (in a probablistic sense) behavior in a specific situation, thereby creating a spurious association between alcohol use and sexual risk behaviors on a particular occasion.

We propose that the viability of this model can be evaluated by estimating the situational association of alcohol use and sexual risk behaviors while controlling for indicators of global alcohol use and sexual risk-taking. If significant effects are obtained after controlling for enduring behavioral patterns, it would indicate that the observed relationships between acute alcohol use and risk-taking on a particular occasion could not be adequately accounted for by more stable or global patterns of drinking and risk-taking behavior.

Alternative Causal Model of Alcohol Use and Risk Behavior Relationship

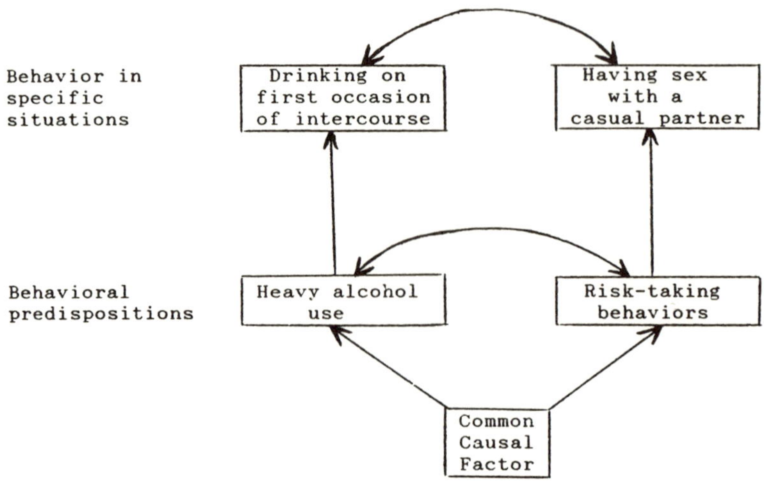

EMPIRICAL EVIDENCE: ALCOHOL USE AND SEXUAL RISK-TAKING AMONG OLDER ADOLESCENTS

We have applied the strategy proposed above to a sample of 165 sexually active older adolescents (Cooper, Skinner, & George, in preparation). To do this we assessed global patterns of alcohol use and sexual risk behaviors, and alcohol use and risk behaviors on three specific sexual occasions: first intercourse, first intercouse with most recent partner and last intercourse.

Our results were consistent with previous research in demonstrating modest associations between global indicators of alcohol use and sexual risk-taking, including more sexual partners and decreased frequency of discussing AIDS risk with potential partners, of using condoms, and of using effective methods of birth control in general. In addition, for first intercourse and first intercourse with most recent partner, those who had been drinking reported a significantly greater number of behaviors that pose serious risk for HIV infection: having intercourse with a casual partner, failing to use a condom and failing to discuss intercourse in advance. These effects were quite robust, with drinkers reporting 1 1/2 to 2 times as many risk behaviors as those who were not drinking.

To evaluate the possibility that these episode-specific effects could be accounted for by dispositional tendencies alone, we re-estimated these equations controlling for average alcohol consumption, total number of sexual partners, and relative frequency of using condoms, of using birth control and of discussing AIDS risk with new partners over the past year. Even after partialing out these indictors of global alcohol use and sexual risk-taking, alcohol use remained a highly significant predictor of the number of AIDS risk behaviors for first intercourse and first intercourse with most recent partner, accounting for roughly 12% and 9% of the variance, respectively. On the basis of these analyses, we concluded that the association between alcohol use and sexual risk behaviors on a given occasion cannot be wholly attributed to predispositions to engage in risky or unconventional behaviors.

ALTERNATIVE INTERPRETATIONS OF THE ALCOHOL USE-SEXUAL RISK BEHAVIOR RELATIONSHIP

Although our data do not support this particular third variable explanation, several alternative explanations can be offered which are consistent with the observed pattern of data. For example, the observed association between alcohol use and risky sexual behavior may reflect the situational availability of both potential sexual partners and alcohol, such as in bars or at parties (Leigh, 1987). This possibility cannot be ruled out at present and requires further study.

If we are nonetheless willing to assume that the relationship between alcohol use and sexual risk-taking is at least partially causal, several alternative causal mechanisms can be identified. Alcohol may disinhibit sexual risk-taking through pharmacologically-induced cognitive impairment (Steele & Southwick, 1985), or through socially learned expectancies that operate largely independent of pharmacological effects (Hull & Bond, 1986). Our data cannot distinguish pharmacological from expectancy effects in that pharmacology and expectancy are unavoidably confounded in naturally occurring drinking situations. Because, however, both processes are thought to disinhibit behavior individually and jointly (Crowe & George, 1989), distinguishing between them may be less important from a strictly pragmatic point of view.

Whether alcohol-induced effects are primarily pharmacological or psychological in nature, both models assume that alcohol-related disinhibition causes sexual risk-taking. However, an alternative hypothesis acknowledges a reverse causal mechanism in which the intention to engage in risky sexual behavior leads to drinking. Thus, an adolescent entering a potentially sexual situation may drink <u>in order to</u> provide an excuse to engage in desired but socially or personally unacceptable sexual behavior. In this scenario, alcohol use does not play a causal role in that consumption does not precede the intention to engage in risky or deviant sexual behavior, but rather follows from it.

Thus, it is not clear in the case of anticipatory excuse drinking that altering drinking behavior would necessarily change risky sexual behavior. Indeed, risky or deviant sexual behavior might occur without the self-protective mantle that drinking provides, thereby leading to additional negative consequences for the adolescent on self-concept and self-esteem. Conversely, if alcohol induces sexual risk-taking, altering drinking behavior should produce the desired effect of decreasing sexual risk-taking.

Although distinguishing among these several interpretations presents a formidable agenda, one may begin to judge the relative adequacy of these alternative causal hypotheses by examining the predictors of drinking proximal to intercourse. If anticipatory excuse drinking is the primary operative mechanism, then adolescents who engage in risky sexual practices while intoxicated should hold a particular constellation of beliefs regarding the excuse-giving properties of alcohol. They should, for example, believe that alcohol promotes uncharacteristic behavior, that one cannot be held accountable for his or her behavior when drinking and that alcohol disinhibits sexual behavior. Moreover, anticipatory excuse drinking in sexual situations should occur disproportionately among adolescents with the strongest need to excuse sexual behavior -- for example, among adolescents who are uncomfortable with their sexuality. Thus, to the extent that anticipatory excuse drinking can account for the situational association of alcohol use and sexual risk-taking, a unique constellation of sexual attitudes and beliefs about alcohol's excuse-giving properties should characterize those adolescents who engage in risky sexual behavior after drinking. If, however, straightforward alcohol-induced disinhibition more adequately accounts for the situational association of alcohol use and sexual risk-taking, one would not necessarily expect this particular constellation of attitudes and beliefs to predict drinking in sexual situations.

CONCLUDING THOUGHTS

We have attempted to highlight several methodological and substantive issues regrading the link between alcohol use and sexual risk-taking. The proposals offered here for addressing these issues are not suggested as final solutions, but as examples that may stimulate more refined approaches to these complex issues. For the purposes of discussion, we have portrayed these various causal processes as mutually exclusive. In reality, however, we expect that different causal processes may operate among different individuals and among the same individuals in different situations. Thus, adequate methodological approaches to the study of underlying causal mechanisms will require that we develop more complex multivariate models that take into account relevant characteristics of the individual and of the situation.

REFERENCES

Bentler PM, Newcomb MD (1986). Personality, sexual behavior, and drug use revealed through latent variable methods. Clinical Psychology Review, 66:366-385.

Cooper ML, Skinner JB, George WH (in preparation). Alcohol and sexual risk-taking among older adolescents.

Crowe LC, George WH (1989). Alcohol and human sexuality: Review and integration. Psychological Bulletin, 105(3):374-386.

Donovan JE, Jessor R (1985). Structure of problem behavior in adolescence and young adulthood. Journal of Consulting and Clinical Psychology, 53(6):890-904.

Ensminger ME (1987). Adolescent sexual behavior as it relates to other transition behaviors in youth. In SL Hofferth & CO Hayes (Eds), "Risking the future: Adolescent sexuality, pregnancy, and childbearing" (Vol. 2). Washington, D.C.: National Academy Press.

Flora JA, Thoresen CE (1988). Reducing the risk of AIDS in adolescents. American Psychologist, 43(11):965-970.

Hull JG, Bond CF (1986). Social and behavioral consequences of alcohol consumption and expectancy: A meta-analysis. Psychological Bulletin, 99:347-360.

Leigh BC (1987, October). Drinking and unsafe sex: Background and issues. Paper presented at the National Institute of Mental Health/National Institute of Drug Abuse Workshop "Women and AIDS," Bethesda, MD.

Mott FL, Haurin RJ (1988). Linkages between sexual activity and alcohol and drug use among American adolescents. Family Planning Perspectives, 20(3):128-136.

Steele CM, Southwick L (1985). Alcohol and social behavior I: The psychology of drunken excess. Journal of Personality and Social Psychology, 48: 18-34.

Zucker R, Battistich VA, Langer GB (1981). Sexual behavior, sex-role adaption and drinking in young women. Journal of Studies on Alcohol, 42:457-465.

Alcohol, Immunomodulation, and AIDS, pages 21–25
© 1990 Alan R. Liss, Inc.

PRELIMINARY RESULTS ON SEXUAL RISK-TAKING IN A GENERAL POPULATION SAMPLE

Karen Trocki, Ph.D.

Alcohol Research Group
Medical Research Institute of San Francisco
1816 Scenic Avenue, Berkeley, CA. 94609

INTRODUCTION

Although the AIDS epidemic is of great concern to those involved in public health, little is known about sexual behavioral patterns in the general population. Most recent studies of sexual behavior have focused on special, high-risk populations such as gays or bisexuals. In order to model the possible spread of the epidemic, it is necessary to know how much 'high-risk' sex there is. Secondly, in order to effectively develop prevention programs, it is necessary to know which subgroups in the population are at highest risk and what activities or factors are associated with risk-taking.

The number of AIDS cases spread through heterosexual contact has been relatively small to date -- estimated at about 5 percent. In addition, most of these cases have been spread through direct contact with bisexuals or IV drug users (Johnson and Murray, 1988). Because of the slow pace of spread in the heterosexual population, most people perceive heterosexual sex as 'safe'. Unfortunately, this complacency fosters continued risk-taking which will eventually lead to a greater build-up of seropositivity among heterosexuals. Johnson and Murray, in reviewing the Shilts' (1988) book, <u>And</u>

the Band Played on, point out how with each wave of the epidemic, there has been a tendency to attribute the disease to 'dark customs and sexual practices' that do not apply to most people and thus does not foster preventive action. We know however, that eventually it will be the everyday practices -- that is, having unprotected sex with another person who in turn has unprotected sex with others -- that will lead to the gradual spread of the disease.

The purpose of this paper is to present some preliminary results from what may well be one of the first recent studies to use rigorous probability methods in surveying people about their sexual practices. Of particular note will be the role that alcohol use plays in risk-taking. Alcohol has long been associated with 'disinhibited' behavior especially disinhibited sexual behavior. But most of this is 'common knowledge' with no hard data based on high quality surveys. A better knowledge of how sexual expectations are associated with alcohol use in general as well as how drinking modifies or enhances these expectations is crucial to containing the spread of AIDS as well as a whole host of other sexually transmitted diseases.

METHODS

The data are from a study of sexual behavior patterns from a probability sample, face-to-face interview conducted in late 1988 and early 1989. The final number of respondents is expected to be 1000, these are preliminary results from the first 550 respondents. All respondents live in a single county in the Bay Area of California. It should be noted that this county is often considered to be a microcosm of American society since it has a wide range of ethnicities as extremely rich subgroups as well as extreme poverty. The lower age limit for participation in the survey was 18 and no upper age limit was set. Thus the patterns represent a good cross-sectional determination of the extent of high risk sex in the general population. Information was collected both on aggregated sexual behavior patterns and several specific situational patterns. Respondents were asked an extensive series of questions about their last sexual encounter as well as their last sexual encounter involving a 'new' partner. The role of alcohol and drug use in high risk sex is explored.

RESULTS

Figure 1 below shows the distribution of sexual risk-taking categories in the county studied. All individuals for whom there was no

FIGURE 1: DISTRIBUTION OF SEXUAL RISK-TAKING GROUPS

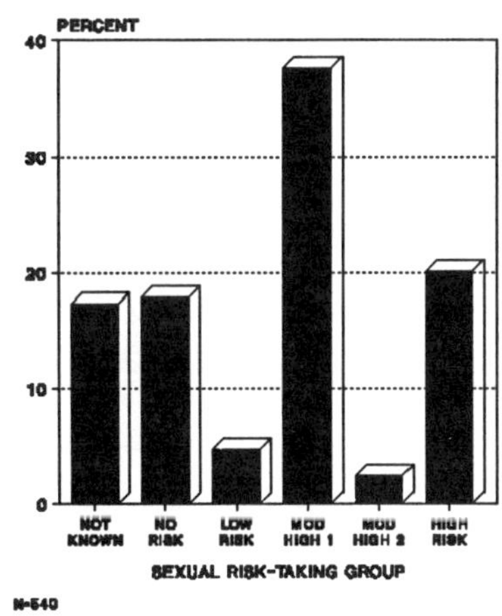

determination on risk are included in a separate category. The other categories are roughly equivalent to categories created in studies of gay populations to estimate risk of converting to HIV positive. The 'not known' category contains those people for whom there was insufficient information to place them in any of the other categories. The 'low risk' (17%) category are those who have been celibate in the last 12 months. The modified low risk category are people who have been in monogamous relationships for the last 12 months and always use condoms (6%). The modified high risk 1 category (38%) are those who are monogamous but do not always use condoms. The modified high risk category 2 (3%) consists of those individuals who are nonmonogamous but always use condoms. Finally, the high risk group (20%) are those who do not always use condoms and have had multiple partners in the last 12 months or who have a partner who has had other sexual partners in the last year.

Figure 2 shows the relationship between overall drinking patterns and these various sexual risk-taking groups (the not known group is excluded). The relationship is a modest but significant one. Of those who are in the 'celibate' group, nearly 50 percent drink only rarely or never. At the opposite extreme, nearly 70 percent of the high risk group falls into the two highest drinking groups.

FIGURE 2: OVERALL DRINKING PATTERNS IN RELATION TO SEXUAL RISK-TAKING GROUP

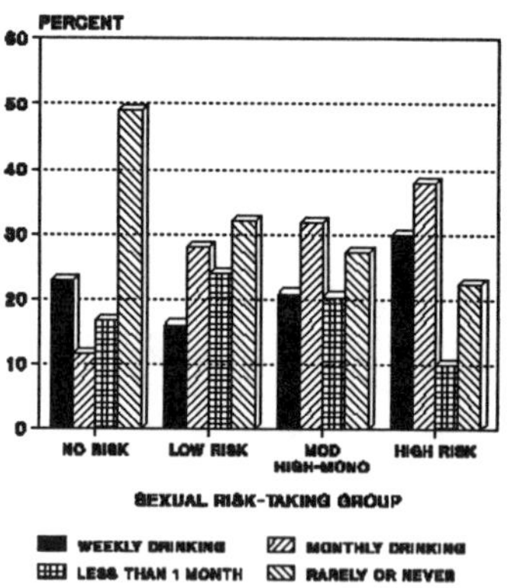

Respondents were also asked about their last sexual experience. Of those whose last sexual experience was with a new or occasional partner

over 60 percent were drinking compared to only 30 percent of those whose last sexual experience was with a regular or 'main partner. It is also noteworthy that only 20 percent of respondents who had a new or occasional partner during the last sexual experience used a condom at that time.

SUMMARY

This preliminary analysis has shown that there is a considerable amount of sexual risk taking among what is largely a heterosexual population. Although it is not likely that people will faithfully use condoms with regular or main partners, only a few people use them with new or occasional partners. The fact that 20 percent of the adult population took some sexual risks in the last 12 months is quite significant from a public health perspective. This is likely a lower bound estimate since adolescents were not included and it is likely that respondents would fail to report liasons rather than inventing ones that did not happen.

The association of alcohol and risk-taking is only looked at in a very globabl sense here. Future analyses will look closely at the entire sexual encounter event and when and under what circumstances alcohol is important. Also in future analyses we will be looking closely at the cultural belief systems which generate this alcohol and risk-taking association to see if there are mechanisms for prevention strategies.

REFERENCES

Johnson, D. and Murray, J.F. AIDS without end. The New York Review of Books, August 18, 1988, pp. 57-63.

Shilts, R. And the Band Played on. New York: Saint Martins Press, 1988.

Alcohol, Immunomodulation, and AIDS, pages 27–34
© 1990 Alan R. Liss, Inc.

DRINKING PATTERNS AND DRINKING PROBLEMS IN A COMMUNITY SAMPLE OF GAY MEN

John L. Martin

Division of Sociomedical Sciences, Columbia University School of Public Health, New York, New York 10032

INTRODUCTION

There is currently great interest in discovering factors responsible for the epidemiologic restriction of AIDS to specific risk groups in the U.S., particularly gay men and IV drug users. Over 90% of all adult cases of AIDS fall into one of these two groups. Drugs of abuse and ethanol have been suggested as feasible determinants of this pattern, possibly acting as both catalysts for high risk sexual and injecting behavior, as well as directly impairing immune competence (Molgaard et al., 1988). This argument, however, assumes that rates of use and abuse of drugs and alcohol are substantially higher among homosexual men and IV drug users compared with the rest of the population. While this assumption appears to be well supported for IV drug users, both in and out of methadone treatment (Turner et al., 1989, ch.3), the situation is not so clear with respect to homosexual men. Considering alcohol use only, the current situation is especially ambiguous.

There is widespread belief that alcohol abuse and problems due to excessive drinking are common in the homosexual population, particularly among homosexual men (Ziebold and Mongeon, 1982). While no consistent definition or measurement of alcoholism or drinking problems have been applied across studies, excessive drinking, dependence, and serious problems due to drinking have been estimated to be on the order of 30% in a number of investigations of gay men (Fifield, 1975; Lohrenz et al., 1978, Saghir and Robins, 1973; Weinberg and Williams, 1974). However, due to the sampling methods employed in each of these studies, this estimate is most likely spuriously inflated. Portions of these samples, (in some cases, the majority of the sample) were drawn from gay bars or mental health treatment facilities. Such sources contain a higher concentration of individuals with drinking problems or other psychiatric disorders than one would expect to find in the general, untreated population, that does not frequent bars. Thus, using such samples as the basis for making estimates about drinking patterns among the larger population of homosexual men is inappropriate. Regarding the question of differences in rates of problem drinking between homosexuals and heterosexuals, it should also be pointed out that the only heterosexual groups appropriate for comparison with these types of homosexual samples are ones that are drawn from similar sources, i.e. bars and mental health treatment facilities, not general population samples. No such comparisons have been made.

One investigation (Stall and Wiley, 1988) of drinking patterns based on a randomly drawn sample of homosexual and heterosexual men residing in the Castro district of San Francisco suggests that there is no difference between gay and non-gay community residents with regard to patterns of usual drinking. The modal consumption category for both groups over a twelve month period was "frequent/light." In addition, the two groups did not differ with regard to the average annual incidence of episodes of heavy drinking. While the measures used in this study cannot be taken as indicators of abuse, dependence, or serious problems due to drinking, the findings suggest that previously described differences between heterosexual and homosexual groups on measures of drinking consumption will diminish when either (a) homosexual samples are drawn from community sources, rather than from treatment sources or bars or (b) both homosexual and heterosexual comparison groups are sampled from the same sampling frame.

The purpose of the present study was to examine trends over time in patterns of usual drinking and alcohol dependence and abuse in a sample of homosexual men drawn from community sources in New York City. Our primary aims were to (1) extend the findings of Stall and Wiley (1988) to a geographically distant sample of gay men drawn from community sources and (2) to examine drinking patterns of this group in terms of both alcohol consumption and diagnosable problems of abuse and dependence.

METHOD

The Sample

In 1985 746 gay male residents of New York City, aged 20 to 70 who did not have AIDS, were recruited through one of two steps in the sampling process. First, an initial pool of 291 men (39%) were recruited directly by the researchers through the following channels: (1) Gay organizations (n = 131), (2) unsolicited volunteers (n = 41), (3) pilot sample referrals (n = 32), (4) the 1985 New York City Gay Pride Festival (n = 72), and (5) a public health clinic (n = 15). The remaining 455 (61%) respondents were recruited through personal referrals to the study by those 291 already interviewed. (See Martin et al., [1989] for a discussion of the sampling methods.)

Three follow-up interviews were conducted with respondents at one year intervals, in 1986, 1987, and 1988. Respondents who failed to complete all four interviews or who developed AIDS during the course of the study were not included in this analysis. As of 1988, 560 respondents (75% of the original sample) had been interviewed four times and had not been diagnosed with AIDS. The panel sample (N = 560) was relatively unchanged compared with the original sample. Respondents were primarily white (89%), college educated (72%), Manhattan residents (74%), with a median income of $30,000 in 1986, and a mean age of 39 in 1988. Forty-four percent of the respondents were coupled with a lover.

Measures

Usual consumption of alcohol was measured as a product of (a) the frequency of drinking in a typical week over the year prior to the interview and (b) the usual number of drinks per episode. These data were collected in all four waves of interviewing. Thus, this measure is available for 1985, 1986, 1987 and 1988.

We adopted a psychiatric diagnostic approach to measuring alcohol abuse and dependence. DSM-III (APA, 1980) criteria for each subtype were employed. The Diagnostic Interview Schedule (DIS: Robins et al., 1981) section on alcoholism was included in the interviews. Using the standard algorithm developed by the St. Louis team, the prevalence of alcohol abuse and dependence disorders were calculated. Annual rates reported here are based on the date of the occurrence of the most recent symptom of abuse and/or dependence. Data on abuse and dependence diagnoses were collected only during wave 2 and wave 3. Thus, diagnostic information is available only for 1986 and 1987.

RESULTS

The means and standard deviations for usual consumption of alcohol are shown for each of four years in Table 1. It can be seen that there is a high degree of stability over time in these scores for the sample as a whole. Overall, the average respondent in this sample consumed three to four drinks per week, during each year from 1985 to 1988. None of the mean differences shown in Table 1 were significantly different, using matched t-test procedures comparing contiguous years.

TABLE 1. Average scores (SD) on an index of usual drinking per week, for four annual time periods.

Year			
1985	1986	1987	1988
3.58	3.64	3.72	3.50
(3.31)	(3.75)	(3.97)	(3.70)

The proportion of the sample abstaining from alcohol in each year was also stable: 15.3% in 1985, 16.1% in 1986,

15,9% in 1987, and 16.1% in 1988. In order to determine the extent to which abstainers reduced the values for typical drinking patterns shown in Table 1, we removed those who reported no drinking each year from the total, and recalculated the means. The overall effect of this procedure was to increase scores by approximately one additional drink per week for the group who drank alcohol at all during a particular year.

Turning now to the question of DIS/DSM-III diagnoses of alcohol abuse and dependence, we found that 12.0% of the sample met diagnostic criteria for one or both of these subtypes of alcoholism in the twelve months prior to the 1986 interview. When the DIS was readministered in 1987, 9.0% met diagnostic criteria for alcohol abuse and/or dependence in the preceding twelve months. These proportions are not significantly different from each other, and they are highly dependent on one another, (chi square [1] = 138.9, $p < .0001$).

DISCUSSION

The present results provide descriptive data over time on alcohol consumption and problems of alcohol abuse and dependence in a community sample of gay men in New York City. We specifically examined patterns of usual drinking and prevalence of problems which may be used as indicators of alcoholism. These data indicate that patterns of typical drinking in this sample are highly stable over time. Among the 85% of the sample who drank at all during a particular year, the average consumption rate was four drinks per week. The modal category for frequency of drinking was twice per week; The modal category for quantity of drinking was two drinks per episode.

These findings are inconsistent with the proposition that homosexual men are typically heavy drinkers. While our methodology does not permit a rigorous comparison with other studies, men in our sample who received a score of 10 or more on the measure of usual drinking would correspond roughly to "frequent/heavy" drinkers identified by Stall and Wiley (1988). Considered in this categorical manner, 5% to 6% of the sample in each year of interviews would qualify as frequent/heavy drinkers. This is in contrast to the 19% of the San Francisco sample categorized at this level. Regardless of which figure one accepts, neither of them can be taken as evidence of high rates of excessive drinking or alcoholism in these community samples of gay men.

Additional support for this conclusion comes from the findings on DIS/DSM-III alcohol abuse and dependence. The present results suggest that the prevalence of problems indicative of alcoholism, at least as defined by one set of criteria, is in the range of 10% per year among gay men, rather than in excess of 30% at any given time. While this rate is certainly higher than the 4% rate suggested by Dohrenwend and colleagues (Dohrenwend et al., 1980, pp. 65-66) in their synthesis of true prevalence studies in the U.S., it clearly indicates that problem drinkers are not typical among gay men, and are unlikely to constitute as much as a third of the homosexual population.

The sample from which the present data come was not a random sample of a specified population. Thus, the descriptive statistics provided here must be viewed cautiously, from the standpoint of their generalizability to the population of homosexual men in New York City. Since one component of this sample is a true random sample drawn from a defined sampling frame of members of gay organizations, we can and will develop more statistically defensible parameters regarding drinking patterns in future work.

Despite the limitations of the sample, the relatively low rates of heavy drinking and alcohol abuse and dependence which we found have implications for other types of research on AIDS and drinking. Specifically, these findings indicate that researchers should not employ community samples of gay men for the purpose of assessing the role of heavy alcohol use in the natural history and progression of AIDS among HIV infected persons; There simply will be insufficient numbers of cases over a specified time period to conduct meaningful analyses. Studies of the role of heavy alcohol use in disease progression should focus on special groups of heavy drinkers in order to obtain sufficiently large samples of such individuals. In addition, the present findings also indicate that investigations of the role of moderate alcohol use in the progression of AIDS would be the type of research useful to the largest numbers of HIV infected gay men, since it appears that the majority of gay men can be considered light to moderate drinkers, not heavy drinkers or alcohol abusers.

The analyses presented here were not designed to address the question of the role of alcohol use in the development of AIDS. Thus, we explicitly excluded respondents who developed AIDS during the course of this study. It is interesting to note, however, that when we examined the 20 men with AIDS on whom we had complete data for at least three years we found that their average level of usual drinking was two drinks per week: A level significantly below that of the non-ill respondents.

The final implication of the present findings which should be noted is that they are not consistent with the proposition that alcohol abuse is responsible for, or plays an important role in, the epidemiologic distribution of AIDS. There appear to be too few heavy drinkers in this community sample of New York, (as well as in San Francisco [Stall and Wiley, 1988]), to support the idea that homosexual men have experienced a disproportionate amount of AIDS because of the pervasiveness of excessive alcohol use in that population. A more parsimonious explanation of the epidemiologic distribution of AIDS and HIV in the U.S. population can be found in patterns of sexual behaviors and drug injecting behavior (Turner et al., 1989).

REFERENCES

American Psychiatric Association (1980). "Diagnostic and Statistical Manual of Mental Disorders: Third Edition." Washington D C: American Psychiatric Association.

Dohrenwend BP, Dohrenwend BS, Gould MS, Link B, Neugebauer R, Wunsch-Hitzig R (1980). "Mental Illness in the United States: Epidemiological Estimates." New York: Praeger.

Fifield L (1975). "On My Way to Nowhere: Alienated, Isolated, Drunk." Los Angeles: Gay Community Services Center.

Lohrenz L, Connelly J, Coyne L, Spare K (1978). Alcohol problems in several midwestern homosexual communities. J Stud Alch 39:1959-1963.

Martin JL, Dean L, Garcia M, Hall W (1989). The impact of AIDS on a gay community: Changes in sexual behavior, substance use and mental health. Am J Comm Psychol 17: in press.

Molgaard CA, Nakamura C, Hovel M, Elder JP (1988). Assessing alcoholism as a risk factor for acquired immunodeficiency syndrome (AIDS). Soc Sci Med 27:1147-1152.

Robins LN, Helzer JE, Croughan J, Ratcliff KS (1981). National Institute of Mental Health Diagnostic Interview Schedule: Its history, characteristics and validity. Arch Gen Psychiat 38:381-389.

Saghir M, Robins E (1973). "Male and Female Homosexuality." Baltimore: Williams and Wilkins Co.

Stall R, Wiley J (1988). A comparison of alcohol and drug use patterns of homosexual and heterosexual men: The San Francisco Men's Health Study. Drug Alch Dependence 22: 63-73.

Turner C, Miller H, Moses L (1989). "AIDS: Sexual Behavior and Intravenous Drug Use." Washington D C: National Academy Press.

Weinberg M, Williams C (1974). "Male Homosexuals." New York: Oxford University Press.

Ziebold TO, Mongeon JE (1982). Alcoholism and the homosexual community. J Homosexuality 7:3-7.

Alcohol, Immunomodulation, and AIDS, pages 35–46
© 1990 Alan R. Liss, Inc.

ALCOHOL AND UNSAFE SEX: AN OVERVIEW OF RESEARCH AND THEORY

Barbara Critchlow Leigh

Alcohol Research Group, Medical Research Institute of San Francisco, 1816 Scenic Avenue, Berkeley, California 94709

Although conventional wisdom and the teachings of our culture tell us that alcohol disinhibits sexual activity, surprisingly, the relationship of drinking and sex has become the subject of empirical research only in recent years. In light of the AIDS epidemic, any link between drinking and sex assumes a great deal of importance. Recent research with homosexual samples in two cities has shown that the use of alcohol in conjunction with sexual activity is strongly related to sexual activities known to be risky in terms of AIDS infection. If drinking does indeed lead to unsafe sexual activity, understanding the dynamics of this relationship can contribute to research, preventive and education efforts to contain the spread of AIDS infection.

In order to examine the effects of drinking on risky sex, one may draw on research and theory from a number of areas, including laboratory studies on the effects of alcohol on sexual arousal, surveys of drinking and sexual behavior, and studies of contraceptive use. High-risk sexual behavior implies the occurrence of sexual behavior per se; therefore, to examine any relationship of drinking to unsafe sex in particular, we must understand the relationship of drinking to sexual behavior in general. This brief overview will summarize research in on the effects of alcohol on sexual activity and risky sexual behavior, and sketch possible explanations for such relationships.

A NOTE ON METHODS

In general, three types of methods have been used in studying the relationship of drinking to sexual activity. In correlational studies, measures of people's drinking habits and their sexual behavior are collected, often by means of a survey, and relationships between these measures are examined. This type of study does not allow a determination of a causal relationship between variables: For any observed relationship, there are a number of possible causal influences. Studies using a diary methodology ask participants to keep daily logs of their activities (including the time at which they occur) over several days, weeks, or months. This method enables an analysis of data on the temporal relationships of drinking incidents and sexual encounters, both within individuals and across individuals. To the extent that individuals may be used as their own controls, this technique institutes an added control over correlational studies. Laboratory studies, in which alcohol is administered to an experimental group and withheld from a control group, make statements of causal influence possible; however, they may suffer from sterility and lack of ecological validity. Each method has advantages and disadvantages in terms of the interpretation of results.

RESEARCH ON THE EFFECTS OF ALCOHOL ON SEXUAL BEHAVIOR

The effects of alcohol on social behavior, including sexual behavior, are entrenched in history, folklore, and popular opinion. Many sources, from opinion polls to literature, tell us that alcohol consumption intrinsically leads to seduction and sex (for review, see Critchlow, 1986; Lang, 1985; Reinarman & Leigh, 1987; Wilsnack, 1984; Wilson, 1981).

Correlational studies

The results of correlational studies are consistent with the contention, that alcohol disinhibits sexuality, but their interpretation is not straightforward. In general, heavier drinking is positively correlated with past sexual experience and current sexual activity in women (see Wilsnack, 1984). Surveys of adolescents have found relationships between alcohol use and sexual activity (Bentler & Newcomb, 1986; Coles & Stokes, 1985; Zabin et Al., 1986; Zucker et al., 1981). However, these relationships are of only moderate strength, and the relationship found may actually be a manifestation of other factors. Note that a relationship of general drinking habits and general frequency of sexual activity does not illuminate the relationship between drinking and sex on the same occasion; thus causal order cannot be determined. Several interpretations are possible, including that 1) drinking disinhibits sexual activity; 2) drinking and sexual activity are both markers of an individual's standing on a general moral continuum; 3) both drinking and sex are symptomatic of personality characteristics such as impulsivity or desire to flout social restraints; 4) both drinking and sexual behavior may be part of a certain "congenial" social lifestyle (Wilsnack, 1984).

Diary studies

Two studies (both with female samples) in which participants kept daily logs of drinking and sexual behavior have suggested that drinking does not necessarily increase sexual activity. Harvey and Beckman (1986) found that women initiated sexual activities more often when they had not been drinking than when they had been drinking any amount. The women's self-ratings of arousal, pleasure and orgasm were not affected by drinking alcohol prior to sexual activity. Lex et al. (1988) report no relationship between alcohol consumption and sexual activity in their sample.

Laboratory studies

Laboratory studies provide the best means to identify the causal influence of alcohol on sexual behavior, while controlling for confounding variables. Experimental work on the effects of alcohol on human behavior is of relatively recent vintage, and its methodology has become a great deal more sophisticated. Recent studies control for the possibility that alcohol effects are due not to alcohol ingestion but to beliefs about alcohol's effects. Using the "balanced placebo" design (Marlatt & Rohsenow, 1980), subjects are given either alcohol or a placebo, and are told that they are receiving either alcohol or plain tonic water. This design, by fully crossing alcohol administration with the belief that one has received alcohol, thus permits separation of the effects of alcohol consumption from the effects of cognitive set or expectation.

A number of balanced placebo studies have shown that for many different social behaviors, including sexual arousal, alcohol ingestion itself has little or no effect on behavior, but the belief that one has consumed alcohol does affect behavior (See Hull & Bond, 1986; also Lang, 1983 for reviews). This placebo effect suggests that although alcohol does have active pharmacological properties, the direction that changes in behavior will take is determined not by this pharmacological action but by circumstances and beliefs about alcohol's effects. Laboratory studies of sexual arousal show that alcohol ingestion per se and belief about ingestion have quite different effects on sexual arousal, and have different effects on men and women (see Lang, 1985; Wilsnack, 1984; Wilson, 1981 for more detailed reviews of this literature).

In men, high alcohol doses are related to decreased tumescence, increased latency to orgasm, and subjective reports of decreased arousal and orgasmic pleasure and intensity (Malatesta et al., 1979). In studies using the balanced placebo design and somewhat lower blood alcohol levels, alcohol itself generally has no effect on sexual arousal in men, but the belief that one has consumed alcohol leads to greater physiological and subjective arousal in response to sexual stimuli (see Wilson, 1981 for review). Like men, women show a depressed orgasmic response with increasing intoxication (e.g., Malatesta et al., 1982). However, women's subjective reports of arousal and orgasmic pleasurability are positively related to increasing blood alcohol levels (Malatesta et al., 1982; Wilson & Lawson, 1976a) and to increasing subjective intoxication (Wilson & Lawson, 1978). The belief that alcohol has been consumed has no effect on arousal (Wilson & Lawson, 1976a; 1978).

Thus, laboratory research suggests that at low to moderate doses of alcohol the belief that one is intoxicated affects physiological arousal to sexual stimuli among men, but not among women. At higher doses, alcohol decreases sexual response in both men and women; however, measures of objective (physiological) and subjective (self-reported) arousal are positively associated in men, but in women they vary in the opposite direction. The reasons behind the sex differences reported are unclear, but explanations have been advanced that take into account differential socialization experiences for men and women, and anatomical differences that lead to varying degrees of difficulty in monitoring physiological arousal (Wilsnack, 1984; Wilson & Lawson, 1978).

Caution is in order when interpreting results of laboratory studies. For practical reasons, most laboratory studies use relatively low blood alcohol levels (.10% or below), which limits their generalizability, particularly if the effects are not linear. Laboratory studies generally measure two classes of variables--physiological and/or psychological arousal responses to sexual stimuli and time spent viewing erotic materials--and it is a large step from these responses to overt sexual behavior. Controlled psychophysiological measures are not necessarily more salient indicators of sexual arousal than subjective feelings; these increased pleasurable feelings may actually be more important in behavior than genital arousal itself (Wilsnack, 1984).

In summary, research on the effects of alcohol on sexual arousal and behavior suggests that sex does not follow drinking in lockstep fashion. Intriguing sex differences appear, and beliefs about drinking and its effects play a large role in any alcohol-induced "disinhibition." Moving from correlational data to the laboratory increases control over confounding variables, but at the expense of realism, and the translation of arousal responses to actual behavior is still an open question.

RESEARCH ON ALCOHOL AND UNSAFE SEX

Existing data on the relationship of alcohol to unsafe sex is based on correlational or diary studies; risky sexual behavior itself obviously cannot be studied in a laboratory.

Correlational studies

A recent study reported that among a cohort of sexually active gay men in San Francisco, using alcohol or drugs with sex is strongly associated with unsafe sexual behaviors (Stall et al., 1986), and th is finding has been replicated in unpublished studies with other samples in Chicago and New York (However, other studies have failed to replicate; e.g., Leigh, 1988). Valdiserri et al. (1988) also report that gay men in their sample who were high on alcohol and/or drugs with more than half of their sexual partners were less likely to use condoms regularly. The findings are based on correlations between general measures of frequency of unsafe behaviors and of drinking before sex, and thus we do not know if the times when the individual was drinking were the same times that he performed risky activities. Causal interprctation is therefore difficult. In addition, very little is known about the relationship of drinking to unsafe sexual activity outside of male homosexual samples.

The sparse literature on drinking and contraceptive use in women is relevant to this issue, since it deals with sexual protection (albeit against a different outcome). A study of college students found that heavier drinkers were less likely to use contraception than were lighter drinkers and abstainers (Zucker et al., 1981), and a study of women visiting a family planning clinic found a similar negative relationship between drinking habits and contraceptive use (Jaccard, 1987). However, a correlational relationship between general drinking behavior and the frequency of unprotected sex does not mean that drinking necessarily has a direct impact on contraceptive use: Drinking and unprotected sex may both be indicators of a constellation of general sensation-seeking or risk-taking activities, or indicative of problems of impulse control.

Diary studies

The only published study to date that has investigated the effects of drinking proximal to intercourse on contraceptive behavior is that of Harvey and Beckman (1986), who asked social-drinking women in stable heterosexual relationships, all of whom used coitus-dependent contraceptives, to keep daily logs of their drinking, sexual activities, and contraceptive use. Among these women, alcohol consumed before intercourse had no effect on the use or non-use of contraceptives (including both the failure to use any method and the use of an ineffective method such as rhythm or withdrawal). The authors note that their sample was rather mature, well-educated, and involved in stable relationships, all of which may have contributed to particularly responsible contraceptive behavior.

Some studies have used a "critical incident" technique, win which survey respondents are asked a number of questions about a specific sexual incident and about the presence or absence of alcohol and risky sex in these events. This procedure is then similar to a diary method, except that information is only gathered on a few incidents. Some of these analyses (e.g., Robertson & Plant, 1988; Trocki, 1988) have suggested that incidence of unsafe sex is higher in events that included alcohol; others (Leigh, 1989) have not found such a relationship.

To summarize, research with gay men has discovered a strong relationship between frequency of alcohol use with sex and frequency of engaging in risky sexual behaviors, a relationship yet to be replicated in heterosexual samples. Results from literature on drinking and contraceptive use are equivocal. In addition, contraception studies are limited to women, and include all contraceptive methods, including those requiring no cooperation by a sexual partner.

THEORETICAL EXPLANATIONS

A number of explanations for a drinking-sex link, or a drinking-unsafe sex link, have been advanced (e.g., Hull & Van Treuren, 1986; Ostrow, 1986; Stall et al., 1986; Wilson, 1981). A traditional disinhibition model, whereby alcohol, by way of pharmacological action, causes the release of behaviors that are normally suppressed, is called into question by both laboratory data and the weight of anthropological evidence (e.g., Mac Andrew & Edgerton, 1969). However, a psychological, rather than physiological mechanism may also produce disinhibited behavior. To the extent that people believe that alcohol causes a loss of control over sexual behavior, drinking may produce a self-fulfilling prophecy whereby increased sexual risk-taking is the result. "Paraphrasing the classic sociological dictum, effects that are believed real are real in their consequences." (Room, 1983, p. 41)

A cognitive version of a disinhibition model relies on evidence suggesting that alcohol per se interferes with people's ability to attend to peripheral cues and behavioral standards, and to foresee the consequences of their behavior (e.g., Zeichner & Phil, 1979; Steele & Southwick, 1985; Steele & Josephs, 1988). Recent theoretical models of the effects of alcohol on social behavior (e.g., Hull & Van Treuren, 1986; Steele & Southwick, 1985) make reference to the ability of alcohol to impair certain cognitive abilities, particularly higher-order encoding and inference processes (e.g., Birnbaum et al., 1980). Under the influence of alcohol, an individual may be less likely to attend to peripheral environmental cues due to a narrowing of attention (see Pernanen, 1976), or be unable to infer behavioral standards from these cues due to information processing decrements (Hull & Van Treuren, 1986). Taking sexual precautions necessitates paying attention to some future possibility of unwanted consequences, a thought not nearly as salient as the sexual impulse of the moment. Alcohol may then increase the probability of sexual risk-taking by adversely affecting an assessment of risk vs. immediate pleasure.

As mentioned above, studies demonstrating only a correlational relationship between drinking habits and sexual behavior are consistent with the hypothesis that certain personality variables underly both drinking and risky sex. Drinking and risky sex may, for example, be parts of a larger constellation of risk-taking or sensation-seeking behaviors (e.g., Adlaf & Smart, 1983; Zuckerman, 1979). These behaviors may occur together not solely because of underlying personality motivations but also as a result of structural forces. These "problem behaviors" (Donovan & Jessor, 1985) may be learned together and be part of a lifestyle structured so that they continue to occur together.

A social learning analysis of alcohol's influence on sexual behavior hypothesizes that people learn through modeling, reinforcement, and cultural experience the appropriate behaviors to display while drinking (Adesso, 1985; Wilson, 1978). In other words, people who have been drinking become more sexual, aggressive, etc. only because they think alcohol makes them more sexual or aggressive. Such a model is supported by laboratory studies showing strong placebo effects of alcohol. The sanctioned use of alcohol is a powerful source of cultural influence, particularly when it offers a period of "time out" from normal social restraints (Mac Andrew & Edgerton, 1969). The use of alcohol as an excuse for behavior that is unacceptable, either to society or to oneself, may lead to increases in behavior that people would otherwise not do (Critchlow, 1983; Lang, 1983).

The combination of drinking and sex may be a function of the setting in which both appear, a social situation with its own idiosyncratic rules of conduct. Much drinking takes place in venues where potential sexual partners are available, thus, alcohol is confounded with sexual opportunity (Carpenter & Armenti, 1971; Wilson, 1981). Drinking and sex may both be part of a culturally-defined romantic scenario, or both may reflect a "fast-lane" lifestyle in which risky sex and alcohol are part of a routine social ritual (Stall et al., 1986).

Finally, it must be emphasized that in this area as in any other, it is unrealistic to propose a single cause of the phenomenon. The relationship of drinking to sex and risky sex must encompass many factors--pharmacological, psychological, environmental, and cultural--and efforts to understand it must attend to research and theory from all of these disciplines.

SUMMARY AND DIRECTIONS

The research summarized here points to the conclusion that we know less than we think we do about drinking and sex. Controlled research on the effects of alcohol on subjective and objective physiological arousal is limited, and more is needed to explain the sex differences so far demonstrated. Liberal sexual habits are correlated with liberal drinking habits, but an understanding of the causal order underlying this relationship is elusive. Drinking does not seem to interfere with use of coitus-dependent contraception for intercourse with steady partners, but research on new sexual partners is lacking. A strong cross-sectional relationship between use of alcohol with sex and risky sexual behavior has been found in gay men, but has not been replicated in other samples. Obviously, many issues surrounding drinking and sex deserve more investigation, and much remains to be done with what <u>is</u> known. In a sense, conventional wisdom is the enemy of scientific progress in this field: If drinking-related sexual disinhibition is taken for granted, then research to examine its parameters and its very existence will not be seen as high priority.

Promising areas emerge from our current knowledge. Controlled research has revealed differences in alcohol and placebo effects on sexual arousal and behavior in women and men; these should be explored. The notion that the divergent results of these studies for men and women are due to different interpretations of arousal based on sex-role appropriateness remains at the level of hypothesis, and is ripe for investigation.

More work is also needed to examine whether drinking affects effective use of contraception or protection. Correlational studies suggest a relationship (Jaccard, 1987; Valdiserri et al., 1988), but the sole non-correlational study examining this topic (Harvey & Beckman, 1986) found no interference of alcohol on the use of coitus-dependent contraceptives. However, Harvey and Beckman's study was limited to women with steady partners, and with unfamiliar partners this picture might change. Because drinking is such a large part of symbolic courtship and the meeting of potential sexual partners, it may play a larger role in sexual encounters between new partners than old. In addition, research on drinking and contraceptive use, focusing as it does on all manner of contraceptive methods, does not provide specific information about condoms.

Studies on the effects of drinking on risky sex need to be expanded beyond the convenience samples used in previous work (Stall et al., 1986; Valdiserri et al., 1988). Researchers at several institutions are currently studying the drinking-sex link in representative samples of adolescents and adults. Generalizing the important findings of research on nonrepresentative samples of gay men to individuals of different ages and sexual orientation is a necessary first step in examining this issue.

Researchers in this area need to attend to research and theory from areas beyond their own in order to have a full understanding of the issue. Jumping disciplinary lines is not always easy, but contributions can be made from researchers in sociology, anthropology, psychology, medicine, public health, many of whom are unaware of promising work in other areas. No one discipline has a lock on this issue, or a claim to the true explanation of the phenomenon.

Finally, it must be remembered that one's view of the cause of a problem determines one's view of its solution. If drinking is associated with increased AIDS risk, preventive and educational efforts to stem the spread of AIDS will vary according to the chosen explanation for drinking-related risk. Stall et al. (1986) have suggested a number of intervention strategies linked several competing explanations for a drinking-risky sex relationship. For example, if drinking is related to sexual risk-taking because alcohol and sexual partners are found in the same places, then making these environments more conducive to safe sex (e.g., by placing condom machines in bars) may be an effective intervention. If, as predicted by a social learning model, alcohol provides an excuse for risky sexual behavior, the changing of community norms that permit such an excuse is in order. The placing of the locus of the problem--on the individual, on the alcohol, or on the environment in which both exist--implies the acceptance of different kinds of actions taken to attenuate it.

REFERENCES

Adesso VJ (1985). Cognitive factors in alcohol and drug use. In Galizio M, Maisto SA (eds.): "Determinants of Substance Abuse," New York: Plenum, pp 179-208.

Adlaf EM, Smart RG (1983). Risk-taking and drug use behavior: an examination. Drug and Alcohol Dependence 11:287-296.

Bentler PM, Newcomb MD (1986). Personality, sexual behavior, and drug use revealed through latent variable methods. Clinical Psychology Review 6:363-385.

Birnbaum I, Johnson M, Hartley J, Taylor T (1980). Alcohol and elaborative schemas for sentences. Journal of Experimental Psychology: Human Learning and Memory 6:293-300.

Carpenter A, Armenti NP (1971). Some effects of ethanol on human sexual and aggressive behavior. In Kissin B, Begleiter H (eds.): "The biology of alcoholism," New York: Plenum Press, pp 509-543.

Coles R, Stokes G (1985). "Sex and the American teenager," New York: Harper & Row.

Critchlow, B (1983). Blaming the booze: The attribution of responsibility for drunken behavior. Personality and Social Psychology Bulletin 9:451-473.

Donovan JE, Jessor R (1985). Structure of problem behavior in adolescence and young adulthood. Journal of Consulting and Clinical Psychology 53:890-904.

Harvey SM, Beckman LJ (1986). Alcohol consumption, female sexual behavior and contraceptive use. Journal of Studies on Alcohol 47:327-332.

Hull JG, Bond C (1986). The social and behavioral consequences of alcohol consumption and expectancy: A meta-analysis. Psychological Bulletin 99:347-360.

Hull JG, Van Treuren RR (1986). Experimental social psychology and the causes and effects of alcohol consumption. Research Advances in Alcohol and Drug Problems 9:211-243.

Jaccard J (1987). When attitudes aren't enough: Issues in understanding consistent contraceptive use. Invited address, 95th Annual Meeting of the American Psychological Association, New York City.

Lang A (1985). The social psychology of drinking and human sexuality. Journal of Drug Issues 15:273-289.

Leigh BC (1988). Drinking and sex: Preliminary survey results. Paper presented at the Annual Meeting of the Kettil Bruun Society for Social and Epidemiological Research on Alcohol, Berkeley, California.

Leigh BC (1989). The relationship of sex-related alcohol expectancies to alcohol consumption and sexual behavior. Manuscript under review.

Lex BW, Palmieri SL, Mello NK, Mendelson JH (1988). Alcohol use, marihuana smoking, and sexual activity in women. Alcohol 5:21-25.

MacAndrew C, Edgerton R (1969). "Drunken Comportment: A Social Explanation," Chicago: Aldine.

Malatesta V, Pollack R, Crotty T, Peacock L (1982). Acute alcohol intoxication and female orgasmic response. Journal of Sex Research 18:1-17.

Malatesta V, Pollack R, Wilbanks W, Adams H (1979). Alcohol effects on the orgasmic-ejaculatory response in human males. Journal of Sex Research 15:101-107.

Marlatt A, Rohsenow D (1980). Cognitive processes in alcohol use: expectancy and the balanced placebo design. In Mello NK (ed.): "Advances in Substance Abuse: Behavioral and Biological Research," Greenwich, CT: JAI Press.

Ostrow D (1976). Barriers to the recognition of links between drug and alcohol abuse and AIDS. In "Acquired Immune Deficiency Syndrome and Chemical Dependency," (DHHS Pub. No. ADM 87-1513) Washington DC: US Government Printing Office, pp. 15-20.

Pernanen K (1976). Alcohol and crimes of violence. In Kissin B, Begleiter H (eds.): "The Biology of Alcoholism: Social Aspects of Alcoholism (Vol. 4)," New York: Plenum, pp 351-444.

Reinarman C, Leigh BC (1987). Culture, cognition, and disinhibition: Notes on sexuality and alcohol in the age of AIDS. Contemporary Drug Problems 14:435-460.

Robertson JA, Plant MA (1988). Alcohol, sex and risks of HIV infection. Drug and Alcohol Dependence 22:75-78.
Room RG (1983). Alcohol and crime: Behavioral aspects. In Kadish SH (ed.), "Encyclopedia of Crime and Justice (Vol. 1)," New York: Free Press, pp 35-44.
Stall R, McKusick L, Wiley J, Coates T, Ostrow, D (1986). Alcohol and drug use during sexual activity and compliance with safe sex guidelines for AIDS: The AIDS Behavioral Research Project. Health Education Quarterly 13:359-371.
Steele CM, Josephs RA (1988). Drinking your troubles away II: An attention-allocation model of alcohol's effect on psychological stress. Journal of Abnormal Psychology 97: 196-205.
Steele CM, Southwick L (1985). Alcohol and social behavior I: The psychology of drunken excess. Journal of Personality and Social Psychology 48:35-46.
Trocki K (1988). Drinking and sex: Examining the situation. Paper presented at the Annual Meeting of the Kettil Bruun Society for Social and Epidemiological Research on Alcohol, Berkeley, California.
Valdiserri RO, Lyter D, Leviton LC, Callahan CM, Kingsley LA, Rinaldo CR (1988). Variables influencing condom use in a cohort of gay and bisexual men. Am J Pub Health 78:801-805.
Wilsnack SC (1984). Drinking, sexuality, and sexual dysfunction in women. In Wilsnack SC, Beckman LJ (eds.): "Alcohol Problems in Women," New York: Guilford, pp. 189-227.
Wilson GT (1978). Booze, beliefs, and behavior: Cognitive processes in alcohol use and abuse. In Nathan PE, Marlatt GA, Loberg T (eds.): "Alcoholism: New Directions in Behavioral Research and Treatment," New York: Plenum, pp 315-339.
Wilson GT (1981). The effects of alcohol on human sexual behavior. In Mello N (ed.): "Advances in Substance Abuse (Vol. 2)," Greenwich, CT: JAI Press, pp 1-40.
Wilson GT, Lawson D (1976). The effects of alcohol on sexual arousal in women. Journal of Abnormal Psychology 85:489-497.
Wilson GT, Lawson D (1978). Expectancies, alcohol and sexual arousal in women. Journal of Abnormal Psychology 87:358-367.
Zabin LS, Hardy JB, Smith EA, Hirsch MB (1986). Substance use and its relation to sexual activity among inner-city adolescents. Journal of Adolescent Health Care 7:320-333.
Zeichner A, Pihl R (1979). Effects of alcohol and behavior contingencies on human aggression. Journal of Abnormal Psychology 88:133-160.
Zucker R, Battistich V, Langer G (1981). Sexual behavior, sex-role adaptation and drinking in young women. Journal of Studies on Alcohol 42:457-465.
Zuckerman M (1979). "Sensation-seeking: Beyond the Optimal Level of Arousal," Hillsdale, NJ: Erlbaum.

Alcohol, Immunomodulation, and AIDS, pages 47–55
© 1990 Alan R. Liss, Inc.

NEUROIMMUNOTOXIC EFFECTS IN OFFSPRING OF PATERNAL ALCOHOL CONSUMPTION

Ernest L. Abel, Linda S. Hazlett, Richard S. Berk and Milton G. Mutchnick
Departments of Obstetrics and Gynecology (E.L.A.), Anatomy (L.S.H.), Immunology/ Microbiology (R.S.B.) and Gastroenterology (M.M.), Wayne State University, Detroit, Michigan 48201

INTRODUCTION

Nearly all studies of prenatal alcohol exposure have focused on in utero exposure. We have been extending these studies to focus on the effects of paternal exposure and in the course of these studies we have found that both paternal and maternal alcohol consumption are associated in rats and mice with an increased susceptibility of offspring to infection which may be related to an increased responsiveness of these animals to stress.

In our studies of paternally-mediated effects, we have been especially concerned about possible sources of confounding and inconclusive findings due to methodological shortcomings noted by Randall et al. (1982) in their critique of work in this area. Our overall treatment/test paradigms are characterized by large numbers of litters per group, at least three concentrations of alcohol, pair feeding to control for alcohol-related undernutrition, testing offspring at different ages, and use of two different species (rats and mice). Since fathers are removed from mothers after conception and never come in contact with offspring, those changes which we see in offspring sired by alcohol-consuming fathers can only be due to some effect of alcohol on the sperm which fertilized mothers.

Our basic protocol for both our rat and mouse studies is almost identical. Male rats are assigned to one of four groups. One group is given ad lib access to a liquid alcohol diet containing 35% ethanol derived calories (EDC). Two other groups receive diets containing 17.5 or 0% EDC and are pair fed to those in the higher group. A fourth group of nontreated animals is fed lab chow as a further control for possible effects of diet restriction associated with pair feeding. Our behavioral test procedures are identical to those we and others use to test offspring of animals born to mothers that consume alcohol during pregnancy (e.g., Abel, 1982; Riley et al., 1979). Our mouse studies have presented diets containing 20 or 25% EDC as the maximum alcohol concentration. Diets are presented for a minimum of one complete cycle of spermatogenesis (53 days in rats, 45 days in mice) (Dixon and Hall, 1981).

Effects on Activity

The most consistent effect on offspring behavior associated with paternal alcohol exposure that we have observed is a <u>decrease</u> in activity in both rats and mice (See Figure 1). This effect on activity is surprising

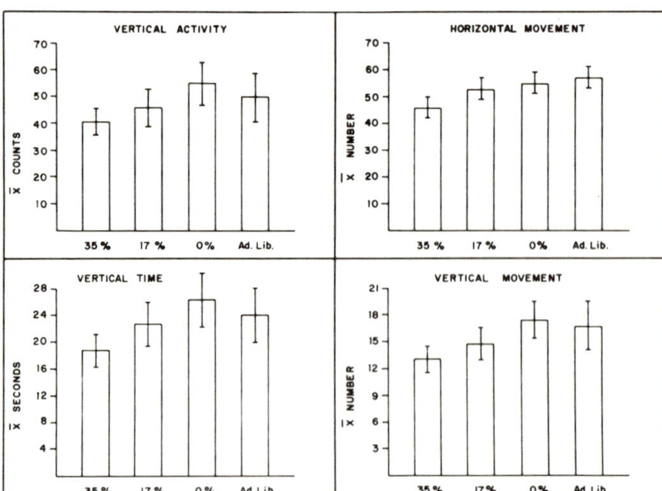

Figure 1. Activity of rat offspring sired by fathers consuming liquid alcohol diets containing 35%, 17.5% or 0% ethanol derived calories (EDC). Ad lib: Nontreated fathers.

because it is opposite to the increased activity in offspring associated with maternal alcohol exposure which we and others have reported (Abel, 1982; Bond and DiGiusto, 1977). We have now replicated this observation in four studies (Abel and Lee, 1988; Abel and Tan, 1988; Abel, 1989a, 1989b). On the basis of our findings in mice, we have now narrowed the threshold concentration for this effect in this species to between 15 and 20% EDC.

Effects on Responsiveness to Stress

A second series of behavioral observations that we have made is that rats sired by alcohol consuming fathers do not adapt to stress as well as controls. Our stress test is Porsolt et al.'s, (1977) inescapable swimming test. The general paradigm for these studies is that animals are placed for 15 minutes in a swimming tank. Twenty-four hours later they are exposed again to the same conditions and total immobility time during a 5 minute period is recorded. The current interpretation of behavior in this test is that the more immobile the animal during testing, the greater its adaptation to an inescapable stressful environment (e.g., Borsini et al., 1986; Hawkins, et al., 1978). In our studies, we have found that rats sired by alcohol-consuming males are <u>less</u> immobile than controls, i.e., they do not adapt to the stress as well as controls:

TABLE 1. Effects of paternal alcohol consumption on immobility in an inescapable swimming task in rats.

x ± SE Immobility Time (Sec)		
35% EDC	17.5% EDC	0% EDC
84 ± 14	112 ± 15	121 ± 12

We have also studied offspring exposed to alcohol *in utero*. As did Nelson et al. (1984), we found that rats so exposed were less immobile in this swimming test (Bilitzke and Abel, 1989). Thus, while maternal and paternal alcohol exposure have different effects on locomotor activity, they have similar effects on swimming behavior. In our paternal model, we also found that imipramine was able to reverse the differences between alcohol-sired animals and controls in the swimming test. In this study, we treated rats with 4 injections of imipramine prior to testing. The results were as follows:

TABLE 2. Effects of imipramine on the immobility response of rats sired by alcohol-consuming fathers.

	Immobility Time (Sec)	
Imipramine	35% EDC	0% EDC
0 mg/kg	67 ± 17	116 ± 19
15 mg/kg	113 ± 16	69 ± 12
30 mg/kg	111 ± 17	69 ± 14

Susceptibility to Infection

A third observation we have made is that rat offspring sired by alcohol-consuming males or exposed to alcohol _in utero_, are more susceptible to infection. In these studies, we scarified the cornea and topically applied _Pseudomonas aeruginosa_, a gram negative opportunistic bacterium. A significantly greater number of offspring sired by alcohol-consuming males and offspring exposed to alcohol _in utero_ had perforated corneas and the days to perforation were shorter (Hazlett et al., 1989) (See Figure 2).

To summarize, four interesting relationships have emerged thus far from our studies, _viz_., animals sired by alcohol-consuming males are: a) hypoactive whereas those exposed _in utero_ are generally hyperactive, b) animals sired by males consuming alcohol do not adapt as well to a stressful situation as controls, and this appears to be true also for animals exposed to alcohol _in utero_, c)

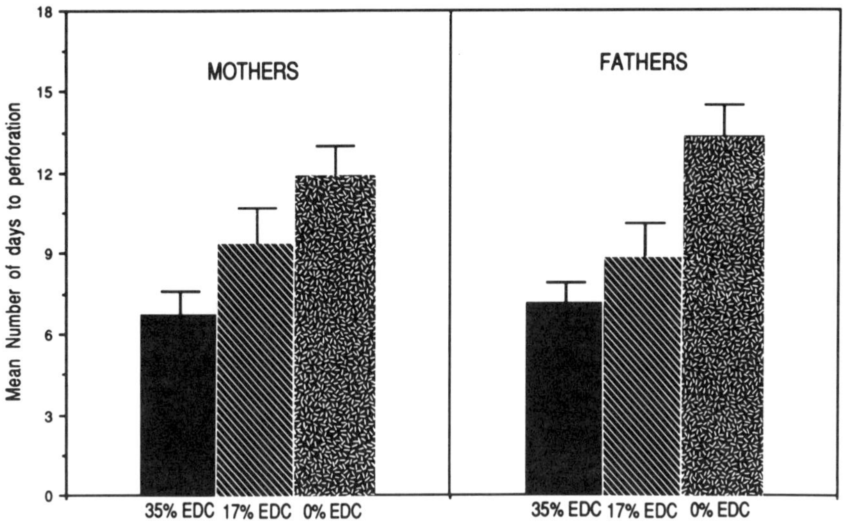

Figure 2. Days to corneal perforation in rat offspring sired by alcohol-consuming fathers.

imipramine reverses this relationship, and d) offspring exposed to alcohol <u>in utero</u>, or via alcohol's effects on father's sperm, are also similar in exhibiting an increased susceptibility to <u>Pseudomonas</u> ocular infection.

Increased susceptibility to <u>Pseudomonas</u> is associated with decreased T-cell-mediated immunity (e.g., Holt and Misfeldt, 1988) raising the interesting possibility that paternal or maternal alcohol consumption affects susceptibility to infection via decreased T cell-mediated immunity. Accordingly, we measured thymosin alpha 1 (TA-1) levels in rat offspring sired by alcohol consuming males, since this peptide is involved in T-lymphocyte maturation and function (Low and Goldstein, 1984) and indeed we found that animals sired by alcohol-consuming fathers did have lower serum TA-1 levels compared to controls (Abel et al., 1989):

TABLE 3. Effect of paternal alcohol consumption on Thymosin Alpha-1 levels of offspring in Long Evans rats (N = 15/group)

0% EDC	17.5% EDC	35% EDC
1964 ± 80 pg/ml	1302 ± 181 pg/ml	1532 ± 96 pg/ml

We do not know as yet if offspring exposed to alcohol in utero, also have lower TA-1 levels.

Changes In Sperm DNA

One of the conceptual difficulties associated with changes in the behavior or physiology of offspring of alcohol-consuming males is the nature of the mechanism by which they are mediated. The obvious candidate is a change in the genetic material in sperm.

One general indication of germ cell damage in males is a change in sperm morphology. Such changes have been interpreted as evidence of sperm cell mutagenesis (Wyrobek et al., 1975). We and others have reported alcohol-induced alterations in sperm cell morphology in humans and animals (Abel and Moore, 1987; Semczuk et al., 1978; Lester and Van Thiel, 1977) suggestive of such damage. If this has in fact occurred, it is not unreasonable to assume that changes have occurred in other genes as well and some of these genes may be involved in the effects we have noted.

Having observed altered sperm cell morphology in alcohol consuming rats, we looked for some way to characterize such damage further. We attempted to do this by removing sperm from the epididymis of alcohol consuming males, extracting DNA from sperm and examining its migration under pulsed field electrophoresis. Our preliminary results (Abel, 1989) showed that DNA from alcohol treated males migrated further than DNA from pair fed controls. Although we cannot attribute any meaningful biological interpretation to this observation, it does suggest alcohol may indeed have altered genomic DNA in a way that may be responsible for our behavioral observations.

A Proposed Model

There is now considerable evidence that stress reactivity and immune function are linked (see review in Solomon, 1987). In animals, increased stress decreases immune reactivity (e.g. Keller et al., 1981; Solomon, 1969); in humans increased stress has been linked to increased activation of latent herpes viruses (Kiecolt-Glasen et al., 1987) and tumorigenesis (e.g. Riley, 1981). Data from our swimming test is tentative evidence for such a paternal influence.

The ability of the CNS to influence immunity was elegantly demonstrated about 15 years ago by Ader and Cohen (1975). Subsequent studies have shown stressful situations initiate a cascade of physiological changes in the CNS. Neurotransmitters and neuroendocrines are quickly released. These substances may then modulate immune responsiveness via the thymus and endocrine glands respectively. Evidence of CNS control over thymus activity is that depletion of CNS catecholamines reduces thymic-dependent immunity (e.g., Cross et al., 1986). Increased turnover of catecholamines may also be associated with decreased lymphocyte activity (Gottesfeld et al., 1989). Serotonin is also known to be involved in immune responsiveness (Devoino and Idova, 1973). Since imipramine is able to reverse the effects of paternal alcohol exposure in our studies, it is conceivable that the stress response and the altered susceptibility to infection in these animals is mediated by catecholamines or serotonin.

Catecholamine depletion also affects ACTH, prolactin and luteinizing hormone levels (Cross et al., 1987). Changes in catecholamine release may therefore affect immune responsiveness indirectly via hormonal factors acting on lymphocytes. It is well known, for instance, that corticosteroids have potent effects on lymphocyte number and function and on neutrophil activity (Arnold et al., 1988).

Our laboratory has been exploring possible risk factors contributing to the adverse effects of prenatal alcohol exposure for many years. The present studies represent an extension of these studies to the realm of paternal influences.

The increased susceptibility to infection on the part of offspring sired by alcohol-consuming males is a new discovery with interesting implications for general impairment of the immune system due to a previously unrecognized congenital source, viz., paternal alcohol consumption.

Our tentative model for explaining the link between paternal alcohol consumption and increased susceptibility to infection is as follows:

Paternal Alcohol Consumption --> Alteration in Sperm DNA --> Increased Reaction to Stress --> Increased NE Turnover -->

Decreased Thymosin A-1 --> Decreased Lymphocyte Activity --> Increased Susceptibility to Infection

REFERENCES

Abel EL (1982). Alc Clin Exp Res 6:369-376.
Abel EL, Lee JA (1988). Alc Clin Exp Res 12:349-355.
Abel EL, Moore C (1987). Alc Clin Exp Res 11:533-535.
Abel EL, Tan SE (1988). Neurotoxicol Teratol 10:187-192.
Abel EL (1989). Alc Clin Exp Res, in press.
Abel EL, Hazlett LD, Berk RS, Mutchnick MG (1989). Al Clin Exp Res, in press.
Ader R, Cohen N (1975). Psychosom Med 37:333-340.
Arnold M, Schrieber L, Brooks P (1988). Drugs 36:340-363.
Bilitzke P, Abel EL (1989). Alc Clin Exp Res, in press.
Bond NW, DiGiusto EL (1977). Psychopharmacology (Berlin) 52:311-312.
Borsini F, Volterra G, Meli A (1986). Physiol Behav 38:385-386.
Cross RJ, Jackson JC, Brooks WH, Sparks DL, Markesberg WR, Roszman TL (1986). Immunology 57:145-152.

Cross RJ, Brooks WH, Roszman TL (1987). J Neuros Res 18:75-81.
Devoino LV, Idova GV (1973). Eur J Pharmacol 22:325-331.
Dixon RL, Hall JL (1981). In Hayes AW (ed): "Principles and Methods of Toxicology," New York: Raven Press, pp 107-121.
Gottesfeld Z, Garcia CJ, Lingham RB, Chromister RB (1989). Neuroscience, in press.
Hawkins J, Hichs RA, Phillips N, Moore JD (1978). Nature 274:512.
Hazlett LD, Barrett RP, Berk RS, Abel EL (1989). Ophthal Res, in press.
Holt PS, Misfeldt ML (1988). Infect Immun 52:96-100.
Kiecolt-Glaser JK, Fisher LD, Ogrocki P, Stout JS, Speicher CE, Glaser R (1987). Psychsom Med 49:13-34.
Keller SE, Weiss JM, Schleifer SJ, Miller NE, Stein M (1981). Science 213:1397-1399.
Lester R, Van Thiel DH (1977). Adv Exp Med Biol 85A:399-414.
Low TLK, Goldstein AL (1984). Thymus 6:27-42.
Nelson LR, Taylor AN, Lewis JW, Branch BJ, Liebeskind JC (1984). Proc West Pharmacol Soc 27:583-586.
Porsolt RD, LePichon M, Jolfre M (1977). Nature 266:789.
Randall CL, Burling TA, Lochry EA, Sutker PB (1982). Drug Alc Depend 9:89-95.
Riley EP, Shapiro NR, Lochry EA (1979). Pharmacol Biochem Behav 11:513-519.
Semczuk M (1978). Zeit Mikroskap-Anat Fors 92:494-508.
Solomon GF (1969). Int Arch Allergy 35:97-104.
Solomon GF (1987). J Neuro Res 18:1-9.
Wyrobek AJ, Heddle JA, Bruce WR (1975). Canad J Genet Cytol 17:675-681.

Alcohol, Immunomodulation, and AIDS, pages 57–66
© 1990 Alan R. Liss, Inc.

INTERACTION BETWEEN ALCOHOL AND HIV IN THE CENTRAL NERVOUS SYSTEM DETECTED BY THE AUDITORY BRAINSTEM RESPONSE: METHODOLOGY

Don L. Jewett, M.D., D.Phil.

Department of Orthopaedic Surgery, University of California-San Francisco, San Francisco, CA 94143-0728

INTRODUCTION

Both alcohol and HIV (Human Immunodeficiency Virus) adversely affect both the immune system and the CNS (Central Nervous System), acutely and chronically. (This parallelism is not surprising when one recalls that parts of the immune system are embryologically derived from neural crest cells and that cells of the CNS and immune system have many similar receptor sites.) Alcohol can affect the likelihood of becoming infected with HIV by increasing risky behaviour, and also by reducing immune system function. Alcohol also may well affect the progression of HIVI (HIV Infection) by either direct effects within the CNS, or indirectly by changes in the immune system.

How might the effects of alcohol on progression of CNS HIV effects be detected? One possibility would be to compare differences between drinkers and abstainers in duration of HIVI before the development of AIDS (Acquired Immuno-Deficiency Syndrome), but such a study presents considerable difficulties: 1) usually the date of infection is not known, 2) the diagnosis of AIDS can be made for non-CNS causes, 3) CNS effects are often silent, there being a higher percentage of CNS lesions at autopsy than are clinically detected before death [Anders et al, 1986], 4) it is difficult to quantify the amount of alcohol consumed over periods of years. A better study would longitudinally follow HIV-infected drinkers and abstainers, recording their alcohol consumption, as well as markers of the progression of CNS effects. What is not known is which markers are the best indicators of progressive damage from HIV, or alcohol; possible measures include 1) clinical neurological examinations, 2) neuropsychological test batteries, 3) evoked responses (e.g. ABR [Auditory Brainstem Response]), 4) Magnetic Resonance Imaging, 5) antigen or antibody from cerebrospinal fluid. It is clear that such a study would be large, expensive, and still have difficulty in isolating alcohol as an independent variable. Another alternative would be to do a cross-sectional comparison using one of the markers, with alcohol consumption as the independent variable, but in such a study quantification of the amount of alcohol consumed still presents considerable methodological problems.

These problems could be avoided by testing the effects of acute alcohol ingestion on CNS function in patients with HIVI. Since both HIV and alcohol produce detectable changes in the ABR, the ABR could be used to quantitatively measure the interaction. It is reasonable to ask whether the HIV and alcohol effects are independent (in which case simultaneous effects will be additive), or whether the damage from alcohol and HIV are synergistic (where the effects of alcohol will be greater in a patient who already has some HIV-related damage). If synergism is proven, then this would suggest that those with HIV should avoid alcohol because of possible synergistic CNS damage, as well as because of possible alcohol effects upon the immune system. Furthermore, if the ABR response to acute alcohol ingestion is abnormal in patients with "normal" pre-ingestion ABRs, then acute alcohol ingestion could be used to detect subclinical CNS abnormalities, i.e. to increase the sensitivity of the ABR in detecting CNS impairment due to HIV. (This idea is directly comparable to the suggestion that the CNS effects of chronic alcohol intake might be detected by the effect on evoked responses of a challenge dose of alcohol [Porjesz & Begleiter, 1985].)

LITERATURE REVIEW

Effect of alcohol on the ABR.

Chronic alcoholics have prolonged latencies of ABR waves after wave I [Begleiter et al, 1981; Chu et al, 1982]. Begleiter et al [1981] hypothesized that the delayed ABR latencies seen in these patients occurs as a result of demyelinization, or as a result of aberrant fluidizing effects upon central membranes. These ABR latency deficits in alcoholics, however, have been shown to recover over about a three month period [see Begleiter & Porjesz, 1988], which would argue against permanent demyelinization, but not against reversible membrane effects. It is uncertain as to whether the chronic effect of alcohol on the ABR is due to the same mechanism as the acute effect of alcohol ingestion.

Acute alcohol administration has been shown to produce prolonged latencies of ABR waves (II - VII) in both humans [Church & Williams, 1982; Squires et al, 1978a] and animals [Chu et al, 1978; Squires et al, 1978b]. Longer latency delays are seen in the later waves of the ABR, which indicates a uniform cumulative action throughout the brainstem auditory pathway. Because wave I of the ABR, which reflects activity of the auditory nerve (peripheral activity), is not affected by alcohol ingestion, the principal effects are central.

A factor confounding clear measurement of the influence alcohol ingestion upon the ABR is the strict inverse relationship between brain temperature and ABR latencies. Several studies have shown a strong correlation between shifts in brain temperature (hyperthermia and hypothermia) and corresponding shifts in ABR latency, in both humans [Marshall & Donchin, 1981; Bridger &

Graham, 1985; Bastuji et al, 1988] and animals [Williston & Jewett, 1982; Rossi & Britt, 1984; Gold et al, 1985]. As brain temperature increases ABR latencies decrease, and conversely as temperature decreases ABR latencies increase. It should be noted that rectal temperature may not correlate with brain temperature; Williston & Jewett [1982] showed that brain temperature (directly measured) correlated with ear-canal temperature, but not with rectal temperature, in rats.

These findings complicate the interpretation of alcohol influences on ABR latencies, as alcohol is known to reduce ear-canal temperature [Church & Williams, 1982]. However, Church and Williams [1982] present evidence that alcohol has an effect on ABR latencies beyond the temperature effect; as they found no dose-dependent effect of alcohol upon tympanic temperature while finding a clear dose-dependent effect on ABR latencies. In addition, they measured an alcohol effect on wave VI of the ABR, even when the temperature had returned to baseline levels. Animal studies indicate that there is an alcohol effect in addition to any secondary temperature effect. Squires et al [1978a] found an alcohol increase of animal ABR latency even when they controlled for a temperature effect. They tested rats wrapped in cloth and found that the rectal temperature did not vary following alcohol treatment, while the latency of the ABR's did increase. They also found that in cats, once rectal temperature had returned to pre-alcohol levels, a latency increase in the ABR was still seen (just as Church & Williams saw with respect to wave VI in humans [1982]). Church et al [1984] were able to replicate these results using rats.

Effect of HIV on ABR.

The ABR is abnormal in from 30 to 47% of those that have AIDS from various causes [Helweg-Larsen et al, 1988, Comi et al, 1988], and the incidence was found to be greater than 50% even when the diagnosis of AIDS was due to a non-CNS cause:

Pneumcystis Carinii Pneumonia (PCP) [Gardi et al, 1989]. There is some direct effect of HIV on the ABR, since even patients who are only HIV seropositive can also show increased latencies [Smith et al, 1988]. The effect of HIV on the ABR may be due to some form of patchy demyelinization, since some of the histological lesions of white matter due to HIV are similar to those of multiple sclerosis [Price et al, 1988]. Since CNS pathology in various forms occurs in 70% of AIDS patients who reach autopsy [Anders et al, 1986], those patients with AIDS and with an abnormal ABR are likely to have histologically-detectable CNS lesions. Certainly since an abnormal ABR is evidence of non-normal brainstem function, patients with AIDS or HIV seropositivity and abnormal ABRs have ABR-detectable CNS pathology. There have as yet been no longitudinal studies to indicate whether ABR abnormalities worsen with progression of HIVI. However, by comparing the ABR studies quoted above, it is likely that there is increase in ABR latency with HIVI progression since the mean latency change of AIDS patients is about twice that of HIV seropositives. For the purpose of discussing the proposed study, Fig. 1 shows a distribution of ABR wave V latencies likely to be found (for specific distributions see Gardi et al, 1989).

PROPOSED METHODOLOGY AND RATIONALE

The following study is designed to determine whether the change in the ABR response due to acute alcohol ingestion in non-alcoholic male patients with HIVI, differs from that of ABR-matched seronegative controls. To be sure that the patients have some ABR-detectable CNS lesions, we propose studying only patients who have a unilateral ABR abnormality, based upon a wave V latency greater than 2 SD of an age-matched control group. This will increase the statistical power of the study since this selection process increases the likelihood that the "normal" side in the patient has already been affected by HIV, as compared with random selection from patients with

HIV, some of whom will have bilaterally unaffected ABRs at the time of testing. The research problem is to study individuals who already have some CNS effects, since no alcohol/HIV interaction can be detected if there is no ABR-detectable CNS lesion. But, if the ABR effects are bilateral, then the only way to determine if a response is excessively prolonged by alcohol is to extrapolate from alcohol responses in normals-- a procedure prone to error. Said in another way: to determine if HIVI affects the ABR response to alcohol, one must compare the responses in normals and HIVI patients who are matched for ABR latency. Thus, in Fig. 1, it is only those that fall between the two vertical dashed lines that can be used in this study. The unilateral ABR abnormality guarantees that a normal-latency ABR is being tested in a patient who has some ABR-detectable HIVI CNS effect. It is likely that the "normal" side is actually also increased in latency, compared with the patient's pre-infection latency; note that in Fig. 1, it is probable that all AIDS patients have increased latencies, i.e. that the entire AIDS distribution is shifted to the right.

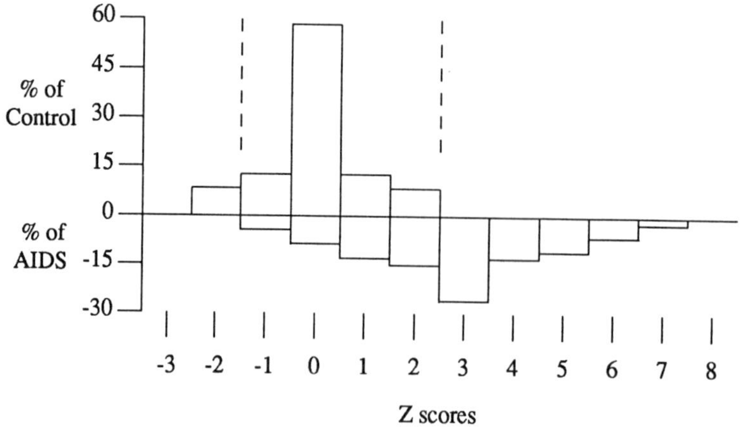

Fig. 1. Hypothetical differences between AIDS patients and controls with respect to Wave V latency in the ABR, expressed as Z scores (i.e. standard deviation units). Percentage of controls plotted as positive numbers, percentage of AIDS patients plotted as negative numbers.

Thus, the dependent variable to be studied is the increase in ABR latency of the response of the patient's "normal" ear, due to a standardized alcohol ingestion, as compared with controls who have about the same latency ABR before ingestion. The pre-ingestion latencies must be matched since the ABR response to alcohol (i.e. that portion of the alcohol effect that is not secondary to a temperature change) may be a function of latency. Since temperature effects are immediate and do not carry-over, the primary measure is the change in latency of wave VI when the body temperature has returned to the level observed during the pre-ingestion recording. This procedure will eliminate all temperature effects except the temperature dependency of the alcohol response itself, as affected by the pre-ingestion temperature. The influence of circadian rhythm temperature differences can be reduced by testing at the same time of day. Wave VI is suggested as the primary measure because this wave has been shown to be increased in latency by alcohol ingestion when temperature is controlled for as described above [Church & Williams, 1982].

The proposed study would follow the testing procedure of Church & Williams [1982]. Subjects would be requested to arrive for testing about 8:00 A.M., having not taken caffeine nor breakfast, having been requested to abstain from alcohol for 24 hrs prior to testing. After a pre-test BAC (blood alcohol concentration via a Breathalyzer) and pre-ingestion recording of the ABR, the subjects would receive the equivalent of 1.0 g of 190 proof ethyl alcohol per kg body weight, which gives, on the average, a blood alcohol level of 100 mg/dl. This is the level that has been found to best dissociate the temperature effects from ABR effects, using wave VI. The ABR and BAC, along with the ear-canal temperature would be taken every 30 min until the ear-canal temperature is 0.2 degrees C above the pre-ingestion level or until the BAC has returned to less than 20 mg/dl. The dependent variable is the latency of the ABR wave VI at the time the temperature has returned to baseline.

The primary research question, whether or not the patients and controls differ in the change in ABR due to ingestion of alcohol, can be answered using a matched pairs t-test applied to the matched patient-control pairs. The null hypothesis is that the population difference is zero between control and patient groups, comparing pre-ingestion to post-ingestion change in the ABR. Should the study prove positive, then it would be reasonable to see if other measures are also abnormal, e.g. the peak latency change after alcohol ingestion, and wave V latencies. With a positive study there would be reason to propose longitudinal studies to determine if progression of ABR changes in HIVI was different in drinkers and abstainers.

REFERENCES

Anders KH, Guerra WF, Tomiyasu U, Verity MA, Vinters HV (1986). The neuropathology of AIDS: UCLA experience and review. Amer J Psych 124:537-58.

Bastuji H, Garcia-Larrea L, Bertrand O, Mauguiere F (1988). BAEP latency changes during nocturnal sleep are not correlated with sleep stages but with body temperature variations. EEG clin Neurophysiol, 70:9-15.

Begleiter H, Porjesz B (1988). Potential biological markers in individuals at high risk for developing alcoholism. Alcoholism: Clinical and Experimental Research 12:488-493.

Begleiter H, Porjesz B, Chou CL (1981). Auditory brainstem potentials in chronic alcoholics. Science 211:1064-1066.

Bridger MW, Graham JM (1985). The influence of raised body temperature on auditory evoked brainstem responses. Clin Otolaryngol 10:195-9.

Chu NS, Squires KC, Starr A (1978). Auditory brain stem potentials in chronic alcohol intoxication and alcohol withdrawal. Arch Neurol 35:596-602.

Chu NS, Squires KC, Starr A (1982). Auditory brainstem response in alcoholic patients.

EEG clin Neurophysiol 54:418-425.
Church MW, Williams HL (1982). Dose- and time-dependent effects of ethanol on brain stem auditory evoked responses in young adult males. EEG clin Neurophysiol 54:161-174.
Church MW, Williams HL, Holloway JA (1984). Brain-stem auditory evoked potentials in the rat: Effects of gender, stimulus characteristics and ethanol sedation. EEG clin Neurophysiol 59:328-339.
Comi G, Medaglini S, Locatelli T, Martinelli V, Canal N, Lazzarin A, Castagna A, Moroni M (1988). Multimodality evoked potentials in acquired immunodeficiency syndrome. In Barber C, Blum T (eds): "Evoked Potentials III," London: Butterworths.
Gardi JN, Morledge DE, Jewett DL, Medina I, Sooy CD, Boccellari A, Dilley JW (1989). Auditory brainstem response (ABR) conduction delays in acquired immune-deficiency syndrome (AIDS). J AIDS [in press].
Gold S, Cahani M, Sohmer H, Horowitz M, Shahar A (1985). Effects of body temperature elevation on auditory nerve-brain-stem evoked responses and EEGs in rats. EEG clin Neurophysiol 60:146-153.
Helweg-Larsen S, Jakobsen J, Boesen F, Arlien-Soborg B, Brun B, Smith T, Ulrich K, Orskov B, Gyldensted C, Permin H, Gaub J, Petersen C, Gerstoft J, Bruhn P, Boysen G, Nielsen JO, Faber V, Trojaborg W (1988) Myelopathy in AIDS. A clinical and electrophysiological study of 23 Danish patients. Acta Neurol Scand 77:64-73.
Marshall NK, Donchin E (1981). Circadian variation in the latency of brainstem responses and its relation to body temperature. Science 212:356-358.
Porjesz B, Begleiter H (1985). Human brain electrophysiology and alcoholism. In Tarter RE, Thiel DH (eds): "Alcohol and the Brain," New York: Plenum.
Price RW, Breu B, Sidtis J, Rosenblum M, Scheck A, Cleary P (1988). The brain in AIDS: central nervous system HIV-1 infection and AIDS dementia complex. Science 239:586-592.

Rossi GT, Britt RH (1984). Effects of hypothermia on the cat brain-stem auditory evoked response. EEG clin Neurophysiol 57:143-155.
Smith T, Jakobsen J, Gaub J, Helweg-Larsen S, Trojaborg W (1988). Clinical and electrophysiological studies of human immunodeficiency virus-seropositive men without AIDS. Ann Neurol 23:295-297.
Squires KC, Chu NS, Starr A (1978a). Auditory brain stem potentials with alcohol. EEG clin Neurophysiol 45:577-584.
Squires KC, Chu NS, Starr A (1978b). Acute effects of alcohol on auditory brainstem potentials in humans. Science 201:174-176.
Williston JS, Jewett DL (1982). The Q10 of auditory brain stem responses in rats under hypothermia. Audiology 21:457-465.

Alcohol, Immunomodulation, and AIDS, pages 67–73
© 1990 Alan R. Liss, Inc.

HUMAN IMMUNODEFICIENCY VIRUS AND HEPATITIS B VIRUS INFECTIONS IN ALCOHOLICS

Jeffrey M. Jacobson, Theresa M. Worner +Henry S. Sacks, Charles S. Lieber
Infectious Diseases Section, (J.M.J.), Alcohol Research and Treatment Center, (T.M.W., C.S.L.), Bronx Veterans Administration Medical Center, New York, and Department of Medicine (J.M.J., H.S.S.) and Department of Biomathmatical Science, (H.S.S.) Mount Sinai School of Medicine, New York

There is a body of literature suggesting that alcoholism is associated with an increased seroprevalence of hepatitis B virus. Mills et al, (1981) prospectively studied 250 Caucasian patients lining in Glasgow, Scotland who had histologically proven chronic liver disease. Alcoholics with cirrhosis, but not those with milder or no liver disease, had a higher prevalence of hepatitis B virus antibodies (34%) than did subjects with other forms of liver disease (13%) or no liver disease (5%). Hislop et al, (1981) surveyed 195 patients with alcoholic liver disease living in 5 cities of Scotland and northern England (Hislop et al, 1981). 15% were hepatitis B surface antibody positive, compared to a 2-3% prevalence in a previous general population survey of Scotland. Those with cirrhosis tended to have a higher seroprevalence, again suggesting a role for hepatitis B virus in chronic alcoholic liver disease. Similar data were duplicated in France (Goudeau et al, 1981); alcoholics, particularly those with cirrhosis, demonstrated a higher hepatitis B virus seroprevalence.

A number of studies have confirmed the finding of hepatitis B infection in alcoholics, but have failed to support the role of the virus in progression of liver disease. In a study in Italy, Basile et al, (1981) found no serological differences between 43 cirrhotics and 32 other alcoholics, although, as a group, alcoholics had more evidence of exposure. Chalmers et al's (1981) study of 110 English alcoholics also revealed no association with liver disease. In a Danish study of 253 alcoholics with liver disease, 4% were positive for HBsAg and 31% for some marker of HBV infection (Orholm et al, 1981). Of the 11 HBsAg positive subjects, 9 had liver biopsies. Only three of the biopsies had histologic features suggestive of an alcoholic etiology. In addition, alcoholics with cirrhosis were not more likely to have evidence of past or present HBV infection than the other alcoholics. 285 English alcoholics with various stages of liver disease were studied for serological evidence of hepatitis B virus infection (Saunders et al, 1983). While a high overall prevalence of HBV markers were found, there was no association between the presence of HBV seropositivity and severity of liver disease. The only risk factors determined for HBV susceptibility were previous residence in a foreign country with a high (72%) prevalence of HBV infection, and previous blood transfusions or parenteral medical therapy.

In short, a number of European studies, as well as reports from Japan (Inove, 1977) and the United States (Chopra et al, 1980), have noted a higher seroprevalence of hepatitis B virus infection in alcoholics. The reasons for this increased frequency of HBV infection remains largely unexplained. Rarely have subjects been actively antigenemic. The usual serological pattern has reflected past exposure and recovery from infection, with surface and/or core antibody positivity. However, viral DNA has been found in liver cells of patients with serum anti-HBS antibody. (Brechot et al, 1982). In addition, more sensitive techniques such as polymerase chain reaction (Sunsky et al, 1988), for detecting the presence of HBV in serum and liver have recently become available and are reviewed elsewhere in these proceedings. While the role of the virus in the progression of alcoholic liver disease is currently debatable, these newer HBV assays could help clarify this issue.

The human immunodeficiency virus, or HIV, is transmitted via parenteral, sexual, and perinatal routes. This resembles hepatitis B virus. Studies in a population of alcoholics at the Bronx Veterans Administration Medical Center (Jacobson, et al, 1988) have found increased prevalence of both HIV and hepatitis B virus infections.
143 consecutive subjects entering alcoholic treatment programs were studied. HIV antibody testing was performed by enzyme-linked immunosorbent assay, with confirmation by Western blot assay. Hepatitis B core and surface antibodies and surface antigen were done by enzyme-linked

immunosorbent assay. During the interview, patients were asked about alcohol and other drug use and risk factors for HIV and hepatitis B virus acquisition.

19 individuals (13%) were HIV positive, with two subsequently developing AIDS. This is an unusually high and unexpected finding. Of the HIV seropositive subjects, 42% used intravenous drugs. Only 4% of the seronegatives gave such a history. 58% had heterosexual encounters with IV drug users, compared to 10% of HIV negatives. HIV positives reported a larger number of sexual partners over the previous three years. There was also more anal hetero-sexual intercourse in the HIV positive group (29%) than in the HIV negatives (10%). These findings were all statistically significant (P <.01). There also tended to be greater heterosexual contact with prostitutes in the HIV positive group. However, this difference did not reach statistical significance. Oral sex, travel, and blood transfusions were not differential factors.

HIV seropositive individuals had a lower mean age (40 vs 49 years old). All the patients in both groups had annual incomes less than $15,000. There were no racial differences between the positives and negatives, with the majority of the study population being black and hispanic.

6 of the 19 HIV positive men gave a history of heterosexual contact with IV drug users and/or prostitutes as their only risky exposure (one had a blood transfusion). Two others had no risk factors.

We also found an unusually high seroprevalence of hepatitis B infection in our alcoholics. Of the 40% hepatitis B seropositives, 4.2% were surface antigen positive, 17.5% positive for both surface and core antibodies, 1.4% for only surface antibody, and 16.8% positive for core antibody alone. Intravenous drug use was the only significant risk behavior for hepatitis B infection. Of the HBV seropositive subjects, 28% were IV drug users, compared to 6% of the seronegatives. The other heterosexual risk behaviors did not reach statistical significance.

The 13% prevalence of HIV infection in our group of Bronx alcoholics is an unusually high finding. This could, in part, reflect current trends in the spread of the virus in the Bronx, where intravenous drug use and heterosexual transmission to partners of IV drug users seem to be of paramount importance. A recent Department of Defense survey of civilian applicants to the military (Burke et al, 1987) demonstrated that the Bronx, New York was the county with the second highest prevalence of HIV infection in the country. The male: female ratio of seropositivity was 1:1. This closely resembles reports from Africa (Laing et al, 1986) and the Caribbean (Pape, 1985), where heterosexual spread is the prime means of HIV transmission. Blacks and hispanic Americans, particularly in poorer, inner-city areas are especially at risk for HIV acquisition.[15] This, in large part, reflects the greater use of intravenous drugs in these populations (Friedland, Klein 1987).

Approximately 40% of the HIV positive alcoholics in our series gave a history of concomitant intravenous drug use. It was the most important risk behavior for HIV acquisition. Heterosexual contact with IV drug using women was the second most important risk behavior for this population. Three-fifths of the HIV-positive cases, including 75% of those without a history of homosexuality or IV drug use, reported such exposure. This finding gives further evidence of the female-to-male sexual transmissibility of the virus. Several studies of heterosexual partners of HIV infected individuals have suggested such transmission. (Fischl it al 1987, Peterman et al 1988). Other high risk heterosexual behaviors, such as multiple partners, prostitute contact, and anal intercourse, were significant (P <.01), but less so.

It is not clear what role alcohol itself may have in affecting susceptibility to HIV infection. The most obvious one would be its disinhibiting effect on risk-taking behavior. Although our study did not show this, other studies have demonstrated a strong association between acute alcohol intake and high risk sexual behavior (Stall, 1987). The exact nature of this relationship remains to be defined.

Alcohol has profound effects on a number of immune functions (MacGregor, 1987). Probably the most important defense against HIV infection is cell-mediated immunity. Alcohol has been shown to reduce the number of circulating T lymphocytes and impair delayed hypersensitivity reactions in human subjects. In vitro studies have demonstrated a suppressive effect on mitogen-induced lymphocyte transformation, cell migration, natural killer cell function, and antibody-dependent cellular cytotoxicity. Alcohol also inhibits macrophage migration, activation, and phagocytosis. These adverse effects are amplified by concomitant malnutrition and liver disease.

Alcohol also suppresses primary antibody responses to new antigens. Alcohol has adverse effects on neutrophil activity, but this is probably unimportant in preventing HIV infection. Bone marrow production is depressed by reduced levels of colony stimulating factors. Furthermore, neutrophil adherence to endothelial cells, and hence delivery to sites of infection, is impaired.

In addition, as a result of the above immune abnormalities, alcoholics are more susceptible to other infections. Conceivably, the more frequently activated CD4 lymphocytes and macrophages may be more receptive to HIV infection.

It is unclear why there should be a high seroprevalence of hepatitis B virus in alcoholics. Our study revealed concomitant intravenous drug use in only a few of the subjects. Saunders et al's, (1981) survey found an association with residence, blood transfusions and other parenteral medical treatment. It would seem likely that heterosexual transmission plays a role with this virus as it does with the human immunodeficiency virus in this population. Our study group may have been too small to have revealed this factor. Another possibility is salivary spread through sharing of bottles and cans. Animal studies have demonstrated infectious hepatitis B virus in saliva (Alter et al, 1977). Institutionalized retarded children are known to be at risk for hepatitis B infection with salivary exposure being implicated (Mosley, 1975).

In summary, many alcoholics appear to be especially susceptible to HIV and hepatitis B virus infection. The contribution of HBV to the development of alcoholic liver disease remains unsettled.

Controlled studies are needed to further characterize the higher prevalence of HIV and hepatitis B virus in alcoholics. The associated risk factors need to be more clearly defined.

ACKNOWLEDGEMENTS

Supported, in part, by the Veterans Administration and DHHS grant #AA 03508

REFERENCES

Alter JH, Purcell RH, Gerin JL (1977). Transmission of hepatitis B to chimpanzees by hepatitis B surface antigen-positive saliva and semen. Infect Immun; 16:928.

Basile A, Vitale G, Macor C, Scudeller G (1981). Hepatitis B virus infection in alcoholic cirrhosis. Br Med J; 282:1705.

Brechot C, Nalpas B, Courouce AM, Duhamel G, Callard P, Carnot F, Tiollais P, Berthelot P (1982). Evidence that hepatitis B virus has a role in liver-cell carcinoma in alcoholic liver disease. N Engl J Med 306:1384-7.

Burke DS, Brundage JF, Herbold JR, Berner W, Gardner LI, Gunzenhauser JD, Voskovitch J, Redfield RR (1987). Human immunodeficiency virus infections among civilian applicants for United States military service, October 1985 to March 1986: demographic factors associated with seropositivity. N Engl J Med; 317:131-136.

Chalmers DM, Bullen AW, Levi AJ (1981). Evidence for previous hepatitis B infection in alcoholic cirrhosis. Br Med J; 282:819.

Chopra S, Tupper JC, Ahn CS, Bayog R, Koff RS (1980). Hepatitis B markers in an alcohol treatment unit. Gastroenterology; 11C.

Fischl MA, Dickenson GM, Scott GB, Klimas N, Fletcher MA, Parks W (1987). Evaluation of heterosexual partners, children, and household contacts of adults with AIDS. JAMA; 257:640-644.

Friedland GH, Klein RS (1987). Transmission of the human immunodeficiency virus. N Engl J Med; 317:1125-1135.

Goudeau A, Maupas P, Dubois F, Coursaget P, Bougnoux P. (1981). Hepatitis B infection in alcoholic liver disease and primary hepatocellular carcinoma in France. Prog Med Virol; 27:26-34.

Hislop WS, Follett EAC, Bouchier IAD, MacSween RNM (1981). Serological markers of hepatitis B in patients with alcoholic liver disease: a multicentre survey. J Clin Pathol; 34:1017-1019.

Inove K (1977). The clinicopathological features of the alcoholic liver injury in Japan and its etiological relationship to hepatitis B virus. Gastroenterol Jpn; 12:230-240.

Jacobson J, Worner T, Sacks H, Lieber C (1988). HIV and HBV infections in an alcoholic populaton. AMSADD meeting, Washington DC.

MacGregor RR (1987). Alcohol and drugs as co-factors for AIDS. Adv Alcohol Subst Abuse; 7:78-88.

Mills PR, Follett EAC, Urguhart GED, Clements G, Watkinson G, MacSween RNM (1981). Evidence for previous hepatitis B virus infection in alcoholic cirrhosis. Br Med J; 282: 437-438.

Mosley JW (1975). Hepatitis types B and non-B. Epidemiologic background. JAMA; 233: 967.

Orholm M, Aldershvile J, Tage-Jensen V, Schlicting P, Nielsen JO, Hardt F, Christoffersen P (1981). Prevalence of hepatitis B virus infection among alcoholic patients with liver disease. J Clin Pathol; 34:1378-1380.

Pape JW, Liautaud B, Thomas F, Mathurin JR, St. Amandd MMA, Boncy M, Pean V, Pamphile M, Laroche AC, Dahovitz J, Johnson WD (1985). The acquired immunodeficiency syndrome in Haiti. Ann Intern Med; 103:674-678.

Peterman TA, Stoneburner RL, Allen JR, Jaffe HW, Curran JW (1988). Risk of human immunodeficiency virus transmission from heterosexual adults with transfusion-associated infections. JAMA; 259:55-58.

Quinn TC, Mann JM, Curran JW, Piot P (1986). AIDS in Africa: an epidemiologic paradigm. Science; 234:955-963.

Saunders JB, Wodak AD, Morgan-Capner P, White YS, Portmann B, Davis M, Williams R (1983). Importance of markers of hepatitis B virus in alcoholic liver disease. Br Med J; 286:1851-1854.

Stall R (1987). The prevention of HIV infection associated with drug and alcohol use during sexual activity. Adv. Alcohol Subst Abuse 7:73-88.

Thiers V, Nakajima E, Kremsdorf D, Schellekens H, Driss R, Wands JR, Sninsky J, Ozawa K, Tollais P, Brechot C (1988). Detection and cloning by the polymerase chain reaction of hepatitis B virus (HBV) DNA sequences in blood samples negative for HBV serologic markers. Lancet ii: 1273-1276.

Alcohol, Immunomodulation, and AIDS, pages 75–78
© 1990 Alan R. Liss, Inc.

ALCOHOL AND IMMUNE SYSTEM: ROLE OF GASTRIC TISSUE

Salwa A. Elgebaly, Robert A. Kozol and
Donald L. Kreutzer*

Departments of Surgery and Pathology*, University of Connecticut Health Center, School of Medicine, Farmington, Connecticut, 06032

INTRODUCTION

A number of studies have shown the association between acute and chronic ethanol intoxication and lowered resistance to infection in these patients (Feliu, 1977; Pickrell, 1938). Impairment in neutrophil chemotaxis (i.e., mobilization) due to the presence of serum inhibitors was suggested as a major mechanism for the increased susceptibility to infection (VanEpps, et. al. 1975; Robbins, et. al. 1987). Cells releasing these inhibitors have not yet been identified. Since gastric tissues are the first to be exposed to ingested ethanol and are exposed to the highest concentrations for a length of time (i.e., minutes), we began testing their capability to release chemotaxis inhibitors. Our hypothesis is that gastric tissues exposed to ethanol release inhibitors for neutrophil chemotaxis. To test this hypothesis, full-thickness gastric tissue obtained from isolated rabbit stomachs were placed in standard Ussing chamber (Kozol, et. al. 1989). Mucosal and serosal sides of control stomachs were incubated with 7ml of phosphate buffered-saline (PBS) in a 5% CO_2/95% oxygen atmosphere for 1 hour. For experimental stomachs, the

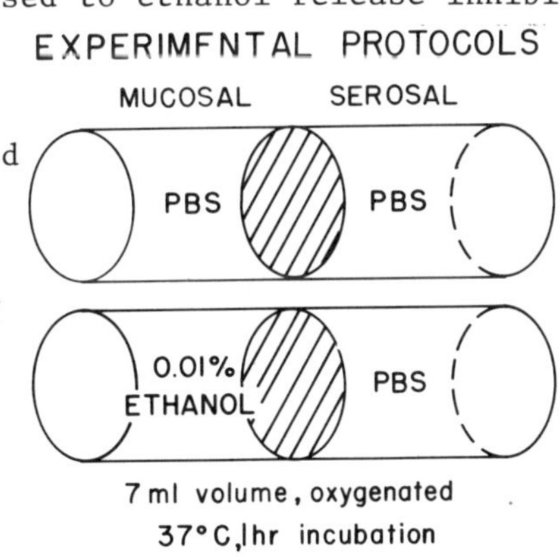

Figure 1: Ussing chamber prep.

mucosal surfaces were incubated with 0.01% ethanol (V/V) while the serosal sides were incubated with PBS under similar conditions described above. Neutrophil chemotactic activity was then determined in supernatant solutions collected from serosal sides of control (PBS) and experimental (ETOH) stomachs using modified Boyden chambers (Elgebaly, et. al. 1987; Elgebaly in press). Rabbit peritoneal neutrophils were used as indicator cells. The standard chemoattractant C5a was the positive control. Cell migration in response to the putative chemoattractants was expressed as % maximum chemotactic response induced by C5a. The chemotactic index (CI) is defined as distance travelled in the filter x cell number at that distance.

$$\%\ \text{maximum chemotactic response}\ (\%\ C5a) = \frac{\text{CI exp.} - \text{CI neg. cont.}}{\text{CI}_{C5a} - \text{CI neg. cont.}} \times 100$$

RESULTS

As can been seen in Figure 2 (a representative experiment) neutrophil chemotactic activity detected in the serosal sides following exposing the mucosal sides to 0.01% ethanol for 60 min was markedly lower than control stomachs indubated with PBS. This observation was further confirmed in an additional eight experiments with an average suppression of chemotaxis of 51% ± 13 (mean I standard error). It should be noted that there was no detectable level of ethanol on the serosal side of these tissues.

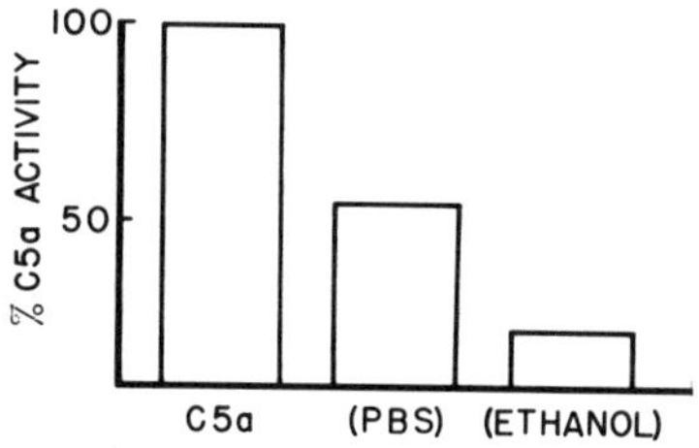

Figure 2: Neutrophil chemotactic activity recovered in serosal supernatants after mucosal exposure to PBS or 0.01% ethanol.

When the serosal solutions of alcohol-treated stomachs were diluted 1:3 and 1:9 in PBS, the recovered chemotactic activity remained quite low in both dilutions (Figure 3).

These data indicate that the above observed reductions in chemotaxis following alcohol treatment is not due to a desensitization effect on neutrophils but rather suggest the presence of inhibitors.

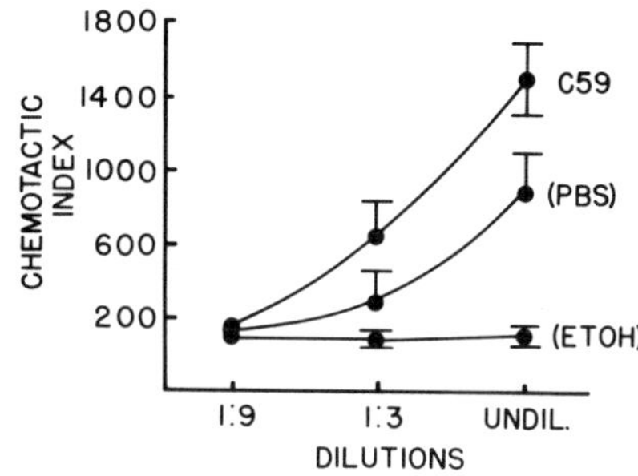

Figure 3: Dilution curves of neutrophil chemotactic activity recovered in serosal supernatants after mucosal incubation with PBS or 0.01% ethanol.

Results of these studies support our hypothesis that gastric tissues exposed to ethanol release inhibitors for neutrophil chemotaxis. The generation of these gastric-derived immunosuppressors following alcohol consumption might increase the susceptibility of individuals to various infections including, possibly, the Human Immunodeficiency Virus (HIV). In summary, these studies support a role for alcohol as a cofactor in immunosuppressive disorders.

REFERENCES

Elgebaly, SA, Herkert N, O'Rourke J, Kreutzer DL (1987). Characterization of neutrophil and monocyte-specific chemotactic factors derived from isolated corneas in response to hydrogen peroxide injury. Am J Pathol 126: 40-50.

Elgebaly SA, Masetti P, Allam M, Forouhar F, Bohn M. Cardiac derived neutrophil chemotactic factors: preliminary biochemical characterization. J Mol Cell Cardiology (in press).

Feliu E, Gougerot M, Hakim J, Cramer E, Auclair C, Rueff B, Boivin P (1977). Blood polymorphonuclear dysfunction in patients with alcoholic cirrhosis. Eur J Clin Invest 7: 571-577.

Kozol RA, Downes RT, Kreutzer Dl, Wentzel S, Rossomando E, Elgebaly SA. Release of neutrophil chemotactic factors from gastric tissues: initial biochemical characterization. Dig Dis Sci (in press).

Pickrell KL (1938). The effect of alcoholic intoxication and ether anesthesia on resistance to pneumococcal infection. Bull Johns Hopkins Hospital 63: 238-260.

Robbins RA, Zetterman RK, Kendall TJ, Gossman GL, Monsour HP, Rennard SI (1987). Elevation of chemotactic factor inactivator in alcoholic liver disease. Hepatology 7: 872-877.

VanEpps DE, Strickland RG, Williams RC (1975). Inhibitors of leukocyte chemotaxis in alcoholic liver disease. Ann Intern Med 59: 200-207.

Alcohol, Immunomodulation, and AIDS, pages 79–91
© 1990 Alan R. Liss, Inc.

SUPPRESSION BY MORPHINE AND ETHANOL OF TUMOR CELL CYTOTOXIC ACTIVITY RELEASED BY MACROPHAGES FROM RETROVIRALLY INFECTED MICE UPON IN VITRO STIMULATION BY BETA CAROTENE

Ronald R. Watson and Tuan H. Nguyen[1]

Department Family and Community Medicine, and
Medical Class of 1992[1], School of Medicine
University of Arizona, Tucson, Arizona 85724

INTRODUCTION

Dietary compounds can modulate disease and tumor resistance. They alter the functioning of macrophages by release of cytotoxic factors including tumor necrosis factor (TNF) lymphotoxin (LT), as well as interferon gamma, and interleukin-1 which have been occasionally reported to have tumor cell cytotoxic activity. We have also recently reported that human monocytes released, upon stimulation by beta carotene, a novel tumor cytotoxic factor (Abril et al., 1989).

Carotenoids including beta-carotene (BC) are recognized as chemopreventive agents, reducing tumor development in animals and possibly in man (Temple and Basu, 1988). Immunological enhancement, including TNF production due to BC consumption, is associated with reduced tumor development in animals (Schwartz et al., 1986; Schwartz, et al., 1988). BC functions as an anti-neoplastic agent in part by providing immunostimulation (Watson and Rybski, 1988). The immunostimulatory activity of BC is suggested by the enhancement of T and B cell mitogen responsiveness, and the increase in the number of circulating $CD4^+$ and $CD3^+$ T-cell subsets observed in humans given oral BC (Alexander et al., 1985). Although BC has some effect on T and B cells little is known about its effects on mononuclear phagocytes. We have recently reported that carotenoids including BC stimulated human monocytes in vitro. Then the monocytes produced a novel cytokine which was cytotoxic for tumor cells (Abril, et al., 1988), and also were activated for direct tumor cell cytotoxicity (Schoen and Watson, 1988).

On the other hand, (Watson, 1988) ethanol consumption is associated with low BC tissue levels (Yahya and Watson, 1987), and both ethanol and morphine use caused increased tumors and also induced immunosuppression. Therefore, we have examined the secretion of tumor cell cytotoxic materials upon in vitro culturing of murine macrophages with BC. We investigated the effects of potentially immunosuppressive drugs of abuse to modify secretion of tumor cytotoxic activity. Our findings indicate that in vitro BC, dietary ethanol, and morphine, as well as retroviral infection, alter secretion of materials cytotoxic for a murine leukemia cell line from mouse monocytes.

MATERIALS AND METHODS

Isolation and Purification of murine splenic macrophages: Murine macrophages were obtained by disruption of the spleen under aseptic conditions followed by a brief water lysis of red blood cells as described previously (Moriguchi et al., 1985). The cells were then centrifuged at 800 x g for 15 min. The cell pellet was then resuspended in 1 ml of Iscove's Modified Dulbecco's Medium (IDM) supplemented with 10% heat inactivated fetal bovine serum, 100 U Penicillin/ml, 100 ug streptomycin/ml, 0.25 ug fungizone/ml and buffered to pH 7.2 with 12 nM sodium Bicarbonate (Gibco Grand Island, NY). Adherent cells were obtained by incubating mononuclear cells in a 100 x 15 mm plastic petri dish (Falcon, Los Angeles, CA) for 1 hr at 37°C. Adherent cells were dislodged with a cell scraper, washed once in HBSS and resuspended in IDM. The cells were added to a 96 well plate at a density of 1×10^5 cells/well suspended in 100 ul of complete medium. Supernatant fluids from mononuclear cells were collected after 48 hr of incubation at 37°C in a humidified incubator and tested for cytotoxicity (Abril et al., 1989).

Mice and Retinyl Palmitate Diet. C57BL/6 female mice, 3-4 weeks old and weighing approximately 15 g, were obtained from Simonsen Laboratories, Inc., Gilroy, CA.

They were routinely provided with Purina laboratory chow and water ad libitum for 1 week. Then half were fed a diet containing 120 IU of retinyl palmitate (RP)/gm as described elsewhere (Watson et al., 1988a). It was a 30-fold excess over the amount of retinol in the control diet AIN 76A, which was otherwise identical and fed to the controls.

Ethanol and Morphine Treatment of Mice: Three to four-week-old C57BL/6 female mice, weighing approximately 15 g, were routinely provided with Purina laboratory chow and water ad libitum. Thirty mice were injected with morphine sulfate intraperitoneally or fed a 7% ethanol liquid diet every day for 7 days during weeks 0, 4, and 8 as described elsewhere (Watson et al., 1986). The morphine was given at a daily dose of 75 mg/Kg body weight by intraperitoneal injection. Controls were injected with saline concommitantly.

LP-BM5 Murine Leukemia Virus (MuLV). The retrovirus mixture, LP-BM5, produces a non-neoplastic, lymphoproliferative disease in adult mice (Watson, 1989). After one week some of the mice fed retinyl palmitate, ethanol, injected with morphine, and those fed the control diet were injected intraperitoneally with 0.1 ml of a LP-BM5 MuLV inoculum which was a kind gift of Dr. R.A. Yetter (Microbiology Research, Veterans Administration Hospital, Baltimore, MD). Mice were sacrificed at 4 and 8 weeks post infection with LP-BM5 MuLV by ether anesthesia.

Cell Lines: Murine L-929s cells were a gift from Dr. Philip Scuderi, Arizona Cancer Center, University of Arizona, Tucson. L-929s cells are sensitive to 1×10^2 U/ml of murine TNF. They were isolated by Dr. Scuderi, and were his kind gift (Abril et al., 1989).

Cytotoxicity Assay: The in vitro cytotoxicity assay with supernatants from BC stimulated human monocytes has been described previously (Abril et al., 1989). Murine macrophages were treated identically. Murine macrophages or human peripheral blood monocytes after isolation and partial purification were incubated in media alone or with BC for 48 hours and then the supernatant media was collected by centrifugation. The cytotoxic activity of culture supernatants was assessed by adding 100 ul of freshly collected culture fluid to the target cells, L-929S. After incubation for 72 hr, the plates were centrifuged at 100 xg for five minutes and the wells were washed once with HBSS. Each well subsequently received 100 ul of substitute containing 5 ug of MTT dye (3-4,5 Dimethylthiazozyl-2-yl-2,5- diphemyltetrazalium bromide (Sigma Inc., St. Louis, MO.). The assay plates were incubated at 37°C for four hours, and the unmetabolized MTT was subsequently removed by aspiration (Abril et al., 1989). The crystalized tetrazalium salt was solubilized by the addition of 100 ul of acidified isoprapanol. Optical density measurement were determined on a Tetertech Multiskan (Four Labs Inc., McLean, VA) at a wavelength of 570 nm. The percentage cytotoxic activyt was calculated as follows:

$$\% \text{ MTT} = \frac{\text{Experimental}}{\text{Tumor Control}} - 1 \times 100$$

<u>In Vitro Incubations of Spleen and Immunomodulators.</u> Beta-carotene (BC), was purchased from Sigma Chemical Co. (St. Louis, MO). Methods to produce BC in culture media with the limited solubility of BC at low concentrations in ethanol and also aqueous media, containing serum have been reported previously (Abril et al., 1989). BC was first prepared as stock solutions of 10^{-3}M by dissolving in absolute ethanol. Briefly, serial dilutions of this stock solution were made in complete medium and human monocytes or murine macrophages were exposed to each compound by adding 100 ul of diluted stock to 100 ul of complete medium containing the cells. As a control for the effects of the solvent some mononuclear cells received ethanol in media diluted as the BC-ethanol solution which did not contain BC or morphine. All solutions used were filter sterilized with 0.22 um filter before addition to cells. In vitro stimulation of macrophages isolated from control mice was done as above except that the media during supernatant development of the 48 hour incubation contained in media BC. They were treated with BC at 1×10^{-8}M for 48 hours. Morphine at 1×10^{-8}M was incubated in vitro for 1 hour, the cells were washed twice with media, and then incubated with media or BC for 48 hours. This resulting supernatant was tested for cytotoxic activity.

Human Monocytes. Human monocytes were collected from peripheral blood of laboratory personnel with informal consent. None were using BC supplements or morphine. They were isolated and treated with BC as previously described (14).

RESULTS

Effects of beta-carotene and morphine in vitro on stimulation of human monocytes to produce supernatants with cytotoxicity for tumor cells.

BC in vitro stimulated human monocytes to produce tumor cytotoxic factor in their supernatant, which was reduced significantly by simultaneous addition of morphine (Table 1). Morphine exposure for 1, 4, 8, and 12 hours followed by removal by cell washing, prior to BC stimulation resulted in reduced stimulation. This was greatest at one hour (data not shown), which was used throughout.

Table 1. Morphine Suppression of Tumor Cytotoxic Factor Activity During In Vitro Beta-carotene Stimulation of Human Peripheral Blood Monocytes

In Vitro Additive	Cytotoxicity (%)[a]
Media	-1.64 ± 0.04
Beta-carotene	31.60 ± 0.57 *
Morphine + beta-carotene	23.80 ± 0.42 *+

a Mean ± S.D. of samples from 5 normal volunteers treated in vitro with morphine prior to BC stimulation

* significantly different from media treated cells ($P<0.05$).

\+ significantly different from BC treatment only($P<0.05$).

Effect of in vitro stimulation of murine macrophages by beta-carotene on production of supernatants cytotoxic for murine L929S leukemia cells. The cytotoxic activity of BC was initially tested on a cytokine sensitive murine cell line. The production of supernatants by murine adherent splenic macrophages with cytotoxic activity in response to BC, was concentration dependent. The optimum BC concentration for the production of supernatant biological activity was observed to be between 10^{-7} and 10^{-9}M. Culturing mouse macrophages from control mice with 10^{-6} to 10^{-10}M BC showed a broad peak of activity. It went from 24.1% MTT released with tumor cell lysis at 10^{-6}M BC to 32.91% at 10^{-10}M BC with a peak at 10^{-7} and 10^{-9}M. However much lower activity was found in media without fetal calf serum. Then the peak activity was at 10^{-7}M (14.3%) with 5.5% and 6.6% at 10^{-6} and 10^{-8}M. Below 10^{-8}M BC, essentially no affect was seen in the accumulation of MTT by L-929 cells without serum in the media. Similar concentrations of BC added directly to L929S cells failed to bring about cytolysis and resulted in their enhanced proliferation and growth as observed previously (9).

Table 2 Morphine Suppression of Tumor Cytotoxic Activity During In Vitro Beta-carotene Stimulation of Murine Macrophages.

	Cytotoxicity (%)[a] produced by cells from mice injected with	
In Vitro Additive	Saline	Morphine
Media	-0.87 ± 0.07	-0.88 ± 0.05
Beta-carotene[b]	24.24 ± 0.65 +	14.10 ± 0.65 *+x
Morphine + Beta-carotene[b]	17.25 ± 2.57 +	3.52 ± 0.91 *ox

a Mean ± S.D.

b BC in media was added to give a final concentration of 10^{-7}M. In vitro morphine treatment was for 1 hour and was removed prior to BC stimulation.

* significantly different from control cell source ($P<0.05$).

\+ significantly different from media treatment in vitro ($P<0.05$).

x significantly different from beta-carotene of control cell source ($P<0.05$)

o significantly different from morphine + beta-carotene of control cell source (<0.05).

BC stimulated murine macrophages to produce tumor cell cytotoxicity (Table 2). However, the combined morphine plus BC in vitro treatment produced significantly less stimulation, then BC alone. In addition, cells from mice treated in vivo with morphine could not be stimulated normally. However, the addition of BC plus morphine in vitro to cells from morphine injected mice almost totally prevented release of tumor cell cytotoxicity activity in macrophage supernatants (Table 2).

Spleen and Body Weights. Evidence of retroviral infection with LP-BM5 was found at 4 weeks of infection when the virally infected mice had larger spleens than uninfected controls with average spleen weights of 0.114 ± 0.006 and 0.074 ± 0.005 gm, respectively. These were significantly different (P 0.05). There were no significant differences between groups based upon bodyweight (data not shown). However, retroviral infection but not RP, ethanol or morphine caused a significant (P 0.05) increase in the spleen/body weight ratio (data not shown). Studies by others show that the increase in cell numbers is due to lymphocytes, not macrophages (Watson, 1989)

Effect of murine retroviral infection and morphine on beta carotene stimulation of secretion by macrophages of tumor cell cytotoxicity. The effect of retroviral infection with murine leukemia virus on the functions of in vitro stimulated macrophages is shown in Table 3. Retroviral infection alone, as did in vitro morphine treatment, yielded significantly less stimulation in vitro by BC, although all BC treated groups were significantly increased over unstimulated cells with only media added in vitro. However, in vivo treatment with morphine did not significantly modify the suppressed response of cells from virally-infected mice upon in vitro BC incubation (Table 3).

Table 3: Action of Morphine on Tumor Cytotoxic Activity Production During In Vitro Beta-carotene Stimulation of Murine Spleen Macrophages from LP-BM5 Retrovirally-infected Cells

	Cytotoxicity (%)[a] Produced by Cells isolated from			
	Uninfected Controls		Retrovirus Infected	
	Injected with		Injected with	
In Vitro Additive	Saline	Morphine	Saline	Morphine
Media	−0.86 ± 0.06	−0.84 ± 0.05	−1.83 ± 0.11	4.63 ± 0.36+
Beta-carotene[b]	24.10 ± 0.55*	14.01 ± 0.64*+	13.21 ± 0.96*	14.54 ± 1.36*

a Mean ± S.D.
b BC in media added to give final concentration of 10^{-7}M.
* significantly different from in vitro media treated cells ($P<0.05$).
\+ significantly different from cells from virally-infected mice untreated with morphine ($P<0.05$).

Table 4: Effect of Dietary Ethanol Followed by In Vitro Beta-Carotene Stimulation of Macrophages from Retrovirally-Infected Mice on Tumor Cytotoxic Activity Production

	Cytotoxicity Produced by Cells From (%)[a]		
	Uninfected		Retrovirus Infected,
In Vitro Additive	Control Diet	Ethanol-fed	Ethanol-fed
Media	0.81 ± 0.05	4.65 ± 0.38	$-11.48 \pm 0.65^{+}$
Beta-carotene[b]	23.98 ± 0.61	$8.28 \pm 0.59^{*}$	$14.79 \pm 0.79^{*+}$

a Mean $\pm$ S.D.
b BC added in media to give a final concentration of 10^{-7}M.
* significantly different from media treated animals' cells ($P<0.05$).
\+ significantly different from cells from uninfected mice fed ethanol ($P<0.05$).

Table 5. Immunomodulation of Vitamin A: Effect on Tumor Cytotoxic Activity Production of In Vitro Beta-carotene Stimulated Spleen Macrophages Isolated from Mice Infected with LP-BM5 Murine Leukemia Virus

	Cytotoxicity (%) Produced by Cells from Mice Fed Vitamin A and	
In Vitro Additive	Saline injected	Retrovirus injected
Media	-37.76 ± 2.17	-4.34 ± 0.25 +
Beta-carotene	23.48 ± 1.52 *	16.38 ± 0.83 *+

a Mean ± S.D.
* significantly different from media treated cells ($P<0.05$).
\+ significantly different from uninfected mice ($P<0.05$).

DISCUSSION

We found that BC stimulated in vitro the secretion of a cytotoxic factor(s) from murine macrophages. These studies confirm in vitro studies done showing that BC caused similar stimulation of human monocytes in vitro (Abril et al., 1989). They are extended by showing that morphine in vitro suppressed the ability of human monocytes to be stimulated by BC and release tumor cytotoxic factor. In vitro BC stimulated human monocytes to produce a novel tumor cytotoxic factor (TCF) at very low levels of BC, 10^{-10}M (Abril et al., 1989). Tumor cytotoxic factor induced by BC was previously shown to not be TNF, LT, gama interferon or interluekin 1 (Abril et al., 1989). Since, BC causes the regression of neoplasias in animals (Schwartz, et al., 1986), a possible mechanism for BC induced antitumor effect is the stimulation of macrophage cytokine production (Abril et al., 1989). In vitro exposure of human macrophages showed (Abril et al., 1989) that only extremely high levels of RP stimulated tumor cytotoxic factor release. Thus, it suggests that the structure of BC, not vitamin A produced from BC is the mechanism of monocyte stimulation. If the mechanism of activation of BC was by conversion to RP, vitamin A, then high dietary RP would be expected to reduce the ability of macrophages to be activated in vitro by BC. This was not seen in cells from mice fed RP.

In vivo and in vitro exposure of mice to morphine reduced significantly production of tumor cell cytotoxicity activity by BC stimulation of macrophages in vitro. This supports studies with morphine administration in mice which caused a profound increase in susceptibility to bacterial and fungal infections (Tubaro et al., 1983). The increased susceptibility was partly due to a decreased reticuloendothelial system activity as well as a reduction in the number of phagocytes and not due to a direct cytotoxic effect of the drug. These observations are in agreement with altered disease resistance in man (Tubaro et al., 1985). The ability of animals to mount a response to tumor challenge was also affected by morphine treatment (Yahya and Watson, 1988). Interferon produced by macrophages as well as a variety of other cell-mediated reactions have also been altered by morphine (Yahya and Watson, 1985). This reduced secretion of tumor cytotoxic activity caused by morphine was present only upon stimulation by BC. Such reductions could affect the tumor resistance capacity adversely, particularly that associated with BC. The information presented suggests that morphine in vitro affected activation of mouse macrophages. This was true whether it was given by injection to the mice prior to cell isolation and stimulation, or given only in vitro after cell isolation. In both cases BC had reduced ability to cause the secretion of cytotoxic materials into solution.

We have previously showed that the number of lymphocytes and macrophages was reduced by dietary ethanol and morphine given by injection (Watson et al., 1988b). The reduction in the number of lymphoid cells with various markers may reduce cytokine modification of immune functions and hence tumor and disease resistence. We showed here that dietary ethanol, and morphine, as well as the retrovirus also reduced the ability of macrophages to function by release of cytotoxicity factors upon in vitro stimulation. Such changes due to the retrovirus are in agreement with reduced lymphoid cell function caused by the virus by others (Watson 1989). Mice also have reduced lymphocyte cell numbers after ethanol exposure (Mufti et al., 1988). Ethanol significantly changes lymphoid cell functions in a variety of studies (Watson 1988). Finally the activation that still occurs in macrophages from morphine, retrovirus or ethanol treated mice by BC in vitro agrees with reports of human monocyte activation by BC (Schoen and Watson 1988, Abril et al., 1989).

Dietary cells from ethanol-fed infected and retrovirally-infected mice had reduced release of cytotoxic activity in vitro upon stimulation by BC. The combination of dietary ethanol plus concommitant retroviral infection did not synergistically suppress cytotoxic release, beyond either treatment alone. As shown in Table 5, macrophages from mice fed RP were still activated by BC in vitro. Alterations of monocyte cytotoxic secretions directly due to drugs of abuse such as morphine or ethanol, or due to dietary changes they cause such as low levels of BC is largely unexplored. The additive effects of retroviral infections may be a critical component of monocyte cell functions. The mouse offers a chance to explore further these parameters.

Acknowledgments. Supported by grants from Wallace Genetics, Inc., and NIH: CA27502, AA08039 and DA04827 grants, support for N.T. from the University Medical Student Research Program.

REFERENCES

Abril ER, Rybski JA, Scuderi P, Watson RR (1989). Beta-carotene stimulates human leukocytes to secrete a novel cytokine. J Leuk Biol 45:255-261.

Alexander M, Newmark H, Miller G (1985). Oral beta-carotene can increase the numbers of OKT4+ cells in human blood. Immunol Lett 9:221-225.

Moriguchi S, Werner L, Watson RR (1985). High dietary vitamin A and cellular immune functions in mice. Immunology 56:169-177.

Moriguchi S, Kohge M, Kishino Y, Watson RR (1988) In vitro effect of retinol and 13-cis retinoic acid on cytotoxicity of human monocytes. Nutr Res 8:255-264.

Mufti SI, Prabhala R, Moriguchi S, Sipes IG, Watson, RR (1988). Functional and numerical alterations induced by ethanol in the cellular immune system. Immunopharmacology 15:85-94.

Schoen DJ, Watson, R.R (1988). Prevention of UV irradiation induced suppression of monocyte functions by retinoids and carotenoids in vitro. Photochem Photobiol 48:659-664.

Schwartz J, (1988). Prevention of experimental and cancer by extracts of Spirulina-Dunaliella algae. Nutr Cancer 11:127-134.

Schwartz J, Suda D, Light G (1986). Beta carotene is associated with the regression of hamster buccal pouch carcinoma and the induction of tumor necrosis factor in macrophages. Biochem Biophys Res Comm 136:1130-1135.

Temple NJ, Basu TK (1988). Does beta-carotene prevent cancer? A critical appraisal. Nutr Res 8:685-701.

Tomita Y. (1987). Augmentation of tumor immunity against syngeneic tumors in mice by beta-carotene. J Nat Cancer Inst 78:679-681.

Tubaro E, Borelli G, Croce C, Cavallo G, Santiageli C (1983). Effect of morphine on resistance to infection. J Infect Dis 148:656-666.

Tubaro E, Avico U, Santiageli C, Zuccaro P, Cavallo G, Pacifici R, Croce C, Borelli G (1985). Morphine and methodone impact on human phagocytic physiology. Int J Immunopharmacol 7:865-874.

Watson RR (1988). Ethanol, Immunomodulation and cancer. Prog Food Nutr Sci 12:189-209.

Watson RR, Yahya MD, Darban MR, Prabhala RH (1988a). Enhanced survival by vitamin A supplementation during a retrovirus infection causing murine AIDS. Life Sci 43:xii-xvii.

Watson RR, Prabhala RH, Darban HR, Yahya MD and Smith TL (1988b). Changes in lymphocyte and macrophage subsets due to morphine and ethanol treatment during a retrovirus infection causing murine AIDS. Life Sci 43:v-xi.

Watson RR (1989). Murine models for Acquired Immune Deficiency Syndrome. Life Sci 44:i-xiii.

Watson RR, Rybski JA (1988). Immunological response modification by vitamin A and other retinoids. Nutrition and Immunology. Chandra, R., ed. Alan R. Liss, New York, 87-99.

Yahya MD, Watson RR (1987). Minireview. Immunomodulation by morphine and marijuana. Life Sci 41:2503-2510.

Alcohol, Immunomodulation, and AIDS, pages 93–102
Published 1990 Alan R. Liss, Inc.

THE SEARCH FOR COFACTORS IN AIDS, INCLUDING AN ANALYSIS OF THE ASSOCIATION OF NITRITE INHALANT ABUSE AND KAPOSI'S SARCOMA

Harry W. Haverkos, M.D.
Clinical Medicine Branch; Division of Clinical Research; National Institute on Drug Abuse; Alcohol, Drug Abuse, and Mental Health Administration; Rockville, Maryland 20857

INTRODUCTION

Some investigators have speculated that drugs of abuse may expedite the disease process of HIV infection or promote specific disease outcomes, such as Kaposi's sarcoma or non-Hodgkin's lymphoma. These hypotheses result from the knowledge that there is a high frequency of AIDS among intravenous drug abusers and homosexual/bisexual men who report abuse of large quantities of drugs before developing AIDS. In fact, the purpose of this conference is to explore the ways in which alcohol may be a "cofactor" in AIDS and how investigators can decipher the role of alcohol, if any, in the pathogenesis of AIDS. In this paper, I will present some general comments on the difficulties encountered by investigators attempting to identify drugs of abuse as cofactors in AIDS and then focus on a discussion of the evidence associating nitrite inhalant abuse with Kaposi's sarcoma in AIDS.

COFACTORS IN AIDS

A cofactor in AIDS is a non-HIV related influence that operates in conjunction with HIV to affect disease progression. There are a number of epidemiological and natural history studies that purport to search for such factors in AIDS. A number of investigators have proposed other viruses as cofactors in AIDS, such as cytomegalovirus and Epstein-Barr virus infections. Drugs of abuse have been proposed by others (Haverkos, 1987).

There are several hypotheses involving drugs of abuse as cofactors in AIDS. Drugs of abuse, such as alcohol and "crack," may increase risk-taking behavior for AIDS when individuals are under their influence or draw individuals into settings where they are likely to meet and consort with HIV-infected individuals. Drugs, such as opiates and alcohol, may directly alter the immune system of HIV-infected individuals and speed the disease process from infection to the development of AIDS and ultimately death. Finally, drugs of abuse may act to increase the likelihood of the development of specific disease manifestations of AIDS, such as Kaposi's sarcoma or non-Hodgkin's lymphoma.

When one considers a drug as a cause of a disease, one generally considers one of two mechanisms. The first is a dose response reaction. The more drug one is exposed to, the more likely the outcome. The outcome may be clinically more severe with increasing exposure to the causative agent or occur sooner following exposure to increased doses than when smaller doses are employed. Secondly, idiosyncratic or hypersensitivity reactions can occur and may only be appreciated by investigators if the outcome rapidly and consistently follows the exposure.

Another important consideration is the timing of the interaction between, drug, virus, and the host. For example, when salicylates are used to treat some viral infections, such as influenza B or varicella-zoster virus infections, during the prodromal phase, the risks for the development of Reye's syndrome increases. Salicylate use at other times does not appear to predict development of this syndrome (Reye et al., 1963; Hurwitz et al., 1987; Pinsky et al., 1988).

There are a number of difficulties one must deal with when trying to establish drugs of abuse as co-factors in AIDS. Confounding is a major problem. Drug abusers generally do not use only one substance. Poly-drug abuse appears to be the rule rather than the exception. In addition, drug abusers are exposed to a variety of potential cofactors, such as infectious diseases, malnutrition, and other environmental factors, that may complicate data analysis. Second, the dosage used by study participants is difficult to measure. Look-alike drugs and impurities are often present in illicit substances. The accuracy of self reported histories of drug abuse may be impaired by the effects of drugs on memory, denial, or fear of legal reprisals when reporting illegal behavior to investigators. Laboratory tests may be used by researchers to measure drug levels, however, these tests may not be helpful quantitating chronic exposure to substances. In fact, the half-life of most substances is too short to make drug testing a definitive tool in many AIDS-related studies (Hawks and Chiang, 1986). Finally, the results of studies addressing similiar hypotheses are not comparable because the wording of the questionnaires or time intervals queried are not equivalent (Haverkos, 1988).

Because of the difficulties inherent in epidemiologic studies, animal models may be an approach to further explore plausible hypotheses concerning cofactors and AIDS. One may wish to employ animal models infected with HIV or other retroviruses, challenge the animals with potential cofactors, and check for outcomes suggestive of AIDS or AIDS-like conditions. However, if the interactions of HIV or other retroviruses with "cofactors" are species-specific, negative studies may not be helpful, and in fact, may be misleading.

AIDS-RELATED KAPOSI'S SARCOMA AND NITRITE INHALANTS

Although there are several hypotheses implicating cofactors in AIDS, most theories are based on laboratory observations and not clinical data. However, there is strong clinical and epidemiological data to suggest the existence of a cofactor in Kaposi's sarcoma in AIDS.

In 1872, Moriz Kaposi described 3 fatal cases of multiple idiopathic pigmented hemangiosarcoma in elderly men in Vienna, Austria. "Classical" Kaposi's sarcoma (KS) has since been described throughout the world. In 1981, an unusual form of KS was reported among young homosexual men in New York, San San Francisco, and

Los Angeles. Although histologically identical, the "epidemic" or AIDS-related KS differs from the classical form is a number of ways. AIDS-related KS occurs more commonly on the upper body, arms, and head, including the nose, and is associated with a low T-helper lymphocyte count and human immunodeficiency virus (HIV) infection. In contrast, classical KS occurs mainly on the arms and legs, is generally associated with normal T-helper lymphocyte counts and patients lack antibody to HIV (Friedman-Kien et al., 1989).

Although associated with HIV infection, HIV alone seems not to cause KS in AIDS patients. KS is concentrated in homosexual men (especially white homosexual men) with AIDS and is rare in others, and the proportion of AIDS cases with KS has been decreasing each year (Des Jarlais et al., 1987; Haverkos et al., 1985a; Haverkos et al., 1988; Rutherford et al., 1989). Furthermore, in transfusion-acquired AIDS from donors in whom KS subsequently developed, KS is rare, suggesting that a specific strain of HIV is not responsible (Peterman et al., 1985).

Specific "cofactors" have been proposed to account for the unique epidemiology of KS in AIDS. In 1981, New York investigators proposed that genetic factors may be important in the etiology of KS in AIDS because of an increased prevalence of clasical KS among Eastern European and Mediterranean men. They initially observed that 10 of 12 homosexual men with AIDS-related KS were positive for HLA-DR5 phenotype, compared with 12 percent of controls (Rubenstein et al., 1984). However, as the size of the study population increased, the association was no longer significant.

Other investigators have suggested that cytomegalovirus (CMV) may be a cofactor in KS. CMV and classical KS were first associated by Gaetano Giraldo and colleagues when they observed herpes type viral particles in five of eight tissue culture cell lines from African patients with KS (Giraldo et al., 1972; Giraldo et al., 1980). San Franciscan investigators have linked AIDS-related KS with CMV infection among homosexual men and demonstrated a decline in CMV seroconversion among gay men paralleling the decline in proprtions of KS (Drew et al., 1988). However, the seroprevalence rates for CMV infection are also high among hemophiliacs and heterosexual intravenous drug abusers, yet KS is rare in those populations. In addition, CMV as the KS cofactor cannot explain the racial distribution of KS among gay men (Haverkos et al., 1988).

Other sexually transmitted agents have been proposed as KS cofactors. One investigator reported seeing the agent on electron microscopy, however, his findings cannot be reproduced (Lo, 1986). One limitation of proposing a second sexually transmitted agent as the KS cofactor is that there is no known sexually transmitted disease that occurs so exclusively among gay men and more commonly among whites than Blacks (Judson, 1981; Judson et al., 1980).

There are several reasons to consider nitrite inhalants as the KS cofactor. First, nitrite inhalants are used more commonly by gay men than others (Centers for Disease Control, 1982), use is on the decline since AIDS was reported (Lange et al., 1988), and use among whites is greater than among Blacks (National Institute on Drug Abuse, 1988). Second, three epidemiologic studies have shown a strong statistical association between the development of KS among gay men with AIDS and the use of large quantities of nitrite inhalants when compared with gay men with AIDS, but without KS (Mather-Wagh et al., 1985; Haverkos et al., 1985a, Osmond et al., 1985). Third, anecdotal reports of the increased frequency of AIDS-related KS on the face and chest, and especially the nose, is consistent with the likely areas of skin most healvily exposed to nitrite vapors when inhaled. Finally, two plausible mechanisms of action for nitrites to be carcinogenic have been proposed (Goedert et al., 1982; Mirvish et al., 1988).

There have been several arguments against nitrite inhalants as the KS cofactor. However, I do not believe that any of these arguments is convincing enough to eliminate nitrites from further consideration. First, a few gay men with KS report never using nitrites. However, passive exposure to nitrites in bars, bath-houses, and other settings is possible. In addition, the use of nitrous oxide, another durg abused by some gay men, should be explored in those patients. Second, some AIDS-related KS cases occur in other risk groups who probably do no use nitrite inhalants, e.g., pediatric patients (Buck et al., 1983). However, a few KS cases reported to CDC among children have not been comfirmed by experienced pathologists upon review of skin biopsies from those children (Personal Communication: D. Porter, UCLA). Nitrite inhalant abuse is not limited to gay men, but many physicians reporting KS cases to CDC have not adequately explored or reported the drug abuse history of their patients. Third, three epidemiologic studies comparing gay men with KS and those with opportunistic infections failed to demonstrate an association between nitrite inhalant abuse and KS (Goedert et al., 1986; Polk et al., 1987; Darrow et al., 1987). A reveiw of the methodologies of those studies, particularly analysis of sample sizes and wording of questionnaires concerning nitrites, raise concerns about the validity of their conclusions (Haverkos, 1988). Finally, NCI investigators have produced KS-like lesions in mice after exposing the mice to retroviral particles or factors generated in cultured KS tissues without exposure of these mice to nitrite inhalants (Salahuddin et al., 1988; Vogel et al., 1988). It may be interesting to see if exposure of these mice to nitrite vapors potentiates the endothelial lesions.

Nitrite inhalants have not been scientifically proven to be the KS cofactor, however, there are sufficient reasons to consider them to be the leading candidate. Identifying the KS cofactor in AIDS could prove valuable for prevention of the most common cancer afflicting AIDS patients. Clarifying the mechanisms by which HIV infection and the KS cofactor produce disease may have implications for other cancers and diseases.

SUMMARY

The identification of cofactors in AIDS is a challenging scientific task. If successful, identifying cofactors could prove valuable in understanding the pathogenesis of HIV infection and AIDS and in the development of strategies to prolong survival and/or prevent complications in HIV-infected individuals. There is sufficient evidence to suggest the existence of a cofactor in KS in AIDS. Nitrite inhalants remain a leading candidate to be the KS cofactor. Until more is known to document or refute this specific virus-drug interaction hypothesis in the pathogenesis of KS in AIDS, clinicians should encourage their patients to avoid use of nitrite inhalants.

This article was prepared by a Federal Government employee as part of official duties; therefore, the material is in the public domain and may be reproduced or copied without permission.

REFERENCES

Buck BE, Scott GB, Valdes-Dapena M, et al. (1983). Kaposi's sarcoma in two infants with AIDS. J Pediatr 103:911-913.

Centers for Disease Control (1982). Epidemiologic aspects of the current outbreak of Kaposi's sarcoma and opportunistic infections. N Engl J Med 306:248-252.

Darrow WW, Echenberg DF, Jaffe HW, et al. (1987). Risk factors for human immunodeficiency virus infection in homosexual men. Am J Public Health 77:479-483.

DesJarlais DC, Stoneburner R, Thomas P, Friedman SR (1987). Declines in proportion of Kaposi's sarcoma among cases of AIDS in multiple risk groups in New York City. Lancet 2:1024-1025.

Drew WL, Mills J, Hauer LB, et al. (1988). Declining prevalence of Kaposi's sarcoma in homosexual AIDS patients paralleled by fall in cytomegalovirus transmission. Lancet 1:66.

Friedman-Kien AE, Ostreicher R, Saltzman B (1989). Clinical manifestations of Kaposi's sarcoma. In: Friedman-Kien AE (editor). Color Atlas of AIDS. W.B. Saunders Company, Philadelphia. Pp. 11-48.

Giraldo G, Beth E, Haguenau F (1972). Herpes-type virus particles in tissue culture of Kaposi's sarcoma from different geographic regions. J Natl Cancer Inst 49:1509-1513.

Giraldo G, Beth E, Huang ES (1980). Kaposi's sarcoma and its relationship to cytomegalovirus (CMV). III. CMV DNA and CMV early antigens in Kaposi's sarcoma. Int J Cancer 26:23-29.

Goedert JJ, Biggar RJ, Melbye M, et al. (1986). Effect of T4 count and cofactors on incidence of AIDS in homosexual men infected with human immunodeficiency virus. JAMA 257:331-334.
Goedert JJ, Neuland CY, Wallen WC, et al. (1982). Amyl nitrite may alter T lymphocytes in homosexual men. Lancet 1:412-416.
Hawks RL, Chiang (1986). Urine Testing for Drugs of Abuse. NIDA Research Monograph 73, U.S. Department of Health and Human Services, PHS, ADAMHA, U.S. Government Printing Office.
Haverkos HW, Amsel Z, Drotman DP, Morgan M (1988). Kaposi's sarcoma in homosexual men with AIDS, by race. Lancet 2:1075.
Haverkos HW, Drotman DP, Morgan M (1985a). Prevalence of Kaposi's sarcoma among patients with AIDS. N Engl J Med 312:1518.
Haverkos HW (1988). Epidemiologic studies - Kaposi's sarcoma vs.opportunistic infections among homosexual men with AIDS. In: Haverkos HW, Dougherty JA (editors). Health Hazards of Nitrite Inhalants. NIDA Research Monograph 83, U.S. Department of Health and Human Services, PHS, ADAMHA. U.S. Government Printing Office, pp.96-105.
Haverkos HW (1987). Factors associated with the pathogenesis of AIDS. J Infect Dis 156:251-257. Haverkos HW, Pinsky PF, Drotman DP, Bregman DJ (1985b). Disease manifestation among homosexual men with acquired immunodeficiency syndrome: A possible role of nitrites in Kaposi's sarcoma. Sex Transm Dis 12:203-208.
Hurwitz ES, Barrett MJ, Bregman D, et al. (1987). Public Health Service study of Reye's syndrome and medication: Report of the main study. JAMA 257: 1902-1911.
Judson FN (1981). Epidemiology and control of nongonococcal urethritis and genital chlamydial infection: A review. Sex Transm Dis 8:S117-S126.
Judson FN, Penley KA, Robinson ME, et al. (1980). Comparative prevalence rates of sexually transmitted diseases in heterosexual and homosexual men. Am J Epidemiol 112:836-843.
Lange WR, Dax E, Haertzen CA, et al. (1988). Nitrite Inhalants: Contemporary patterns of abuse. In: Haverkos HW, Dougherty JA (editors). Health Hazards of Nitrite Inhalants. NIDA Research Monograph 83, U.S. Department of Health and Human Services, PHS, ADAMHA. U.S. Government Printing Office, pp.86-95.

Lo SC (1986). Isolation and identification of a novel virus from patients with AIDS. Am J Trop Med Hyg 35:675-676.
Mathur-Wagh U, Mildvan D, Senie RT (1985). Follow-up at 4-1/2 years on homosexual men with generalized lymphadenopathy. N Engl J Med 313:1542-1543.
Mirvish SS, Ramm D, Babcock DM (1988). Indication from animal and chemical experiments of a carcinogenic role of iso-butyl nitrite. In: Haverkos HW, Dougherty JA (editors). Health Hazards of Nitrite Inhalants. NIDA Research Monograph 83, U.S. Department of Health and Human Services, PHS, ADAMHA. U.S. Government Printing Office, pp.39-49.
National Institute on Drug Abuse (1988). National Household Survey: Main indings 1985. U.S. Department of Health and Human Services, PHS, ADAMHA, DHHS Publication No. (ADM) 88-1586, U.S. Government Printing Office, Washington, D.C., p. 56.
Osmond D, Moss AR, Bachetti P, et al. (1985). A case-control study of risk factors for AIDS in San Francisco. In: International Conference on Acquired Immunodeficiency Syndrome (AIDS), Atlanta, Georgia, April 14-17, 1985.
Peterman TA, Jaffe HW, Feorino PM, et al. (1985). Transfusion-associated acquired immunodeficiency syndrome in the United States. JAMA 254:2913-2917.
Pinsky PF, Hurwitz ES, Schonberger LB, Gunn WJ (1988). Reye's syndrome and aspirin: Evidence for a dose-response effect. JAMA 260:657-661.
Polk F, Fox R, Brookmeyer R, et al. (1987). Predictors of the acquired immunodeficiency syndrome developing in a cohort of seropositive men. N Engl J Med 316:62-66.
Reye RDK, Morgan G, Baral J (1963). Encephalopathy and fatty degeneration of the viscera: A disease entity in childhood. Lancet 2:749-752.
Rubenstein P, de Cordoba S, Oestricher R, et al. (1984). Immunogenetics and predisposition to Kaposi's sarcoma. In: Groopman J (editor). Acquired Immune Deficiency Syndrome. Alan J. Liss, New York, pp. 309-318.
Rutherford GW, Schwarcz SK, Lemp GF, et al. (1989). The epidemiology of AIDS-related Kaposi's sarcoma in San Francisco. J Infect Dis 159:569-572.

Salahuddin SZ, Nakamura S, Biberfeld P, et al. (1988). Angiogenic properties of Kaposi's sarcoma-derived cells after long-term culture in vitro. Science 242:430-433.

Vogel J, Hinrichs SH, Reynolds RK, et al. (1988). The HIV tat gene induces dermal lesions resembling Kaposi's sarcoma in transgenic mice. Nature 335: 606-611.

Alcohol, Immunomodulation, and AIDS, pages 103–111
© 1990 Alan R. Liss, Inc.

ALCOHOL AND IMMUNE FUNCTION IN HIV-1 SERONEGATIVE, HTLV-I/II SERONEGATIVE AND POSITIVE MEN ON METHADONE

Nancy G. Klimas, Robert Morgan, Nancy T. Blaney, Dale Chitwood, J. Bryan Page, Karen Milles and Mary Ann Fletcher

Center for the Biopsychosocial Study of AIDS, University of Miami School of Medicine and the VA Medical Center, Miami, Florida 33101

INTRODUCTION

Nearly one-third of AIDS cases in this country are drug related. In a call for more attention to drug abuse to curb AIDS, Dr. James Curran of the CDC has said that we may be at the later stages of spread among the gay population, at an intermediate stage, still spreading phase among IV drug abusers and at the beginning stage of the spread among heterosexuals (Curran, 1988).

IV drug users are the primary source of heterosexual and perinatal transmission in the U.S., with most of the cases among women resulting from sexual contact with an HIV positive IV drug user (IVDU), or IV drug use itself. Most of the cases in children result from perinatal transmission via a pregnant HIV-1 positive IVDU or a woman infected by a drug user (Des Jarlais and Freidman, 1988; Conviser and Rutledge, 1988).

Methadone maintenance programs for heroin addicted individuals clearly are behavior modifying. Unfortunately treatment programs in the United States are hampered by long waiting lists, poor funding, and increasing numbers of cocaine and crack addicted individuals, who require more intensive and often inpatient rehabilitation. However, public policy is shifting, with more funding for treatment programs planned. Therefore, this opiate is being used with increasing frequency in a population at high risk for exposure to HIV-1. Animal studies, as well as <u>in vitro</u>

studies with human cells, indicate that opiates, including heroin, have immunosuppressive potential (Gungor et al., 1980, Donahoe et al., 1986). Klimas et al. (1984) reported that 200 Of 200 IVDUs in a methadone treatment program had evidence of B cell dysfunction and polyclonal B cell activation.

In addition to having a high frequency of exposure to HIV-1, IVDUs may have a compromised immune system prior to encounter with this immunosuppressive virus (Klimas, et al., 1986, Donahoe and Falek, 1988; Klimas, et al, 1989). They are reported to have an increased incidence of opportunistic infections and cancer (Harris and Garret, 1972). Immune function may be impaired due to a number of possible factors - the illicit drugs' direct effect, repeated exposures to infectious agents, malnutrition, and concurrent use of alcohol and other drugs.

The present report is part of a larger longitudinal study designed to assess the role of pre-existing immune dysfunction as related to psychosocial factors, behavioral factors including polydrug use, and nutritional factors, in the elevated HIV-1 disease risk among methadone-maintained IVDU. In previous reports, the presence of immune dysfunction has been documented in anti-HIV-1 negative methadone subjects (Klimas et al., 1988). This dysfunction included pertubations in the distributions of CD4 subsets and elevations of numbers of T cells bearing activation markers Ta1 and I2. Immunoglobulins G and M were elevated. Lymphocyte response to the plant mitogens, phytohemagglutinin (PHA) and pokeweed (PWM) were significantly reduced as was the natural cell mediated (NK) cytotoxicity against a tumor cell target. This dysfunction could not be ascribed to infection with HTLV-I/II (Klimas, et al., 1989). The purpose of the present report is to examine the relationship between alcohol use and immune function in a cohort of men who were anti-HIV-1 negative.

METHODS

Subjects were 25 men enrolled in the outpatient Drug and Rehabilitation Unit of the Miami VA Medical Center between June 1987 and June 1988.. All of these were anti-HIV-1 negative and 26% were anti-HTLVI/II positive. Subjects were aged 30-66 ($\underline{M}$=39.8) and were predominantly Anglo, but with both black and hispanic men included. A panel of immunologic tests was selected which intended to measure the functional potential as well as phenotype of immune system cells from patients in the study. The whole blood methodologies employed for these measurements have been previously described (Baron, et al, 1985; Fletcher et al., 1987, Fletcher, et al., 1989). Alcohol and drug use behaviors were gathered with a pre-coded structured interview schedule that included sociodemographics, migration history, medical history, drug use history, and self-report of behaviors known to be risky for HIV infection. The interview concentrated on IV drug use and sexual behavior as the primary risk behaviors. The alcohol and drug use items have been used in previous studies of IVDUs (Chitwood, 1985; Chitwood et al., 1988). Spearman rank order correlations were used to determine the degree of association between the drug use data and the immunological parameters.

RESULTS

Descriptive data for the alcohol and drug use behaviors (frequencies and percentages) are shown in TABLE I. Results of the correlational analyses of lymphocyte phenotypes are given in TABLE II.

TABLE I. SELF-REPORTED ALCOHOL AND DRUG USE IN IV DRUG USERS IN METHADONE TREATMENT

Frequency	Alcohol	Cocaine	Heroin	Speedball
never	11(45.8%)*	15(62.5%)	9(37.5%)	16(66.7%)
few times	2(8.3%)	2(8.3%)	3(12.5%)	1(4.2%)
<1/month	1(4.2%)	3(12.5%)	1(4.2%)	2(8.3%)
<1/week	3(12.5%)	2(8.3%)	2(8.3%)	2(8.3%)
1/week	1(4.2%)	0	1(4.2%)	0
<1/day	1(4.2%)	1(4.2%)	0	2(8.3%)
daily	1(4.2%)	0	2(8.3%)	1(4.2%)
>daily	4(16.7%)	2(8.3%)	5(20.8%)	0
Total	24	24	24	24

*Percent of total given in parenthesis.

Of the T lymphocyte subsets related to alcohol use, only

the CD2+Ta1+ subset absolute number showed a significant correlation ($r=-.44$, $p<.05$) with alcohol use related to less activation. Two additional T lymphocyte subsets were marginally associated with alcohol use: CD4+CDw29+ subset ($r=-.37$, $p<.06$) and CD4+CD45R+ subset ($r=-.40$, $p<.06$). The inverse direction of association suggests that alcohol use in this sample was associated with decreased number of the lymphocytes (CD4+CD45R+) which induce activation of T cytotoxic/suppressor cells as well as of the lymphocytes (CD4+CDw29+) activating B cell response to antigen.

TABLE II: CORRELATIONS OF REPORTED ALCOHOL USE WITH LYMPHOCYTE PHENOTYPES.

Measure (cells/mm^3)	r	N
CD4	-.24	24
CD8	-.36*	24
CD4/CD8 ratio	-.10	24
CD2+Ta1+	-.44**	21
CD4+CDw29+	-.37*	23
CD4+CD45R+	-.40*	24
CD8+I2+	-.11	23
NKH.1	-.41**	24
CD20	-.31	23
CD21	-.35	23

All correlations Spearman rank order correlations.
*.05<p<.10; ** p<.05

For natural killer (NK) cells, the absolute number of NK cells (though not percentage of total lymphocytes) was significantly correlated with alcohol use ($r=-.42$, $p<.05$). In contrast to the decline seen in numbers of effector cells, alcohol was positively correlated with an index of NK cell function, the lytic index ($r=.48$, $p<.02$) (TABLE III).

There was no significant association between alcohol use and response of lymphocytes to PHA and PWM (TABLE IV). Alcohol use was marginally correlated with decreased number (not percentage) of total lymphocytes ($r=.35$, $p<.10$) but was unrelated to the overall white blood cell count. Among serum immunoglobulins, only IgM was significantly associated with alcohol use (r=.61, p,.04, N=12).

TABLE III: CORRELATIONS OF REPORTED ALCOHOL USE WITH NATURAL KILLER CELL CYTOTOXICITY[b]

Measure	r	N
lytic index	.48**	24

[b]against K562 tumor cell targets ** $p<.05$

TABLE IV: CORRELATIONS OF REPORTED ALCOHOL USE WITH LYMPHOCYTE RESPONSE TO PLANT MITOGENS

Measure	r	N
response to PHA (net cpm)	-.33	15
response to PWM (net cpm)	-.31	15

An additional question addressed by the present research was the relationship between alcohol and the use of other drugs--heroin cocaine and speedballing-- as well as shooting frequency. As can be seen from the correlations in TABLE V, alcohol use was essentially unrelated to both shooting frequency and the use of other drugs. Only for cocaine was there any correlation, and that was marginal and inverse (r=-.35, p<.08). In this sample of methadone maintained IV drug users, at least, there is no evidence that alcohol is a disinhibitor that is associated with other drug use. On the other hand, use of other drugs seemed to cluster together: heroin, cocaine, and speedballing were all associated with one another, as they were with shooting frequency. As can be seen in Table 1, this cohort reported a relatively high frequency (29%) of daily or more than daily heroin use. However, there appeared to be no association either between alcohol use and heroin use (r=.16, p:ns), or between heroin use and any of the immunological parameters.

TABLE V: CORRELATIONS OF ALCOHOL USE WITH OTHER DRUGS OF ABUSE AND SHOOTING FREQUENCY

	heroin	cocaine	speed-ball	shooting freq.
alcohol	.17 25	-.36* 25	.12 25	-.18 24
heroin	1.00 25	.43** 25	.50** 25	.58*** 24
cocaine		1.00 25	.41** 25	.49** 24
speedball			1.00 25	.72**** 24
shooting frequency				1.00 24

All correlations are Spearman rank order correlations. Ns are shown below each correlation.
* .05<p<.10, ** p<.05, *** p<.01, **** p<.001

DISCUSSION

Results of the correlational analyses suggest that alcohol cannot explain the immunosuppression previously reported (Klimas et al., 1988 and Klimas et al., 1989) in these HIV-1 seronegative methadone maintained IVDU. Alcohol use was associated with diminished numbers of NK cells but with elevated NK cell activity against tumor cell targets as expressed by lytic index. This is compatible with the reports of low numbers of NK cell in alcoholic liver disease (Watson et al, 1985) and of increased NK cell activity (Saxena et al., 1980). It is in contrast to the overall elevation in numbers of NK cells but decreased activity per NKH.1 positive cell in this group as compared to age and sex matched controls. Alcohol use did not explain the significant depression in lymphocyte response to mitogens observed in the methadone group. The cohort has numbers of CD4 cells which are not different from the expected for gender and age group and no effect of alcohol was observed on total numbers of CD4 cells. In the cohort as a whole, there is significant elevation of a subset of CD 4 cells, CD4+CDw29+, which furnish help for B cell response to antigen. Alcohol use correlated marginally with a decrease in this CD4 subset. In the methadone treatment group there was a significant increase in CD8 cells and in CD8 cells expressing the class II antigen I2. Numbers of T cells expressing an alternate pathway of activation marker, Tal also increased in the population as a whole. In contrast, alcohol use correlated significantly with a decrease in CD2+Tal+ cells and marginally with a decrease in CD8 cells. No effect of alcohol use was seen on expression of the I2 activation marker on CD8. Elevated IgM was significantly correlated with alcohol. In the methadone group both IgG and IgM are elevated compared to controls. These findings suggest that in most measures, alcohol may have contrary effects to those of opiates (ie. methadone). Thus one might conclude that both alcohol and methadone effects on the immune system may be rather powerful, but may tend to off-set each other in this cohort.

Also warranting comment is the relative frequency that alcohol and other drugs are used by this methadone treatment sample in comparison to a non-treatment sample of street IV drug users (under study at the University of Miami Center for the Biopsychosocial Study of AIDS). The same interview protocol and interviewers were used with both samples to gather the substance use data. Results showed that alcohol as well as other drugs were used at a substantially lower rate in the methadone as compared to the street users sample. For example, over 58% of the methadone sample reported infrequent alcohol use in the prior year (i.e. from never to less than once a month) compared to only 16% of the street users) In contrast, frequent alcohol use (i.e., at least daily to several times a day) was reported by 21% of the methadone sample, compared to 57% of the street users. Use of other drugs evidenced parallel patterns, with infrequent use characterizing the methadone sample, and frequent use characterizing the street users. These data indicate that the methadone and street user samples differ in the degree to which alcohol and drug use may be cofactors in regard to immunocompetence. Studies are in progress to delineate the effects of street drugs, treatment modalities, and drug withdrawal on immune function, and other potential factors such as health, psychosocial and nutritional status. (Supported by grant P50-MH/DA-42455 from NIMH).

REFERENCES

Baron, GC, Klimas, NG, Fischl, MA and Fletcher, MA (1985) Decreased natural cell-mediated cytotoxicity per effector in acquired immunodeficiency syndrome. Diag. Immunol. 3:197-204.

Chitwood, DD (1985) Patterns and consequences of cocaine use. In NJ Kozel and EH Adams (Eds), Cocaine use in America: Epidemiologic and clinical perspectives. NIDA Research Monograph No. 61, US Government Printing Office: Washington, DC.

Chitwood, DD, Comerford, M, McCoy, CD, Trapido, EJ, Page, JB, McBride, DC, and Inciardi, J (1988) Epidemiology of HIV among intravenous drug users in South Florida. IV International Conference on AIDS, Stockholm, Sweden.

Conviser, R and Rutledge, JH (1988) The Need for Innovation to Halt AIDS Among Intravenous Drug Users and Their Sexual Partners. IV International Conference on AIDS, Stockholm, Sweden June.

Curran, J (1988). Editorial: Health officials urge more attention to drug abuse to curb AIDS. US Medicine 8:Feb.

Des Jarlais, DC and Freidman, SR (1988) HIV Infection Among Persons who Inject Illicit Drugs: Problems and Perspectives. J of AIDS, 1:267-272.

Donahoe, RM, Nicholson, JK, Madden, JJ, Donahoe, F, Shafer, DA, Gordon, D, Bokos, P, and Falek, A (1986) Coordinate and independent effects of heroin, cocaine, and alcohol abuse on T-cell E-rosette formation and antigenic marker expression. Clin. Immunol. Immunopathol., 41:254-264.

Donahoe, RM and Falek, A (1988) Neuroimmunomodulation by opiates and other drugs of abuse: Relationship to HIV infection and AIDS. Adv. Biochem. Psychopharmacol., 44:145-158.

Fletcher, MA, Baron, GA, Ashman, M, Fischl, MA and Klimas (1987). Use of whole blood methods in assessment of immune parameters in immunodeficiency states. Clin Diag Immunol 5:69-81.

Fletcher, MA, Azen, SP, Adelsberg, B, Gjerset, G, Hassett, J, Kaplan, J, Niland JC, Odom-Maryon, T, Parker, JW, Stites, DP, Mosley, JW, and the Transfusion Safety Study Group. (1989) Immunophenotyping in a multicenter study: The Transfusion Safety Study experience. Clin Immunol Immunopathol, in press.

Gungor, M, Genc, E, Sagduyu, H, Eroglu, L and Koyuncuoglu, H (1980) Effect of chronic administration of morphine on primary immune response in mice. Experientia, 36:1309-1310.

Harris, PD and Garret, R (1972) Susceptibility of addicts to infection and neoplasia. N Engl J Med, 287:310.

Klimas, NG, and Fletcher, MA (1984) Polyclonal B Cell Activation in IV Drug Users. Clin. Res., 42:350.

Klimas, NG, Blaney, NT, Milles, K and Fletcher, MA (1988) Immune Abnormalities in anti-HIV negative Methadone Patients. IV International Conference on AIDS, Stockholm, Sweden.

Klimas, NG, Blaney, N, Morgan, R, Simoneau, J and Fletcher, MA (1989) Immunologic abnormalities in anti-HIV-1 negative and HTLV-I/II negative and positive IV drug abusers on methadone. V International Conference on AIDS, Montreal.

Saxena, QB, Mezey, E and Adler, WH (1980) Regulation of natural killer activity in vivo.II. The effect of alcohol consumption on human peripheral blood natural killer activity. Int. J. Can. 26:413-417.

Watson, RR, Jackson, JC, Hartmann, B, Sampliner, R, Mobley, D and Eskelson, C. (1985) Cellular immune functions, endorphins, and alcohol consumption in males. Alcoholism: Clin. Exp. Res. 9:248-254.

Alcohol, Immunomodulation, and AIDS, pages 113–122
© 1990 Alan R. Liss, Inc.

ETHANOL MODULATATION OF THE EFFECTS OF PLATELET-ACTIVATING FACTOR ON HUMAN PLATELETS AND A MACROPHAGE CELL LINE

Rodney C. Baker

Department of Pharmacology, University of Colorado Health Sciences Center, Denver CO, 80262

INTRODUCTION:

The interaction between the biologically active phospholipid 1-O-alkyl-2-acetyl-*sn*-glycero-3-phosphocholine (Demopoulos, *et al.*, 1979) which was referred to previously as platelet-activating factor (PAF) (Benveniste *et al.*, 1972) and ethnaol is considered. The pharmacological responses attributed to PAF are species dependent but, in general, the response to exogenous PAF resembles anaphylactic shock. PAF, injected intravenously, elicits hypertension, thrombocytopenia and in most species bronchoconstriction. However, in the rat, PAF is a very potent hypotensive agent and the thrombocytopenia observed in the quinea pig is not observed following intravenous PAF. (Braquet *et al.*, 1987). Activation of various cell types, including platelets and macrophages, by PAF has been reported. The response of platelets to PAF treatment includes; the release of [^{3}H]serotonin from [^{3}H]serotonin preloaded platelets and release of arachidonic acid derived inflammatory mediators (Braquet *et al.*, 1987). Activation of isolated macrophages upon exposure to exogenous PAF is indicated by calcium mobilization and production of both prostaglandin E_2 and thromboxane B_2. (Pernhan and Leyck, 1983).

The synthesis of PAF, or assumed synthesis based on the presence of PAF in isolated preparations, has been demonstrated in a variety of cell types including platelets and macrophages (Braquet *et al.*, 1987). It was first described as a component released from pig leukocytes which activated rabbit platelets (Benveniste *et al.*, 1972). The synthesis of PAF has since been attributed to many cell types including: rabbit basophils, rat and mouse mcarophages, rabbit neutrophils, human platelets and endothelial cells. Two pathways have been proposed for the synthesis of PAF, one pathway is considered to be linked to the response to infection or hypersensitivity and a second pathway is proposed to play a role in blood pressure control under non-pathological conditions (Snyder 1987). The synthesis of PAF as a component of inflammation is characterized by activation of phospholipase A_2 which produces 1-O-alkyl-2-lyso-*sn*-glycero-3-phosphocholine (lyso-PAF) from 1-O-alkyl-2-acyl-*sn*-glycero-3-phosphocholine. The product, lyso-PAF, is acetylated by a acetyl-CoA dependent reaction to yield PAF. The second pathway, implicated in homeostasis, referred to as the *de novo* pathway is analogous to the Kennedy-Wise pathway of phospholipid synthesis. This pathway is distinguished by transfer of phosphocholine to 1-O-alkyl-2-acetyl-*sn*-glycerol from CDP-choline to yield PAF (Braquet *et al.*, 1987; Snyder, 1987).

Ethanol has the potential of perturbing PAF function either through effects on PAF metabolism or by interfering with PAF mediated responses. Ethanol could affect PAF synthesis in activated cells by altering phospholipase A_2 activity and /or acetyl-CoA concentration. Ethanol inhibition of phospholipase A_2 has been indicated in a variety of preparations including isolated platelets (Fenn and Littleton, 1983). The concentration of acetyl-CoA would most likely be enhanced by the metabolism of ethanol. How the increased concentration of acetyl-CoA would then influence the production of PAF has not been directly addressed. Ethanol was reported to partially replace the protective action of CV 3988, a PAF antagonist, following endotoxin treatment of rats, suggesting that ethanol may also interfere with the pharmacological properties of PAF (Chang *et al.*, 1987) as well as synthesis of this lipid mediator of inflammation.

The effect of ethanol on the synthesis of PAF in a clonal macrophage cell line and the effect of ethanol on the function of exogenous PAF in isolated human platelets is addressed in this report. Two synthetic pathways of PAF production are suggested by these studies, one stimulated by ethanol and a second pathway which is inhibited by the presence of ethanol. The results of these studies addressing the effect of ethanol and PAF function demonstrated an inhibition of PAF-induced platelet aggregation but do not suggest that ethanol interferes with interactions of PAF and a specific receptor.

MATERIALS AND METHODS:

1-O-hexadecyl-2-acetyl-*sn*-glycerol-3-phosphocholine (PAF), 1-O-hexadecyl-*sn*-glycerol-3-phosphocholine (lyso-PAF), phosphatidylethanolamine (PE), phosphatidylcholine (PC) were purchased from Avanti Polar Lipids Birmingham AL. 1-O-[^{3}H]hexadecyl-2-acetyl-*sn*-glycerol-3-phosphocholine prepared from synthetic 1-O-hexadec-9,10-enyl-2-lyso-*sn*-glycerol-3-phosphocholine (22) was supplied by Robert L. Wykle, Bowman Gray School of Medicine. 1-O-hexadecyl-2-[^{3}H]acetyl-GPC was purchased from Dupont NEN Research Products, Boston, Prepared thin layer plates (silica gel G) were purchased from Analtech Inc., Newark DL.

The experiments were carried out using either a macrophage clonal cell line (RAW 264) established from murine tumors induced with Abelson leukemia virus (Raschke *et al.*, 1978) or plateltets obtained from healthy human volunteers. Human blood (250 ml) collected in 3.8% w/v trisodium citrate (1 vol) was centrifuged at 150

X g for 20 min at 25° and the platelet rich plasma (PRP) was isolated. Platelet studies were carried out using PRP.

PAF was measured by two methods, the incorporation of [^{3}H] acetate into PAF and a direct gas chromatography/mass spectrometry analysis. Identification of [^{3}H]acetate labeled material as PAF was based on the following: 1) A phospholipid fraction was isolated by TLC which co-migrated with PAF. 2) The material was hydrolysed with phospholipase C and the diglyceride isolated. 3) Alkyl-2-acetyl-*sn*-glycerol was separated from other neutral lipids by TLC. A similar isolation procedure was used for GC/MS PAF measurements with the exception that pentafluorbenzoyl esters of the diglycerides were made and 1-O-alkyl-[^{3}D]acetyl-*sn*-glycerol was added as internal standard. The ratio of 555/552 was used for quantitation of PAF. The molecular anion of 1-O-alkyl-2-acetyl-pentaflurobenzoate is at m/z 552 for the hexadecyl species of 1-O-alkyl-2-acetyl-pentaflurobenzoate and 555 for the [D_3] analogue.

Phagocytosis was measured by adding unopsonized zymosan, 10 particles per macrophage, directly to the culture dishes. The number of cell associated zymosan particles was determined by direct light microscopy. The results are expressed as the percentage of cells which had taken up one or more particles. Platelet aggregation was monitored photometrically with a Payton aggregation module. Thromboxane B_2 (TxB_2) concentration were measured using an immunoassay (Fitzpatrick, 1982).

RESULTS:

In cells stimulated with zymosan ethanol caused a significant decrease in cell associated PAF, measured either by the incorporation of [^{3}H]acetate or GC/MS. Cells incubated for one hour in the presence of 10 zymosan particles/cell contained 68 $\pm$ 8 ng of PAF /1.1 X10^7 cells, as measured by GC mass spectrometry. PAF levels of 37 ng/1.1 X 10^7

cells, and less than 10 ng/1.1 X 10^7 cells were recovered from cells treated with zymosan plus 20 mM or 100 mM ethanol respectively. The incorporation of [^{3}H]acetate into PAF followed the same pattern, ethanol inhibited the zymosan stimulated production of PAF and inhibited the phagocytosis of zymosan particles.

Figure 1. The effect of ethanol on zymosan stimulated synthesis of PAF and phagocytosis of zymosan particles.

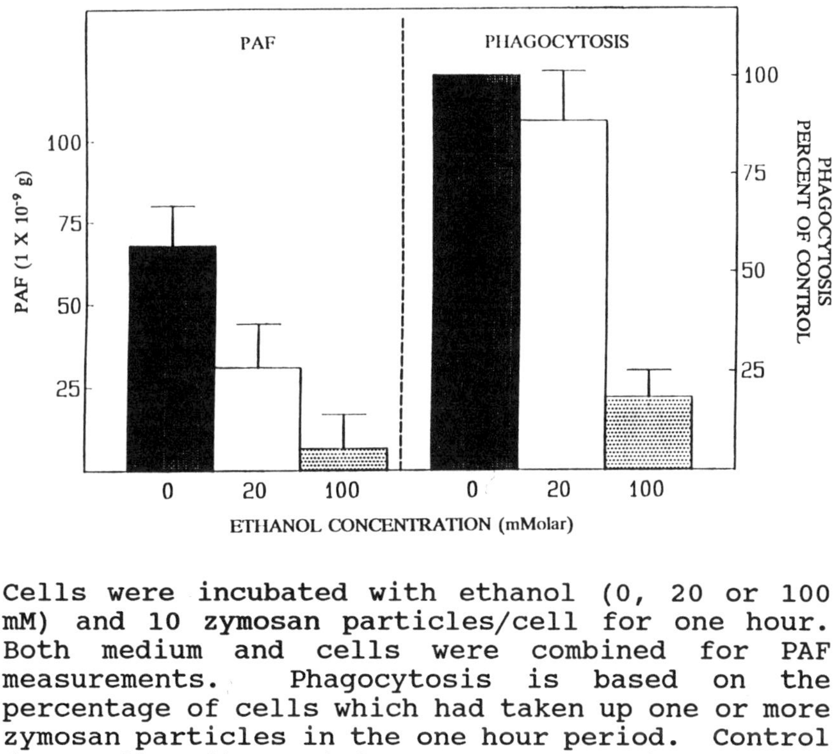

Cells were incubated with ethanol (0, 20 or 100 mM) and 10 zymosan particles/cell for one hour. Both medium and cells were combined for PAF measurements. Phagocytosis is based on the percentage of cells which had taken up one or more zymosan particles in the one hour period. Control (0 mM ethanol) was taken as 100 percent.

Ethanol appeared to have the opposite effect on the production of PAF without any known or added cell stimuli. Cell associated PAF was measured by GC/MS after one hour exposure of the macrophage cell line to 0, 25, 50 or 100 mM ethanol. A level of 1-7 ng/ 1.0 X 10^7 cells was measured in the non-ethanol treated cells. Significant increases in the recoverable PAF were observed after one hour exposure to ethanol.

Figure 2. Effect of ethanol on the production of PAF in non-stimulated cells.

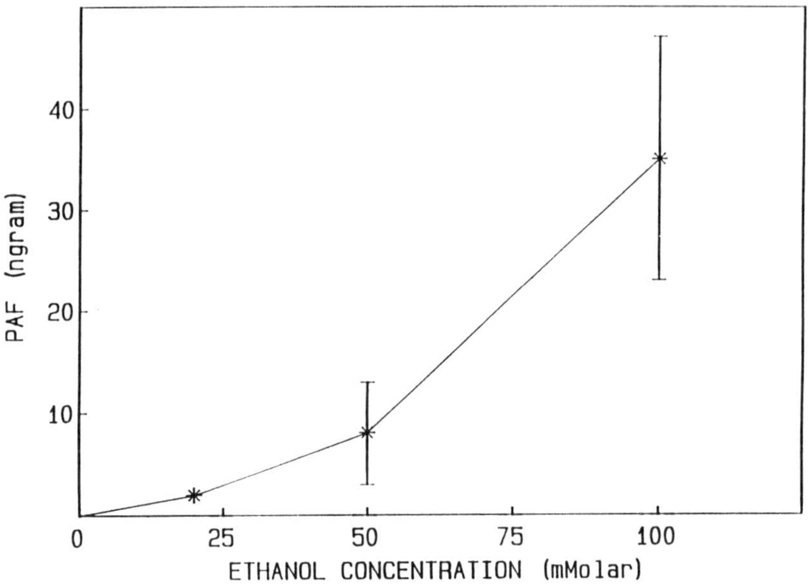

PAF determinations were made following a one hour incubation period in the presence of 0-100 mM ethanol. Medium and cells were combined for PAF measurements.

The aggregation of platelets by PAF is characterized by distinct primary and secondary responses (Miller *et al.*, 1982). Ethanol at concentrations of 20-100mM inhibited the secondary, arachidonic acid dependent wave of PAF induced aggregation. Ethanol had a marginal effect on the initial or primary wave of PAF stimulated platelet aggregation.

Figure 3. The effect of ethanol on the secondary, and primary wave of PAF induced platelet aggregation.

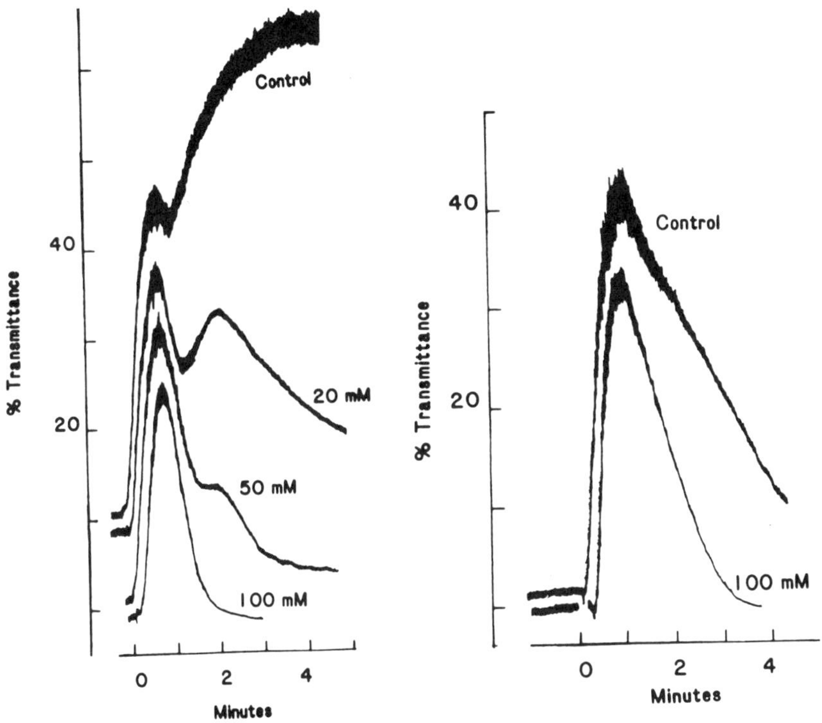

Effects of ethanol on PAF induced aggregation of human platelets (right) and aggregation; of aspirin treated platelets (left). Platelets were stirred for two minutes with 0, 20, 50 or 100 mM ethanol before the addition of 0.5 nmoles of PAF /ml.

Ethanol also inhibited TxB_2 formation in a concentration dependent manner. TxB_2 concentrations declined from their control value of 8.6 $\pm$ 2.5 ng/ml to 3.2 $\pm$ 0.5 ng/ml and 1.5 $\pm$ 0.3 ng/ml in the presence of 50 mM and 100 mM ethanol, respectively.

DISCUSSION:

Ethanol decreased the recoverable PAF in zymosan stimulated macrophages and increased the amount of recoverable PAF in cells not stimulated with zymosan. The decrease in PAF and inhibition of zymosan phagocytosis by ethanol could be due to several interactions including: 1) PAF is required for phagocytosis and the inhibition of PAF synthesis by ethanol stops phagocytosis. 2) Ethanol inhibit zymosan phagocytosis which is the stimuli for PAF production. An unequivocal choice between these two possibility is not afforded by the results of this study. If ethanol only inhibits the synthesis of PAF, the addition of exogenous PAF should restore phagocytic activity. The addition of exogenous PAF did not reverse ethanol inhibition of zymosan phagocytosis suggesting that ethanol inhibits phagocytosis and as a consequence PAF production is decreased. However ethanol antagonized the response to PAF (Rand *et al.*, 1989: Chang *et al.*, 1987), thus if ethanol interferes with PAF action the addition of exogenous PAF may not restore PAF activity.

The recovery of PAF was enhanced by exposure to ethanol in non-stimulated cells as opposed to decreasing recoverable PAF in the presence of the phagocytic stimuli zymosan. Synthesis appears to be responsible for the increase in PAF concentration as ethanol did not stimulate or inhibit the the activity of cell free acetylhydrolase. The divergent effect of ethanol on PAF production is most consistent with the presence of two pathways of PAF biosynthesis, one activated by phagocytic stimuli and a second not dependent on cell activation. Two such pathways have been described (Snyder 1987). The stimulus linked pathway is dependent on the production of 1-O-alkyl-2-lyso-GPC presumably by phospholipase A_2 activity and acetylation of 1-O-alkyl-2-lyso-GPC by the activatable enzyme, 1-O-alkyl-2-lyso-GPC acetylCoA:acetyltransferase The second pathway is characterized by the transfer of phosphocholine to 1-O-alkyl-2-acetyl-*sn*-glycerol. The maintenance of physiological levels of PAF has been proposed to be dependent on this pathway (Snyder, 1987). One might suggest that the *de novo* or phosphocholine transferase dependent pathway is stimulated by ethanol and the second pathway, characterized by the acetylation of 1-O-alkyl-2-lyso-GPC, is inhibited by ethanol.

Ethanol was found to selectively inhibit the second wave of the biphasic aggregation response initiated by PAF, a potent pro-aggregatory phospholipid mediator. Our results are most consistent with a reduction in arachidonic acid availability, rather than with ethanol effects on receptor-agonist interactions. For instance, diminished thromboxane B_2 formation corresponded with the inhibition of aggregation. Effects of ethanol were minimal when aspirin treated platelets were aggregated by PAF or U-46619. Since ethanol inhibited only the second wave of platelet aggregation, it is unlikely that ethanol interferes with binding of PAF to its receptor.

It appears from this study that ethanol may interact with PAF in several ways. A decrease in the stimulated synthesis of PAF was observed, but an increase in non-stimulated PAF synthesis by ethanol was also observed. Two pathways of PAF synthesis are suggested by the results, but divergent pathways have not been demonstrated.

The effect of ethanol on platelet aggregation suggests ethanol inhibits PAF function indirectly, in this case possibly through inhibition of phospholipase A_2 activity.

ACKNOWLEDGEMENTS: The work was presented at Alcohol and Aids Network Conference, April 237-29, Tucson, Arizona. Supported by National Institute on Alcholo Abuse and Alcoholism Grant #AA07157 and National Institute of Health Grant HL34303. The information is included in manuscripts submitted for publication.

REFERENCES:

Benveniste, J., Henson, P. and Cochrane, C. Leukocyte dependent histamine release from rabbit platelets: the role of IgE, basophils and a platelet activating factor. J. Exp. Med. 136:1356-1377 (1972).

Braquet, P., Touqui, L., Shen, T.Y. and Vargaftig, B.B. Perspectives in platelet activating factor research. Pharmacol. Rev. 39:97-145 (1987).

Demopoulos, C., Pinckard, R. and Hanahan D. Platelet activating factor: Evidence for 1-0-alkyl-2-acetyl-*sn*-glyceryl-3-phosphorylcholine as the active component (a new class of lipid chemical mediators). J. Biol. Chem. 254:9355-9358 (1979).

Chang, S-w, Feddersen, C.O., Henson, P.M. and Voelkel, N.F. CV 3988, a platelet activating factor antagonist and ethanol protect against endotoxin-induced hemodynamic alterations in rats. In *New horizons in platelet activating factor research* C.M. Winslow and M.L. Lee eds. John Wiley & Sons Ltd. 293-301. (1987).

Fenn, C.G. and Littleton, J. The human blood platelet as a model for studying interactions of ethanol with membrane lipids. Alcoholism Clin. Expt. Res. 7:59-64 (1983).Fitzpatrick, F. A radioimmunoassay for thromboxane B_2. Methods in Enzymology 86:286-296 (1982).

Pernham, M.J. and Leyck, S. Imflammatory and macrtophage stimulating actions of PAF-acether in normal and immunologically challenged rodents. In *Platelet-activating Factor and Structurally related Ether-lipids.* Benveniste J., and Arnoux, B. eds., Elsevier Sci Pub, pp. 187-194, 1983.

Raschke, W.C., Baird, S., Nakoinz, I. and Ralkph, P. Functional macrophage cell lines transformed by Ableson leukemia virus. Cell 15:261-267 (1978).

Snyder, F. The significance of dual pathways for the biosynthesis of platelet activating factor: 1-O-alkyl-2-lyso-*sn*-glycero-3-phosphate as a branchpoint. In *New horizons in platelet activating factor research* C.M. Winslow and M.L. Lee eds. John Wiley & Sons Ltd. 293-301. (1987).

Alcohol, Immunomodulation, and AIDS, pages 123–133
© 1990 Alan R. Liss, Inc.

EVALUATION OF INTERFERON SYSTEM AMONG CHRONIC ALCOHOLICS

Kailash C. Chadha, Robert B. Whitney, Michael K. Cummings, Marilyn Norman, Michael Windle and Istvan Stadler
Roswell Park Memorial Institute (K.C.C., M.K.C., M.N., I.S.), Erie County Medical Center (R.B.W.) and Research Institute on Alcoholism, Buffalo, NY

INTRODUCTION

Alcoholism is the most common form of drug abuse in the United States where at least half of the adult population are consumers (Halsted, 1980). It has been adequately documented that prolonged and excessive consumption of alcohol results in suppressed or altered host defense mechanisms, thus increasing risk of infections from pathogenic and opportunistic organisms (Eichner et al., 1972; MacGregor, 1986; Smith and Palmer, 1976). Acquired immune deficiency syndrome (AIDS) is also an expression of a profound defect in humoral as well as cellular immunity, resulting in many degenerative and neoplastic diseases (Fauci et al., 1983; Gottlieb et al., 1983). Human immunodeficiency virus (HIV) has been considered as the etiological agent for AIDS (Gallo et al., 1984). In spite of this likelihood, AIDS is now being considered to be more complex and involves noninfectious cofactors such as alcohol and other recreational drugs (Goedert, 1984; Levy and Ziegler, 1983; Shearer and Levy, 1984).

Recently, interferons have received a substantial degree of attention primarily because of their broad range of immunoregulatory, antiviral and antiproliferative effects (Friedman, 1977; Gresser and Tovey, 1978). Interferons constitute one of the earliest defense mechanisms marshalled to protect the host from infections (Hung et al., 1973). In spite of interferon's immunoregulatory role and documented immune suppression among chronic alcoholics, there is still insufficient knowledge regarding status of the interferon system in this group of individuals. In our studies, we have found that chronic alcoholics have compromised interferon system. These individuals have interferons and interferon inhibitors in their blood circulation, and their lymphocytes responded poorly to interferon alpha and gamma inductions in *in vitro* studies when compared to controls.

MATERIALS AND METHODS

Selection of Participants

Three groups of individuals were selected for this study: 1) *chronic alcoholics* - these individuals were selected from those admitted to the Detoxification Clinic at the Erie County Medical Center. Selection was based upon their score on the Michigan Alcohol Screen Test (MAST). Average MAST score was over 15.0. Individuals with a history of drug abuse other than alcohol were not included in the study; 2) *heavy cigarette smokers* - these individuals were selected on the basis of guidelines provided by the National Cancer Institute. They smoked a minimum of 25 cigarettes each day for at least 10 years. The majority of these individuals either never drank alcohol or were very moderate drinkers. Since nearly all chronic alcoholics are also heavy cigarette smokers, it is rather essential to include this category of individuals; 3) *control individuals* - these are healthy individuals who by and large never smoked cigarettes or drank alcohol. Participants in all three categories were asked to fill out a detailed questionnaire regarding their smoking and drinking habits and other demographic data. Attempts were made to match participants for age, sex, and race in each category.

Blood Collection and Lymphocyte Isolation

Twenty milliliters of venous blood was obtained from each subject in sodium heparinized vaccutainers and another 5 ml as clotted blood. Heparinized blood was used for isolation of lymphocytes by gradient centrifugation on Ficoll-Paque (Pharmacia, Piscataway, NJ) as described by Boyum (1968). The lymphocytes were washed twice in 6-8 fold excess of RPMI 1640 medium and finally resuspended in the same medium containing 10% fetal calf serum. These lymphocytes were used for interferon alpha and gamma inductions as well as for the natural killer cell activity assay. The clotted blood was allowed to stand overnight at 4°C, and the serum was collected by centrifugation. The serum was used for interferon and interferon inactivator assays.

Interferon Alpha (HuIFN-α) Induction

Lymphocytes at a density of $5x10^6$ cells/ml in RPMI 1640 medium containing 10% fetal calf serum were infected with 100 HAU of Sendai virus for interferon alpha production. Twenty hours after Sendai virus infection, the supernatant was collected first by low speed centrifugation to remove the cellular debris and followed by high speed centrifugation to remove Sendai virus (Chadha, 1985). Antiviral activity was determined in the supernatant fluid.

Interferon Gamma (HuIFN-γ) Induction

Lymphocytes at a density of $2x10^6$/ml were induced with 1 μg/ml of Staphylococcal enterotoxin-B (Sigma Chemical Co., St. Louis, MO) for interferon gamma synthesis. Seventy-two hours later, supernatant was harvested by low speed centrifugation and dialyzed overnight against 0.02M phosphate buffered saline.

Interferon Antiviral Assays

Interferon antiviral activity was assayed on human foreskin cells using VSV as a challenge virus according to method of Finter (1969).

Interferon Inactivator Assays

For interferon inactivator assays, approximately 50 reference units of HuIFN-α produced by the lymphocytes from normal subjects were mixed with serum, allowed to incubate for 2 hr at 37°C, and then the remaining interferon antiviral activity was assayed on human foreskin cells (Chadha et al., 1987). All appropriate controls were included. A unit of interferon inactivator is the quantity that destroys 5 ref. units of HuIFN-α.

Natural Killer (NK) Cell Activity

NK cell activity was measured using the ^{51}Cr release method (Reynold et al., 1981). NK sensitive human erythroleukemia (K-562) cells were used as target cells. Briefly, 50 μl medium containing 10^4 ^{51}Cr-labeled target cells and 100 μl medium containing various concentrations of effector cells (1:25, 1:50, 1:100) were incubated in triplicate in round bottom microtiter plates. At the end of 14 hr of incubation, plates were spun at 250 xg for 10 min and supernatant counted in an autogamma scintillation spectrometer. Spontaneous release was determined by incubating the target cells with medium alone and usually ran no more than 10% of total release. The percent cytotoxicity was determined as follows:

$$\% \text{ cytotoxicity} = \frac{\text{CPM experimental release} - \text{CPM spontaneous release}}{\text{total CPM incorporated into cells}} \times 100$$

RESULTS

Consent for participation in the study was obtained from all participants. Forty chronic alcoholics, 28 heavy cigarette smokers and 40 control subjects were included in this study. Heavy cigarette smokers were included in our study to serve as one of the controls for chronic alcoholics. In our survey, we found that nearly all chronic alcoholics are heavy cigarette smokers. Smoking alone can have a significant influence upon the host's immune system. To our surprise in the majority of studies dealing with alcohol and the immune system, cigarette smoking has not been considered as one of the important cofactors in alcohol induced immune suppression. The demographic characteristics and substance use data for all participants in three groups are listed in Table 1. As can be seen from Table 1, control subjects were non-smokers and either abstained from alcohol use or drank lightly to moderately; heavy cigarette smokers also either abstained or drank lightly to moderately, and chronic alcoholics were heavy both with respect to drinking and cigarette smoking.

TABLE 1. Demographic Characteristics and Substance Use for Chronic Alcoholics, Heavy Cigarette Smokers and Control Subjects

Variables	Chronic Alcoholics (n=40)	Heavy Cigarette Smokers (n=28)	Controls (n=40)
Age (in years)	35.88 (SD=9.48)	42.11 (14.88)	47.02 (11.93)
Gender	Males (80%)	Males (39%)	Males (48%)
Race	White (77%) Black (23%)	White (93%) Black (4%) Hispanic (4%)	White (90%) Black (8%) Other (3%)
Educational Level	11.50 yrs(SD=2.21)	--	--
Percent Unemployed	59%	--	--
Number of Years Smoking	19.96 (SD=9.67)	24.93 (14.43)	85% never smoked or quit > 15 yrs ago
MAST Score	17.15 (SD=3.84)	2.10 (SD=4.60)	0.97 (SD=1.16)
Drinker Status[1]	Abstainers 0% Drinkers 100%	Abstainers 70% Drinkers 30%	Abstainers 55% Drinkers 45%
Average Number of Heavy Drinking Days[2] for:			
Beer	14.74	0.48	0.32
Wine	3.67	0.05	0.00
Hard Liquor	11.31	0.57	0.24

[1]Abstainers were defined as persons who reported no alcoholic beverage consumption in the 30 days preceding the assessment.
[2]Heavy drinking days were defined as the number of days in the last month in which S's reported drinking six or more cans/bottles of beer, 5 or more glasses of wine, or 5 or more drinks of hard liquor.

A score of 5 or above on the MAST has generally been used as a cut-off point indicative of alcohol problems. All of the chronic alcoholics scored above the cut-off point, and all of the control and heavy cigarette smokers scored below the cut-off point. There were some gender discrepancies in the representation of subjects in each of the three samples; however, gender differences of a low-to-moderate magnitude were found only for serum interferon levels. Similarly, differences between white and minority subjects were minimal, with minorities obtaining somewhat higher scores on serum interferon levels. Age was low-to-moderately correlated with the outcome variables related to immune system functioning. However, using age as a covariate in the analysis of variance models that were conducted did not alter the substantive findings regarding group differences.

Serum Interferon Levels

Among 3 study groups, a maximal serum interferon level was detected among the chronic alcoholics (6.7 ref. units). This level was significantly higher from other two groups (Table 2). No significant differences in serum interferon level were seen among heavy cigarette smokers and the control subjects. A high level of serum interferon is indicative of a weaker immune system among the chronic alcoholics.

TABLE 2. Oneway Anovas for Interferon Parameters Among Chronic Alcoholics, Heavy Cigarette Smokers and Control Subjects

Variables	Interferon Titers ref. units			F-test	Post hoc Comparisons[1]
	Chronic Alcoholics n=40	Heavy Cigarette Smokers n=28	Controls n=40		
Serum Interferon	7	3	<2	28.59*	1,2;1,3
Interferon α	1168	1687	5483	27.85*	1,2;1,3;2,3
Interferon γ	143	144	556	51.33*	1,3;2,3

[1]Post hoc comparisons were made using Scheffe's procedure. The numbers displayed correspond to chronic alcoholics (1). Heavy cigarette smokers (2), control subjects (3). The numbers listed represent statistically significant pairwise comparisons for each variable.
*p=<.001.

Interferon Alpha (HuIFN-α)

The ability of the lymphocytes to produce HuIFN-α in response to Sendai virus infection among all 3 study groups was significantly different. The lymphocytes from chronic alcoholic subjects made an average of 1168 ref. units of HuIFN-α as compared to 1687 ref. units by heavy cigarette smokers and 5483 ref. units by control subjects. Evidently, both heavy cigarette smoking and chronic alcoholism can suppress HuIFN-α production. The maximal suppression of HuIFN-α production was seen among chronic alcoholics. This is perhaps due to additive suppressive effects of both heavy drinking as well as heavy cigarette smoking in this group of individuals (Table 2).

Interferon Gamma (HuIFN-γ)

Lymphocytes from chronic alcoholics as well as heavy cigarette smokers produced significantly lower levels of HuIFN-γ when compared to control subjects (Table 2). However, no significant differences were seen in levels of HuIFN-γ produced by lymphocytes from cigarette smokers and chronic alcoholics (Table 2). This suggests that for HuIFN-γ, maximal suppression can be induced both by heavy cigarette smoking as well as by chronic alcoholism.

Interferon Inactivators

In the majority of control subjects, no detectable levels of interferon inactivators were seen. In some control subjects, very low levels of interferon inactivators were seen, and this may be due to very low levels of subclinical infection in a few participants which remained undetectable during routine examination. Nearly a 500% increase in level of interferon inhibitor was seen among heavy cigarette smokers and an 850% increase among chronic alcoholics in comparison to control subjects (Table 3). The differences in the level of interferon inactivators among heavy cigarette smokers and chronic alcoholics were also significant (Table 3).

TABLE 3. Oneway Anovas for Interferon Inactivators Among Chronic Alcoholics, Heavy Cigarette Smokers and Control Subjects

Subjects	Interferon Inactivators (units)*
Chronic alcoholics (1)	16.4
Heavy cigarette smokers (2)	9.5
Controls (3)	2.0
F-test	103.58**
Post hoc comparisons	1,2;1,3;2,3

Post hoc comparisons were made using Scheffe's procedure. The numbers listed under post hoc comparisons represent statistically significant pairwise comparisons for each variable.
*One unit is the quantity that can inactivate 5 ref. units of HuIFN-α.
**p=<.001.

Natural Killer (NK) Cell Activity

NK cell activity of the lymphocytes isolated from heavy cigarette smokers was significantly reduced when compared to control subjects. Although chronic alcoholics are also heavy cigarette smokers, significant suppression of NK cell activity in this group of individuals was not seen when compared to controls (Table 4).

TABLE 4. Oneway Anovas for Natural Killer Cell Activity Among Chronic Alcoholics, Heavy Cigarette Smokers, and Control Subjects

Smokers	Natural Killer Cell Activity* (% cell killing)
Chronic alcoholics (1)	46
Heavy cigarette smokers (2)	31
Controls (3)	49
F-test	23.78**
Post hoc comparisons	1,2;2,3

Post hoc comparisons were made using Scheffe's procedure. The numbers listed under post hoc comparisons represent statistically significant pairwise comparison for each variable.
*NK cell activity was determined at target to effector cell ratio of 1:25.
**p=<.001.

DISCUSSION

In our study, we have clearly documented that chronic alcoholics have suppressed interferon systems. Since nearly all chronic alcoholics are heavy cigarette smokers and smoking and drinking habits can independently influence the interferon system, we felt rather strongly that a group of individuals who are heavy cigarette smokers with essentially no drinking habits must be included in this study. Therefore, the interferon system was evaluated in the following 3 groups of individuals: 1) chronic alcoholics, 2) heavy cigarette smokers, and 3) control individuals with essentially no smoking and drinking habits (Table 1). Normal healthy (control) individuals had virtually no interferon or interferon inactivators in their plasma, and their lymphocytes produced normal levels of interferon alpha and gamma. In contrast, chronic alcoholics were found to contain significantly higher levels of interferon and interferon inactivators in plasma, and their lymphocytes produced significantly lower levels of both interferons, alpha and gamma (Tables 2 and 3) as compared to controls. The presence of interferon and interferon inactivators is generally indicative of a weaker immune system. Although heavy cigarette smokers also showed increased levels of serum interferon and interferon inactivators in their plasma as compared to controls, these levels were significantly higher among the chronic alcoholics. The highest levels of inhibition of NK cell activity were seen among heavy cigarette smokers. NK cell activity of controls and chronic alcoholics was not significantly different in spite of the fact that chronic alcoholics are also heavy cigarette smokers. The overall weaker interferon system among chronic alcoholics may be responsible for their increased susceptibility to a variety of infections. We have earlier reported in *in vitro* studies that anti-inflammatory drugs, like meclomen, can significantly boost the interferon system (Mahafzah et al., 1989). Since interferons play a significant role in the fight against infections, it is suggested that drugs like meclomen may be useful in the overall management of chronic alcoholics.

ACKNOWLEDGEMENTS

This work was supported by a grant from the National Institute on Alcohol Abuse and Alcoholism and the State of New York. We appreciate excellent secretarial efforts of Marcia Held.

REFERENCES

Boyum A (1968). Separation of leukocytes from blood and bone marrow. Scand J Clin Lab Invest 21, Suppl 97.

Chadha KC (1985). Acid labile human leukocyte interferon. In Dianzani F, Rossi GB (eds): "The Interferon System", Raven Press, NY, pp 35-41.

Chadha KC, Ambrus JL, Ikossi MG (1987). Interferons and interferon inactivators in AIDS, ARC and in cancer patients. In Cantell K, Schellekens H (eds): "The Biology of Interferon System 1986", Martinus Nizhoff Publishers, Boston, p 423-427.

Eichner ER, Buchanan B, Smith JW et al. (1972). Variations in the hematologic and medical status of alcoholics. Amer J Med Sci 263:35-42.

Fauci AS, Macher AM, Longo DL et al. (1983). Acquired immunodeficiency syndrome: epidemiologic, clinical, immunologic and therapeutic considerations. Ann Intern Med 100:92-106.

Finter NB (1969). Dye uptake methods of assessing viral cytopathogenicity and their application to interferon assays. J Gen Virol 5:419-425.

Friedman RM (1977). Antiviral activity of interferon. Bact Rev 41:543-563.

Gallo RC, Salahuddin SZ, Popovic M et al. (1984). Frequent detection and isolation of cytopathic retroviruses (HTLV-III) from patients with AIDS and at risk for AIDS. Science 224:500-502.

Goedert JJ (1984). Recreational drugs: relationship to AIDS. Ann NY Acad Sci 437:192-199.

Gottlieb MS, Groopman JE, Wienstein WM et al. (1983). The acquired immune deficiency syndrome. Ann Intern Med 99:208-220.

Gresser I, Tovey MG (1978). Antitumor effects of interferon. Biochem Biophys Acta 516:231-237.

Halsted CH (1980). Alcoholism and malnutrition. The American J Clinical Nutrition 33:2705-2708.

Hung CY, Lefkowitz SS, Geber WF (1973). Interferon

inhibition by narcotic analgesics. Proc Soc Exp Biol Med 142:106-111.

Levy JA, Ziegler JI (1983). Acquired immunodeficiency syndrome is an opportunistic infection and Kaposi's sarcoma results from secondary immune stimulation. Lancet i:78-81.

MacGregor RR (1986). Alcohol and immune defense. J Am Med Assoc 256:1474-1479.

Mahafzah M, Stadler S, Ambrus JL, Chadha KC (1989). Effect of meclomen on production and action of human interferon alpha. Acta Virologica, in press.

Reynold CW, Brunda MJ, Holden HT et al. (1981). Role of macrophages in in vitro augmentation of rat, mouse and human natural killer activities. J Natl Cancer Inst 66:837-842.

Shearer GM, Levy RB (1984). Non-infectious cofactors in susceptibility to AIDS: possible contributions of semen, HLA alloantigens and lack of natural resistance. Ann NY Acad Sci 437:49-57.

Smith FE, Palmer DL (1976). Alcoholism, infection and altered host defenses: a review of clinical and experimental observations. J Chron Dis 29:35-39.

Alcohol, Immunomodulation, and AIDS, pages 135–143
© 1990 Alan R. Liss, Inc.

THE EFFECT OF ETHANOL ON SIGNAL TRANSDUCTION IN THE RAT ALVEOLAR MACROPHAGE

Raymond J. Dorio

Division of Neonatology and Pediatric Pulmonology, Department of Pediatrics and the Department of Pathology and Laboratory Medicine, Childrens Hospital of Los Angeles and University of Southern California, Los Angeles, California 90027

The alveolar macrophage is the first line of defense against bacterial infection in the lower respiratory tract of the uninfected lung (Green and Kass, 1964a). One of the mechanisms utilized to kill foreign pathogens is the production of superoxide ($O_2^{\cdot -}$). The importance of superoxide production is evident in those individuals with chronic granulomatous disease who have a defect in the ability to produce superoxide (Segal et al., 1982). These individuals suffer recurrent bacterial infections. The underlying hypothesis of this work is that agents which depress the ability of macrophages to produce superoxide may lead to an impaired ability to deal with infections.

Alcoholics also have an increased risk of developing bacterial infections. Pneumonia, in particular, is common in alcoholic populations. The reasons for this increased susceptibility have been ascribed to various factors such as malnutrition and aspiration. However, another possibility is that ethanol acutely suppresses macrophage function. This paper will describe the effects of ethanol upon signal transduction pathways involved in superoxide production in the rat alveolar macrophage.

The importance of the alveolar macrophage in

antibacterial activity in vivo was described by Green and Kass. They used a murine model to show that aerosolized P. mirabilis and S. aureus are killed rapidly in the lung (Green and Kass, 1964a). Following aerosolization, bacteria are found in alveolar macrophages. Neutrophils are not present in alveoli. Therefore, the bacterial killing is due to the antibacterial action of alveolar macrophages. In a second study, the effect of ethanol, in vivo, on killing of aerosolized bacteria was examined (Kass and Green, 1964b). Ethanol inhibits the ability of the mice to kill bacteria in a dose dependent fashion. Significant inhibition of bacterial clearance is not observed until the animals are ataxic or stuporous. Concentrations of ethanol which induced stupor are most effective, resulting in a 50% inhibition of bacterial killing. Therefore, it appears that acute ingestion of ethanol impairs the ability of macrophages to kill bacteria in vivo. These studies emphasize that the levels of ethanol required for inhibition of bacterial clearance are high.

Superoxide is produced by an oxidase on the cell surface of macrophages and neutrophils in response to a variety of stimuli. Stimulation is mediated through two pathways, one dependent upon intracellular calcium mobilization and the other dependent on activation of protein kinase C, figure 1. In general, agonists which bind to surface receptors, lead to activation of phospholipase C. Phospholipase C acts on phosphatidyl 4,5-bisphosphate to produce inositol 1,4,5-trisphosphate (IP_3) and diacylglycerol. IP_3 causes release of intracellular calcium. Diacylglycerol activates protein kinase C. Both these signals lead, either separately or in combination, to the activation of the oxidase responsible for O_2^- production. Experimentally, the cell surface receptors can be bypassed by activation of the system by stimulating protein kinase C directly with phorbol ester (PMA) or by causing the influx of calcium with a calcium ionophore. The phosphoinositide and protein kinase C systems are common to many cells. The pathways may differ in their organization and feedback regulation, from cell to cell.

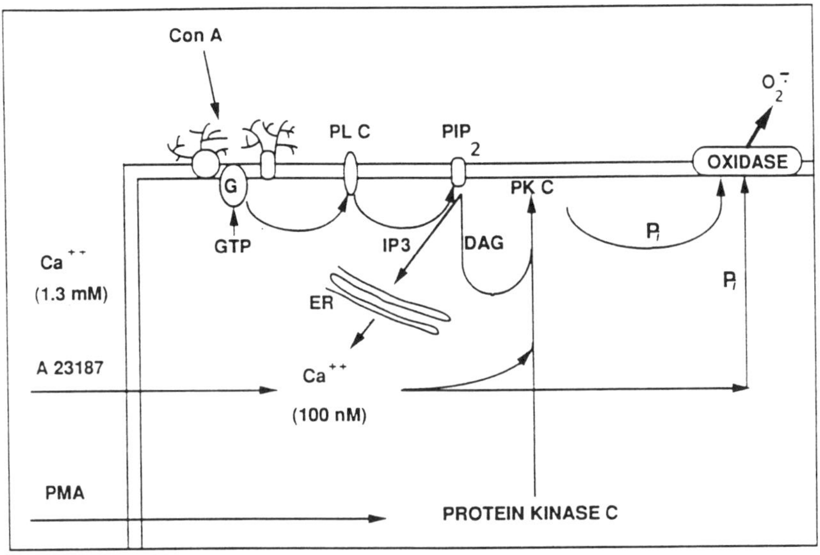

Figure 1. Signal transduction pathways in macrophages: Abbreviations: PMA, phorbol 12-myristate 13-acetate; Con A, concanavalin A; PLC, phospholipase C; PIP_2, phosphatitylinositol 4,5-bisphosphate; IP_3, inositol 1,4,5-trisphosphate; DAG, diacylglycerol; PKC, protein kinase C; G, G proteins (Gi or G_s) (from Dorio et al., 1989, reprinted by permission of the publisher)

We have found that ethanol has several effects on this activation system in alveolar macrophages. Ethanol alone stimulates a small amount of $O_2^{\bar{\cdot}}$ production, raises intracellular calcium acutely and, most importantly, inhibits $O_2^{\bar{\cdot}}$ production by more potent agonists.

When ethanol is added to alveolar macrophages there is a dose dependent production of superoxide. However, the amount of $O_2^{\bar{\cdot}}$ produced by 300 mM ethanol is 2% of that produced by maximal concentrations of the most potent agonist, phorbol ester. This amount of superoxide is probably not significant in terms of anti-bacterial activity.

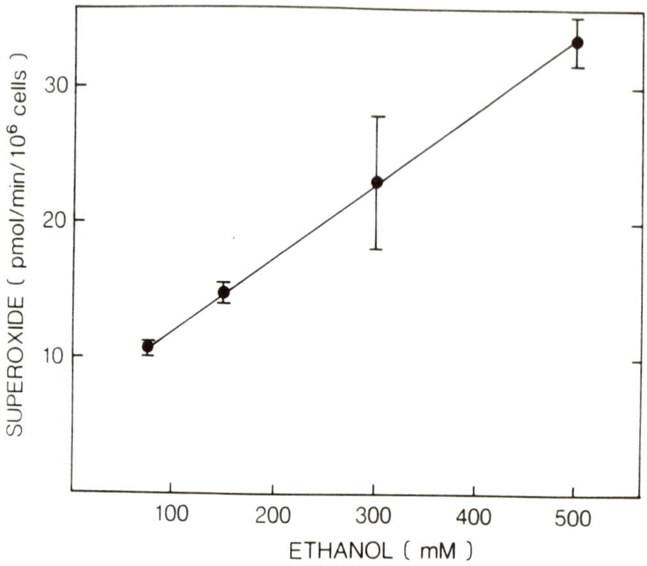

Figure 2. Ethanol stimulation of superoxide production: Superoxide production was measured in 10^6 cells/ml by following the superoxide dismutase inhibitable reduction of ferricytochrome c following ethanol addition (from Dorio, 1988a with permission of the publisher).

One of the pathways which results in superoxide stimulation is activated by elevation of intracellular calcium. The calcium ionophore, A23187, allows extracellular calcium to enter the cell and results in a slight stimulation of superoxide production (Dorio et al., 1987). Ethanol also causes an elevation of intracellular calcium, figure 3. The cells in figure 3 are loaded with the calcium indicator fura-2. Following addition of ethanol, the intracellular fluorescence of fura-2 loaded cells increases. The rise in intracellular calcium with 300 mM ethanol is approximately 50 nM. The rise in intracellular calcium is observed down to ethanol concentrations in the 75 mM range. The internal calcium remains elevated as long as we have made measurements, at least 20 minutes. There is also some elevation observed in the presence of EGTA, although the response is attenuated. Thus, some of the rise in intracellular Ca^{2+} arises from internal calcium stores, possibly as a consequence of IP_3 generation.

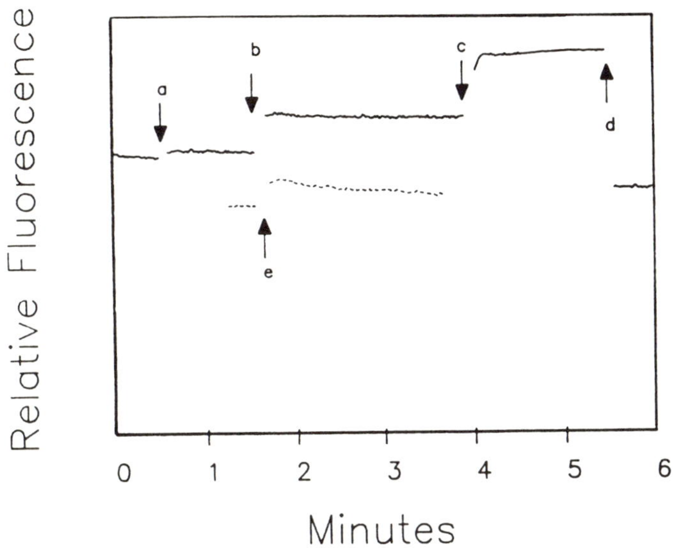

Figure 3. Effect of ethanol on free intracellular calcium in alveolar macrophages: Solid lines: fura-2 loaded cells suspended at 5 x 10^6 cells/ml in the presence of 1.3 mM Ca^{2+} Key: a) stirring control, b) 300 mM ethanol, c) 20 μM ionomycin d) 5 mM EGTA. Dotted lines: cells stored in calcium-free buffer plus 30 μM EGTA Key: e) 300 mM ethanol (from Dorio, 1988a with permission of the publisher)

Support for the idea of release of internal calcium stores by ethanol is given by Diez et al. (1988) who demonstrate that ethanol alone induces phosphoinositide turnover in cultured murine peritoneal macrophages. This turnover may result in the production of IP_3 and the release of intracellular calcium. Ethanol-induced stimulation of phosphoinositide turnover and calcium mobilization has also been demonstrated in the rat liver (Hoek et al. 1987).

Ethanol, thus, acts as a weak agonist for $O_2^{\overline{\cdot}}$ production and mobilizes intracellular calcium. The most dramatic effect ethanol has is the ability to desensitize the cell to stimulation by more potent agonists such as phorbol ester and concanavalin A.

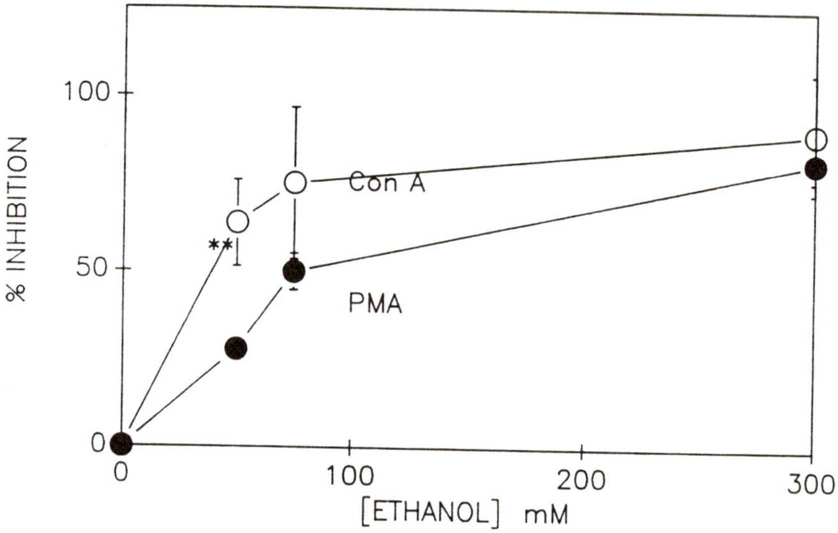

Figure 4. Inhibition of concanavalin A (Con A) and phorbol ester (PMA)-induced $O_2^{\overline{\cdot}}$ production by ethanol: Macrophages (10^6 cells/ml for Con A and 0.2×10^6 cells/ml for PMA stimulation) were preincubated in various concentrations of ethanol for 15 minutes at 37°C. before addition of maximally stimulating concentrations of PMA (10ng/ml) or Con A (250 µg/ml) Values are ± S.D., n=3. Error bars not shown are within the points *p < 0.01 for inhibition for PMA vs Con A. (from Dorio et al. 1988b with permission from the publisher)

We postulate that the mechanism responsible for the ethanol-related inhibition of superoxide production may be related to the rise in intracellular calcium (Dorio et al., 1987). Other agents which elevate intracellular calcium modulate superoxide production. The calcium ionophore A23187 is similar to ethanol in that it is a weak stimulant of superoxide production, raises intracellular calcium, and inhibits phorbol ester induced superoxide production (Dorio, et al. 1988a,b) In other experiments (figure 5), the addition of concanavalin A, which leads to a rise in intracellular calcium, limits PMA-induced superoxide production. When concanavalin A is added to macrophages, $O_2^{\cdot-}$ production is stimulated for a few minutes, then the rate gradually diminishes. In contrast, when phorbol ester is added alone, $O_2^{\cdot-}$ production continues in a linear fashion for as long as we have continued the measurements (up to 20 minutes). Concanavalin A is only about 25% as potent as phorbol ester. However, when PMA and concanavalin A are added simultaneously, there is an initial synergistic increase in the rate of $O_2^{\cdot-}$ production, but the rate subsequently decreases and finally ceases. The presence of concanavalin A seems to superimpose a measure of restraint on PMA-induced $O_2^{\cdot-}$ production (figure 5).

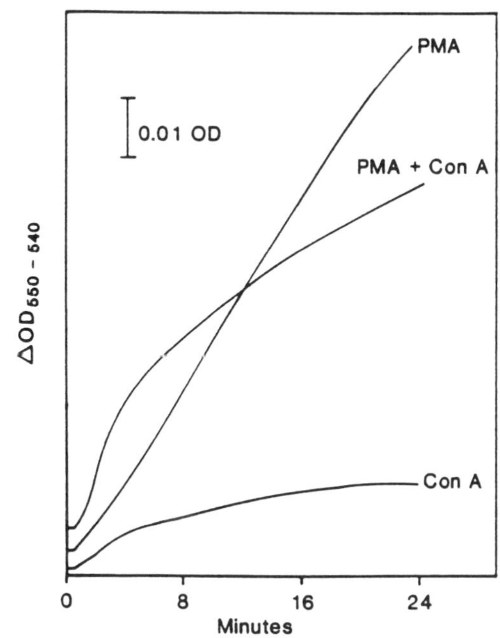

Figure 5. Concanavalin A superimposes a limit on PMA-induced $O_2^{\cdot-}$ production: PMA or Con A were added at time zero to 2 x 10^5 cells in the presence of ferricytochrome c (from Dorio et al. 1987, with permission from the publisher).

The effect of ethanol on the alveolar macrophage is not a toxic phenomenon. Trypan blue staining is not increased. Secondly, if the ethanol is diluted to non-inhibitory concentrations (25 mM) before phorbol ester is added, a normal rate of PMA-induced $O_2^{\bar{\cdot}}$ is observed.

In summary, we have used superoxide production in alveolar macrophages as a model system to study signal transduction. Ethanol causes an acute rise in intracellular calcium, stimulates a small amount of $O_2^{\bar{\cdot}}$ production and inhibits concanavalin A and phorbol ester induced $O_2^{\bar{\cdot}}$ production. Inhibition of $O_2^{\bar{\cdot}}$ production with these agonists is observed at 50 mM ethanol or 0.23% (figure 4), which is within the physiological range. Furthermore, it is those individuals who have extremely high blood alcohol levels that are predisposed clinically to the development of infection. The seemingly contradictory findings that a rise in intracellular calcium can either stimulate or inhibit $O_2^{\bar{\cdot}}$ production, depending upon the conditions, might be explained by the presence of different intracellular calcium pools.

There is also the possibility that the down-regulation of superoxide production in alveolar macrophages and other inflammatory cells may play a physiological role. The alveolar macrophage, in contrast to the neutrophil is a long-lived cell. Regulation of $O_2^{\bar{\cdot}}$ production following stimulation by pathogens may be essential to limit potential local tissue damage. The cell needs to reduce production of toxic radicals when traversing normal structures such as basement membrane. The ability to down-regulate $O_2^{\bar{\cdot}}$ production may be an intrinsic part of the cellular organization. For instance, Hoffstein et al. (1985) demonstrate that when neutrophils adhere to surfaces, the cells become refractive to stimulation by soluble stimuli. Alveolar macrophages also become less sensitive to phorbol ester stimulation after adhering to plastic for two hours (unpublished results). On the other hand, one might speculate that if such a down-regulation pathway is intrinsic to the cell, then, pathogenic organisms might develop mechanisms to exploit this pathway for their own purposes. One hypothesis is that the AIDS virus and mycobacteria can reside in macrophages because they can interfere with the normal cellular defense mechanisms of these cells.

ACKNOWLEDGEMENT

This work was supported by grant AA07312 from the N.I.A.A.A.

REFERENCES

Diez, E, Balsinde, J, Aracil, M, Schüller, A (1987), Ethanol induces release of arachidonic acid but not synthesis of eicosanoids in mouse peritoneal macrophages, Biochim. Biophys. Acta, 921, 82.

Dorio, RJ, Nelson, J, Forman HJ (1987), A dual role for calcium in regulation of superoxide generation by stimulated rat alveolar macrophages, Biochim. Biophys. Acta, 928, 137-143.

Dorio, RJ, Hoek, JB, Rubin, E, Forman HJ (1988a), Ethanol modulates rat alveolar macrophage superoxide production, Biochem. Pharm., 37, 3528-3530.

Dorio, RJ Forman, HJ (1988b), Ethanol related pneumonia: inhibition of superoxide production in rat alveolar macrophages, Ann. Clin. Lab. Sci., 18, 190-194.

Dorio, R.J.(1989, in press), Alcohol and the Macrophage, in Drugs of Abuse and Immune Function, Watson, RR (ed) CRC Press

Green, GM, Kass, E (1964a), The role of the alveolar macrophage in the clearance of bacteria from the lung, J Exp Med, 119, 165-175.

Green, GM, Kass, E (1964b), Factors influencing the clearance of bacteria by the lung, J Clin Invest, 43, 769-776.

Hoffstein, ST, Rennario,DE, Manzi,RM (1985) Surface contact inhibits neutrophil superoxide generation induced by soluble stimuli, Lab Invest, 52, 515-522.

Segal, AW, Cross,AR, Garcia,RC, Borregaard, NB, Valerius,NH, Soothill, JF, Jones, OTG (1982), Absence of cytochrome b_{245} in chronic granulomatous disease. A multicenter European evaluation of its incidence and relevance New Eng J Med, 308, 245-51.

Alcohol, Immunomodulation, and AIDS, pages 145–153
© 1990 Alan R. Liss, Inc.

IN VITRO EFFECTS OF ETHANOL AND ACETALDEHYDE ON CELL-MEDIATED CYTOTOXICITY

Amrik S. Walia and E. W. Lamon

V.A. Medical Center and Department of Surgery,
University of Alabama School of Medicine,
Birmingham, Alabama 35294

INTRODUCTION

Chronic alcohol consumption has been associated with a variety of immunologic abnormalities. (Gluckman et al, 1977; Liu, 1980; Jerrells et al, 1988). In vitro studies have shown that, in the presence of ethanol, blastogenic transformation is depressed (Roselle and Mendenhall 1982). However, some studies have indicated that in vitro effects can only be seen at concentrations of alcohol well above that are compatible with continued life in vitro.

Acetaldehyde is the first oxidized product of ethanol. A number of studies have indicated that acetaldehyde may play a role in the toxic effects of ethanol consumption. (Nomura and Lieber, 1981; Gaillis, 1975; Gaines et al, 1977; Ristow and Obe, 1978). Lymphocytes preincubated with acetaldehyde were found to have increased cytotoxicity for autologous liver cells (Kakumu and Leevy, 1977). We also found potentiation of lysis in antibody-dependent cell-mediated cytotoxicity (ADCC) experiments at lower concentrations of acetaldehyde. Ethanol produced a progressive inhibition of cell-mediated cytotoxicity which seems to be taking place by a calcium-dependent mechanism.

MATERIALS AND METHODS

Pathogen free, young C3H/HEN mice of both sexes were used as source of lymphocytes. RPMI-1640 (Flow Laboratories, McLean, Virginia) with 100μg/ml gentamicin and 10% heat-inactivated fetal calf serum (FCS) was used for all dilutions. Calcium free medium was specifically prepared by Flow Laboratories for these studies. IgG anti-ox red blood cells (ORBC) was used for sensitizing ORBC. P815, mastocytoma cells grown intraperitoneally in DBA-2 mice of H-2^d origin (Jackson Laboratories) are resistent to NK activity and extremely susceptible to alloimmune CTL (Cytotoxic-T-Lymphocyte) activity. YAC is an NK-susceptible Moloney lymphoma target cell derived from A/sn mice.

Murine spleen cells as effector cells and antibody (IgG) sensitized red cells as target cells were prepared, sensitized and incubated as previously described (Lamon et al, 1977, 1978, 1981; Walia et al, 1977, 1981, 1987). After the incubation, the cells were centrifuged and the pellets and supernatants assayed for ^{51}Cr activity in a well-type gamma counter. The maximum releasable counts were determined by lysing nonsensitized target cells with 2 ml of distilled water.

YAC tumor cells, which were susceptible to NK activity, and P815, which are susceptible to T cell activity, were used as target cells. Spleen cells from C3H mice (high NK strain) were used for the NK assay. Alloimmune cytotoxic T cells (CTL) were generated in C3H mice by two i.p. injections of 10^7 P815 cells 11 days apart. Three days following the second injection, spleen cells were harvested from these mice and used as effectors against P815 as previously described (Walia et al, 1987).

Loss of ethanol by evaporation from the incubation mixture was estimated by the measured loss of ethanol from PBS with a carle gas chromatograph. The loss of acetaldehyde at different time intervals was evaluated by an enzymatic method. The concentration of calcium in the FCS and RPMI (Ca^{++} free medium) was evaluated by atomic absorption (Willis, 1963). The concentrations of Ca^{++} in the assay tubes were monitored by calcium electrode (Amman et al, 1979).

RESULTS AND DISCUSSION

ADCC, NK and CTL activity were all inhibited by ethanol (Table 1). There was a progressive decrease in lysis as

Table 1

THE EFFECT OF ETHANOL ON ADCC, NK AND ALLOIMMUNE CTL ACTIVITY

	% Lysis Mean ± S.D.		
ETHANOL (mM)	ADCC	NK	CTL
0	33 ± 2	57 ± 3	42 ± 3
22	30 ± 3	51 ± 1	N.D.
44	22 ± 1	N.D.	37 ± 0.5
88	18 ± 2	32 ± 1	33 ± 1
176	10 ± 1	12 ± 1	26 ± 3

ADCC: Effector cells: C3H mouse spleen cells
Target cells: Antibody sensitized ox red blood cells
E:T ratio: 8:1
Incubation time: 18h
Loss of ethanol approximately 30%

NK: Effector cells: C3H mouse spleen cells
Target cells: YAC
E:T ratio: 128:1
Assay: 4 h

CTL: Effector cells: Spleen cells obtained from mice previously injected with P815 cells.
Target cells: P815
E:T ratio: 128:1
Assay: 4 h

N.D. = not done

the concentration of alcohol was increased. The inhibitory activity of ethanol was found to be reversible (Walia et al, 1987). The ADCC data were analyzed using a mathematical model. An inhibition constant (K_I) of 373 mM^{-2} when two ethanol molecules interact with the site of inhibition was calculated. Fifty percent inhibition of lysis was produced by 52mM (0.24%) ethanol.

Acetaldehyde appeared to have a biphasic effect on the lysis of antibody-sensitized erythrocytes by murine spleen cells. Concentrations less than 1mM acetaldehyde modestly potentiated ADCC. Concentration > 1mM produced a progressive decrease in lysis (Table 2). The inhibitory effects of acetaldehyde were found to be at the effector cell level and were partially irreversible. Preincubation experiments showed that inhibition of ADCC was both concentration and time dependent (Walia et al, submitted). NK activity and alloimmune CTL-mediated lysis were also inhibited by acetaldehyde (Table 2).

Table 2

THE EFFECT OF ACETALDEHYDE ON ADCC, NK AND ALLOIMMUNE CTL ACTIVITY

Acetaldehyde Concentration		% Lysis Mean ± S.D.		
Initial	Final	ADCC	NK	CTL
0	0	25 ± 2	40 ± 5	60 ± 2
40μM	5μM	*32 ± 2	35 ± 5	43 ± 5
1mM	130μM	*29 ± 2	37 ± 2	35 ± 4
10mM	1.3mM	12 ± 3	15 ± 1	6 ± 1
40mM	5mM	9 ± 2	15 ± 3	3 ± 2

*Significant potentiation P< 0.05.

Concentrations of acetaldehyde up to 20mM did not significantly decrease lymphocyte viability as determined by trypan blue exclusion.

Acetaldehyde was lost from the reaction mixture by first order kinetics with a rate constant of 0.5/hr.

Details about effector and target cells of ADCC, NK and CTL are given in Table 1).

It has previously been shown that calcium is required for the lytic step in cell-mediated cytotoxicity (Perlmann and Cerottini, 1979). To evaluate whether excess calcium could reverse ethanol mediated inhibition of lysis, we studied the effect of extra calcium (1-16mM) into the reaction mixture containing antibody sensitized target and effector cells in the presence of ethanol. As shown in Figure 1, the inhibition of ADCC by different concentrations of ethanol (44mM, 88mM and 176mM) was completely reversed by the addition of 16mM Ca^{++} (Walia and Lamon, in press). We have also found that excess Ca^{++} can reverse the inhibitory effects of acetaldehyde in ADCC (data not shown). The addition of 1μM calcium ionophore (A23187) to ethanol treated cells partially reversed the inhibition also (Table 3). This represents a significant

Table 3

INHIBITION OF ADCC BY ETHANOL AND PARTIAL RECOVERY BY CALCIUM IONOPORE (A23187)

CONCENTRATION OF ETHANOL (mM)	% LYSIS MEAN ± S.E. IONOPHORE 0	1μM	% RECOVERY
0	27 ± 3	28 ± 5	---
88	15 ± 3	21 ± 1	41
176	8 ± 2	14 ± 2	31

Mean ± S.E. of three experiments
1μM Ionophore A23187 is not toxic to lymphocytes as determined by trypan blue exclusion.

Effector cells: C3H spleen cells
Target cells: Antibody sensitized ox red blood cells (ORBC)
E:T ratio: 8:1
Assay: 4 h. Percent recovery was calculated by the formula shown in Figure 1.

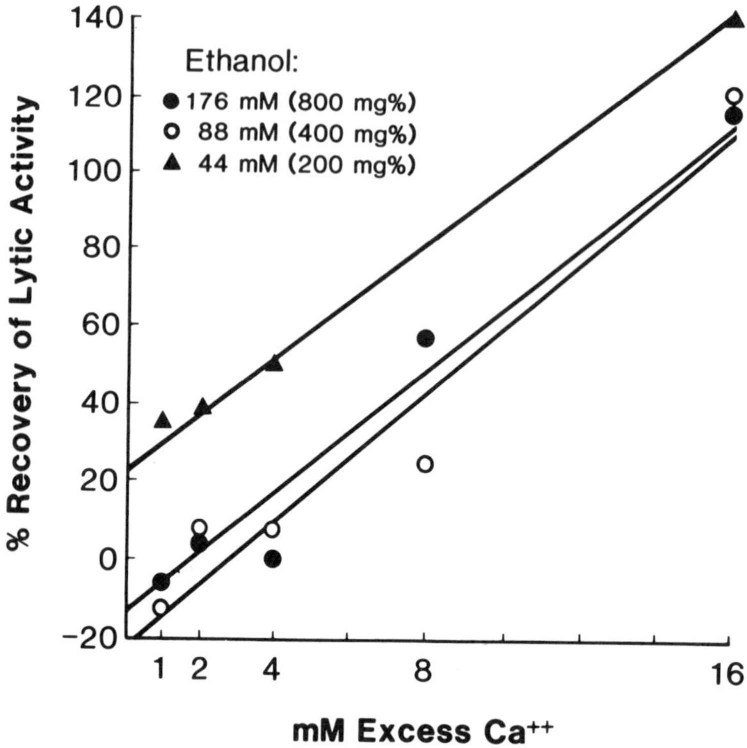

Figure 1

Figure 1 shows percent recovery of ADCC activity by addition of excess calcium. Percent recovery was calculated by the following formula.

$$100 - \frac{100 \text{ X } \% \text{ of inhibition B}}{\% \text{ of inhibition A}}$$

Where A is inhibition by ethanol and B is inhibition by calcium. Data points in this figure were calculated using the % lysis in the amount of excess calcium indicated but in the absence of alcohol as the control values.

The data shown, represents mean values from three experiments.

reversal effect, though the reversal caused by excess extracellular calcium is of much greater magnitude. By trypan blue exclusion, the concentrations of calcium, ionophore and ethanol used in these experiments were not toxic to lymphocytes.

Our data suggest that ethanol and acetaldehyde inhibit ADCC at a calcium dependent step. This carries a broader significance, in terms of the cell biology of ethanol and acetaldehyde mediated toxicity, than a single in vitro model of cell mediated lysis of antibody sensitized target cells. ADCC provides a convenient model for evaluation of the alcohol mediated alteration of a Ca^{++} dependent function. The receptor ligand requirements for initiation of this lytic event are well-defined, i.e., Fc-Fc receptor interaction. The lytic event occurs rapidly following combination of lymphocytes and sensitized target cells; lysis can be detected within 15 minutes and proceeds to plateau levels within 8 hours (Fuson et al 1978). Also the stoichiometry of the alcohol mediated inhibition of ADCC has been defined (Walia et al 1987). Finally, the calcium dependent lytic event is quantifiable by ^{51}Cr-release and many of the requirements for binding, triggering and lysis are known.

Acknowledgements: This work was supported by Alcoholism Research Program of the Veterans Administration and Grants 1P01CA34968 and R01CA38008 from the NIH. We thank Ms. Gwen Marshall for technical assistance and Ms. Judy Mitchell for her expert secretarial assistance.

REFERENCES

Amman D, Meier PC, Simon W. Design and use of calcium-sensitive microelectrodes (1979). In CC Ashley and AK Campbell (eds): "In detection and measurement of free Ca^{++} in cells," Elseiver/North-Holland, Amsterdam, pp 117-129.

Gluckman SJ, Dvorak VC, MacGregor RR, (1977). Host defenses during prolonged alcohol consumption in a controlled environment. Arch Intern Med 137:1539-1543.

Jerrells TR, Marietta CA, Boone G, Weight FF and Eckardt MJ (1988). Ethanol-associated immunosuppression. Physiological neuropsychiatric and substance abuse aspects of AIDS, edited by T Peter Bridge et al. Raven Press, New York, pp 173-185.

Kakumu S, Leevy CM (1977). Lymphocyte cytotoxicity in Alcoholic Hepatitis. Gastroenterology 75:594-597.

Lamon EW, Williams BR, Fuson EW, Whitten HD, Walia AS (1978). Murine T-cells that lyse antibody-sensitized target cells. I. Kinetics and dose-response studies of control and cortisone-resistant thymocytes. J Immunol 1209:244-248.

Lamon EW, Williams BR, Fuson EW, Walia AS, Zwerner RK, Pretlow TG (1981). Murine T cells that lyse antibody-sensitized target cells. II. Enrichment of K cells from normal thymus by isokinetic density centrifugation. Cell Immunol 57:517-523.

Lamon EW, Shaw MW, Goodson S, Lidin B, Walia AS, Fusion EW (1977). Antibody-dependent cell-mediated cytotoxicity in the Moloney sarcoma virus system: Differential activity of IgG and IgM with different subpopulations of lymphocytes. J Exp Med 145:302-313.

Liu YK (1980). Effects of alcohol on granulocytes and lymphocytes. Semin Hematol 17:130-136.

Perlmann P, Cerottini JC (1979). Cytotoxic lymphocytes. In: Sela M, Ed. The antigens, New York Academia Press, Vol V, pp 173-281.

Ristow H, Obe G (1978). Acetaldehyde induces cross-links in DNA and causes sister chromatid exchange in human cells. Mutation Res 48:115-119.

Roselle GA, Mendenhall CL (1982). Alteration of in vitro human lymphocyte function by ethanol, acetaldehyde and acetate. J Clin Lab Immunol 9:33-37.

Walia AS, Lamon EW (1977). Immune response to polyoma tumor cells in mice. I. Magnitude and specificity of the in vitro cellular cytotoxicity elicited by immunization with graded number of tumor cells. J Natl Cancer Inst 58:1671-1675.

Walia AS, Lamon EW (1981). Cell-mediated and humoral antibody responses to virally induced tumors. Ind J Med Res 73:410-419.

Walia AS, Pruitt KM, Rodgers JD, Lamon EW (1987) In vitro effect of ethanol on anti-dependent cell-mediated cytotoxicity by murine spleen cells. Immunopharmacology 13:11-24.

Walia AS, Pruitt KM, Dillehay DL, Marshall GM, Lamon EW (1989). In Vitro effect of acetaldehyde on cell mediated cytotoxicity by murine spleen cells. Alc Clin & Exp Res (submitted).

Walia AS, Lamon EW (1989). Ethanol inhibition of cell-mediated lysis of antibody-sensitized target cells at a calcium dependent step. Proc Soc Exp Biol Med (In press).

Willis JG (1963). Analysis of biological materials by atomic absorption spectroscopy. Met Biochem Anal 11:1-67.

Alcohol, Immunomodulation, and AIDS, pages 155–163
© 1990 Alan R. Liss, Inc.

EFFECTS OF VARIOUS ALCOHOLS APPLIED IN VITRO ON HUMAN LYMPHOCYTE SUBTYPES AND MITOGENESIS

Rao H. Prabhala[1] and Ronald R. Watson

Department of Family and Community Medicine
University of Arizona Health Sciences Center,
Tucson, AZ 85724

[1]Current Address: Department of Physiology
Dartmouth Medical School, Hanover, NH 03756

INTRODUCTION

Chronic, high ethanol intakes cause major changes in cellular physiology including immune functions (Watson, 1984, and Darban and Watson, 1988). Lymphocytes of patients with alcohol induced cirrhosis have impaired mitogen response attributed to both lymphocyte and circulating factors (Thestrap-Pedersen et al., 1976, Young et al., 1979). In patients with severe liver injury, these changes could occur via undernutrition which is immunosuppressive, alterations in immunoregulatory hormones, direct changes in lymphocyte function or development causes by alcohol, or effects of liver disease (Darban and Watson, 1988). Studies in humans suggest that altered hormone levels as well as the direct effects of ethanol or its metabolites change T-cell functions could explain the immunosuppression.

However, there is only limited information that ethanol causes changes directly in lymphocytes. Sorrel and Leevy (1972) showed that there was increased lymphocyte mitogenesis upon addition of ethanol or acetaldehyde to cell cultures in vitro. To better understand the direct effect of ethanol, structurally related alcohols and metabolites, human lymphocytes were treated in vitro. Some structurally related ethanol analogues were also employed to study the actions on cellular immune mitogenesis and cellular numbers of modest structural changes in ethanol while retaining the alcohol functional group.

MATERIALS AND METHODS

Human Subjects. Laboratory personnel, 20-31 years of age, were used for cell sources and they gave informed consent. All samples were collected between 8:30 - 9:30 a.m. Subjects were either abstainers or consumed small amounts, about 0.7-2.0 gm of alcohol/day.

Lymphocyte Separation and In Vitro Incubation. Peripheral blood was collected in sodium heparinized vacutainers. Lymphocytes were separated by density gradient (specific gravity 1.077) centrifugation procedures similar to those previously described (Hicks et al., 1983) Briefly, blood (21 ml) was carefully layered over 9 ml of Ficoll-Hypaque (FH) or Lymphocyte Separating Media (LSM) (Litton Bionetics, Kensington, Maryland) and centrifuged at 22°C for 20 min at 400 x g with the brake off. After removing the plasma, the discrete band of cells at the plasma/FH or LSM interface was aspirated with a Pasteur pipette and transferred to another tube. The cell suspension was then washed in a 6 to 8-fold volume of RPMI 1640 medium (400 x g centrifugation for 30 min) and resuspended in the same medium for subsequent testing. For in vitro studies the lymphocyte preparations were incubated with media alone (control), ethanol, propanol, methanol, acetic acid and acetaldehyde in media at final concentrations ranging from 0.1% to 1.0% for 48 hours at 37°C. Then the cells were washed and assayed.

T-Lymphocyte Subset Analysis. T-cell subpopulations were quantitated by indirect immunofluorescent using monoclonal antibodies specific for T-cells ($CD3^+$), T-helper cells ($CD4^+$) and T-suppressor ($CD8^+$) cells (OKT3, OKT4 and OKT8 respectively; Ortho Diagnostics, Raritan, NJ) as described previously (Prabhala et al., 1989). For each subject, the cell preparation (200 ul) is incubated for 30 minutes with appropriate dilution of monoclonal antibody. After removing unbound primary antibody, cells were then incubated for another 30 minutes with fluorescent-labeled goat anti-mouse immunoglobulins. Then cells were fed into an EPICS V flow cytometer (Coulter, FI). The relative number of T-cells, and of helper and suppressor T-cells were determined as a percentage of the total lymphocyte populations (OKT11 positive).

Lymphocyte Mitogenesis. Mitogenesis of T-cells stimulated by non-specific mitogens showed the relative ability of the cells to respond, grow and divide. A 1:20 dilution of phytohemagglutinin (PHA) (Gibco, Grand Island, NY), a 1:50 dilution of concanavalin A (ConA) (Calbiochem., San Diego, CA) and a 1:20 dilution of pokeweed mitogen (PWM) (Gibco, Grand Island, NY) were used and was done as described elsewhere (Hicks, 1983). The dilution was determined by dose-response curves, which gave maximum transformation response. In triplicate, 0.2 ml of each lymphocyte suspension (1×10^6 lymphocyte/ml) was cultured in Costar 96 well plates along with PHA, ConA or media alone. The mixtures are incubated at 37°C for 4 days with humidified 5% CO_2. Twenty-four hours before the end of incubation, 1 uCi of ^{3}H-thymidine is added to each culture well. After incubation, the cells are harvested onto glass fiber filters with a Brandel cell harvester. The ^{3}H-thymidine level on each filter paper is determined in a Packard liquid scintillation spectrometer.

RESULTS

Effects of ethanol, its analogs and a metabolite, acetaldehyde, on the T-lymphocyte subpopulations: The percentage of total T-lymphocytes measured by OKT11 antibody was decreased by ethanol, its analogs and its metabolites in PBMC after in vitro incubation of 2 days in comparison with control samples. However, the percent of T-helper cells were increased by ethanol and its analogs but not by its metabolite, acetaldehyde, compared to controls. The helper/suppressor ratios changed correspondingly to the T-helper cell increase. The percent of NK cells were decreased by ethanol, its analogs and acetaldehyde in comparison with controls. Results showed that ethanol decreased the T-lymphocytes, and NK cells and caused transient imbalances in helper/suppressor cell ratios as shown in Table 1.

Table 1

Effects of Various Alcohols on Human T-Lymphocyte Subpopulations In Vitro

Alcohol Additives (1.0%)	% Cells with surface markers[a]				
	Helper ($CD4^+$)	Suppressor ($CD8^+$)	Helper / Suppressor Ratio	Total T-cells ($CD3^+$)	NK ($CD16^+$)
None	20.0	9.6	2.1	78.3	9.3
Methanol	34.3*	5.3	6.5*	57.6	5.3
Propanol	34.3*	7.3	4.7	56.0*	4.2*
Ethanol	32.6*	7.2	4.5	64.3*	4.6*
Acetaldehyde (0.01%)	21.0	6.4*	3.3	50.3*	2.2*

a Mean values of three or more experiments containing several samples

* Significantly different from media treated cells (P less than 0.05).

Effects of Ethanol, Its Analogs, and Acetaldehyde on Mitogenesis: ConA and PWM induced mitogenesis of PBMC was inhibited by ethanol, its analogs, and its metabolite as shown on Table 2. Whereas, LPS induced mitogenesis was not affected by these compounds except acetaldehyde, more than 50% inhibition was observed. So, results clearly indicate that the increase in T-helper cells did not yield increased mitogenesis.

Table 2

Effects of Various Alcohols In Vitro on the Mitogenesis of Human Peripheral Blood Mononuclear Cells

	Mitogens[a]		
Alcohol Additives (1.0%)	Concanavalin A (cpm x 10^{-3})	Lipopoly-saccharide	Pokeweed mitogen
None	199.9± 4.1	100.4±13.5	47.6±5.9
Methanol	82.4±14.8*	91.5± 6.4	21.2±1.1*
Propanol	94.0± 4.9*	99.2± 4.0	18.3±3.1
Ethanol	110.5± 4.6*	100 ±13.4	23.3±2.0*
Butanol	81.2± 6.2*	93.3± 5.2	22.0±4.2*
Acetic acid	92.3± 4.4*	102.3± 3.2	27.0±5.8
Acetaldehyde (0.01%)	22.2±18.7*	47.5± 4.1*	11.1±2.3*

a Mean ± S.D. of three or more experiments containing cells from several donars

* Significantly different from media treated cells (P less than 0.05).

DISCUSSION

Our work here shows that ethanol affects lymphoid subsets rapidly during in vitro incubation. This occurred in the absence of changes in serum hormones such as corticosteroids or thymic factors which may change with in vivo use of ethanol. A modest decrease in the number of T-cells with ethanol use by humans has been observed (Watson, 1985). A report of children with fetal alcohol syndrome showed increased life-threatening bacterial infections, decreased E-rosette forming cells, and in vitro decreased lymphocyte mitogenesis (Johnson et al., 1981, Lang et al., 1980). Our data with in vitro treatment of lymphocytes (T-lymphocytes) confirms several in vivo studies showing suppressed E-rosettes.

Ethanol reduced the percentage of cells with NK markers. We have found previously that low, but not high levels of ethanol (greater than 0.1%) add in vitro, stimulated NK activity (Mufti et al., 1988). However, high levels of ethanol in vitro suppressed NK cell functions. Enhanced NK activity at very low levels of ethanol was found with several ratios of target:effector cells. Others have shown higher NK activity in mice (Saxena et al., 1981) and humans (Saxena, 1980) consuming low, but not high levels of alcohol. It has been postulated that such changes in vivo could occur via changes in thymic hormones or serum corticosteroids (Watson et al., 1985). Beta endorphin has been shown to enhance NK activity (Kay et al., 1984). However, endorphins should not be produced by lymphocytes in culture in vitro, and so would not explain the higher NK we observed. Animal studies with varying alcohol intakes in drinking water confirm these human studies (Saxena, 1980). NK activity was significantly higher after 2 weeks in animals given 2, 4, 8, or 16% alcohol in their drinking water. These changes presumably occurred prior to nutritional deficiencies or liver damage, so would be due to interactions of dietary alcohol and the cellular immune systems. A direct stimulatory effect of alcohol on NK cells was thought unlikely in view of the long induction phase which precedes the effect of alcohol feeding.

Sorrell and Leevy (1972) showed that increased lymphocyte mitogenesis upon addition of ethanol or acetaldehyde to cell cultures in vitro. Cells from alcoholics with inactive cirrhosis did not produce increased mitogenesis upon addition of ethanol. We found in the present study that acetaldehyde suppressed T-cell mitogenesis at very low concentrations using cells from abstainers or low alcohol consumers in contrast to the observations of Sorrel and Leevy (1972). They may not have seen these changes if acetaldehyde was allowed to evaporate. We have previously shown that alcohol consumption did not significantly change T-cell mitogenesis using cells from alcohol abusers without liver disease (Watson et al., 1985). In humans advanced liver disease is associated with prolonged, excessive ingestion of ethanol, impaired phagocytic capacity (Schopf et al., 1985) and decreased cell metabolic activity in the liver's reticuloendothelial system. In vitro, ethanol also impairs granulocyte chemotaxis, adherence, and phagocytosis (Mufti et al., 1988). We recently reported that activated macrophages were decreased in ethanol fed mice than in control mice (Watson et al., 1988a,b). In vitro, at high concentrations of ethanol and its analogs decreased mitogenesis by T-cells mitogens not by B-cell mitogens. We did also notice a slight increase in T-helper cells after incubation. This suggests that alcohol may modify helper T-cells.

All the alcohols tested generally had similar effects on mitogenesis and lymphocyte subsets, so some changes may be influenced by the alcohol molecules, and not metabolites.

Clearly cirrhosis due to high, prolonged alcohol intake is immunosuppressive, which may account for increased disease (Young et al., 1979) It is less clear that more moderate intakes of alcohol profoundly affect as many immune systems. However changes do occur resulting in altered lymphocyte sensitivity to alcohol in vitro, and cell development. Medical complications related to the ingestion of large amounts of alcoholic beverages is a major health-care problem and may influence lymphocytes. The direct, in vitro effects we have seen in these preliminary studies of ethanol and acetaldehyde on lymphocytes suggest that they can directly affect lymphocyte surface development as shown by surface markers and activation or mitogenesis. Lymphoid numbers, types and activation of lymphoid cells affected by ethanol could increase targets for retroviral infection or reduce resistance to them afterwards. On the other reduced mitogenesis may produce fewer targets for HIV infection, and reduce progression to AIDS. Such work showed that numerical and functional lymphocytes occurred due to alcohol exposure directly, and might have an important role in increased risk of pathogenesis and carcinogenesis, especially AIDS.

Acknowledgments. Supported in part by specialized Alcohol Research Center, NIH P50AA-8039, and DA04827. Appreciation is expressed to Dr. M.J. Hicks for assistance with flow cytometry analysis.

REFERENCES

Hicks, MJ, Jones, JF, Cole, A, Thies, AC, Weighle, KA, Minnich, LL (1983). Age-related changes in mitogen induced lymphocyte function from birth to old age. Amer J Clin Path, 80:159-163.

Johnson, S, Knight, R, Marmer, DJ and Steele, RW (1981). Immune deficiency in fetal alcohol syndrome. Pediatr Res, 15:908-911.

Kay, N, Allen, J, and Morley, JE (1984). Endorphins stimulate normal human peripheral blood lymphocyte natural killer activity. Life Sci, 35:53-49.

Lang, JM, Ruscher, H, Hasselmann, JP, Grandjean, P, Bigel, P and Mayer, S (1980). Decreased autologous rosette-forming T-lymphocytes in alcoholic cirrhosis. Int Arch Allergy Appl Immun, 61:337-343.

Mufti, SI, Prabhala, RH, Monguchi, S, Sipes, IG, and Watson, RR (1988). Functional and numerical alterations induced by ethanol in the cellular immune system. Immunopharm, 15:85-94.

Prabhala, RH, Maxey, V, Hicks, MJ, Watson, R.R. (1989). Enhancement of the expression of activation markers on human peripheral blood mononuclear cells by in vitro culture with retinoids and carotenoids. J Leuk Biol, 45:249-254.

Saxena, QB, Mezey, E and Adler, WH (1980). Regulation of natural killer activity in vivo. II. The effect of alcohol consumption on human peripheral blood natural killer activity. Int J Cancer, 26:413-417.

Saxena, QB, Saxena, RK and Adler, WH (1981). Regulation of natural killer activity in vivo: Part IV. High natural killer cell activity in alcohol drinking mice. Ind J Exp Biol, 19:1001-1006.

Schopf, RE, Trompeter, M, Bork, K, and Morsches, B (1985). Effects of ethanol and acetaldehyde on phagocytic functions. Arch Dermatol Res, 277:131-137.

Sorrell, MF, and Leevy, CM (1972). Lymphocyte transformation and alcoholic liver injury. Gastroenterology, 63:1020-1025.

Thestrup-Pedersen, K, Ladefoged, K, and Andersen, P (1976). Lymphocyte transformation test with liver-specific protein and phytohemagglutinin in patients with liver disease. Clin Exp Immunol 24:1-8.

Watson, RR (1984). Alcohol and Immune Functions. In: Nutrition, Disease Resistance, and Immune Function. (M. Dekker, Inc.) 35-52, New York.

Watson, RR, Jackson, JC, Hartmann, B, Sampliner, R, Mobley, D and Eskelson, C (1985). Cellular immune functions, endorphins, and alcohol consumption in humans. Alcoholism: Clin Exp Res, 9:248-254.

Watson, RR, Darban, H. (1988). Alcohol and immunosuppression. Clin Immunol, 9:129-131.

Watson, RR, Prabhala, RH, Abril, E, Smith, T (1988). Changes in lymphocyte subsets and macrophage functions from high, short-term dietary ethanol in C57/BL6 mice. Life Sci, 43:865-870.

Watson, RR, Prabhala, RH, Darban, HR, Yahya, DM, and Smith, TL (1988). Changes in lymphocyte and macrophage subsets due to morphine and ethanol treatment during a retrovirus infection causing murine AIDS. Life Sci, 43:5-11.

Young, GP, Van der Weyden, MB, Rose, IS, Dudley, FJ (1979). Lymphopenia and lymphocyte transformation in alcoholics. Experientia, 35:268-269.

Alcohol, Immunomodulation, and AIDS, pages 165–172
© 1990 Alan R. Liss, Inc.

EFFECTS IN VITRO OF ETHANOL AND ACETALDEHYDE ON NATURAL KILLER ACTIVITY FROM RATS

Olcay Yeralan and Joe M. Jones

Departments of Microbiology/Immunology, and Pathology, University of Arkansas for Medical Sciences, Little Rock, Arkansas 72205

INTRODUCTION

Exposure of humans and other animals to ethanol (ETOH) is known to interfere with normal immune responses in a manner that may contribute to increased susceptibility to malignancy and infectious agents (Jerrells et al., 1986, Watson et al.,1988, MacGregor, 1986). Some influences of ETOH may be due in part to direct effects on cells of the immune system; this possibility can be most easily tested by in vitro studies. The present studies focused on natural killer (NK) activity because NK cells represent a first line defense against viral and malignant diseases and are rapidly responsive to exogenous and endogenous influences (Herberman, 1984, Djeu et al., 1979). The studies included acetaldehyde (ACHO), the first metabolite of ETOH. Although seemingly small amounts of ACHO occur in vivo, it is highly reactive (Lieber, 1988) and has effects on cellular organelles such as microtubules that would be predicted to influence NK activity (Carpen et al., 1981).

METHODS

Male F344 rats (6 to 8 weeks old) known to exhibit high NK activity (Oehler et al., 1978) were tested. For some tests, rats were injected i.p. with 250 µg polyriboinosinic-polyribocytodilic acid (poly-IC) 18 hours before assay. NK activity was measured by release of ^{51}Cr from labeled YAC-1 cells as previously described (Hioe and Jones, 1984) using spleen cells, nylon wool-nonadherent spleen cells (NWNA) or NWNA fractionated on discontinuous Percoll density gradients (modified from Timonen et al., 1982). Fractions from 44.2%

to 52.5% Percoll (bands 2 to 4) were collected (LGL). For some tests, amounts to be indicated of ETOH (v/v) or ACHO (v/v) were added into the assay. For other tests, recombinant rat interferon (IFN)-gamma (AMGen, Thousand Oaks, CA) or purified mouse IFN-alpha + beta (Lee Biomolecular, San Diego, CA) was added during the assay. To prevent evaporation, when ETOH or ACHO was used, the microwell plates were sealed inside Tupperware chambers that were equilibrated with an environment containing the tested amounts of ETOH or ACHO and that had the air replaced with 5% CO_2.

RESULTS

The NK cytotoxic activity of spleen cells from untreated rats and from rats injected with poly-IC are shown in Table 1.

Table 1. Influence of poly-IC on NK activity of rat spleen cells

	In vivo treatment and percent specific release[b]	
E:T ratio[a]	Saline	poly-IC[c]
25	12.8 ± 0.01	24.8 ± 0.02
50	19.2 ± 0.01	35.7 ± 0.01
75	25.8 ± 0.01	46.1 ± 0.05
100	25.8 ± 0.01	48.6 ± 0.02

a) $2x10^4$ ^{51}Cr-YAC-1 cells incubated in 250µl RPMI-1640 medium with indicated effector:target (E:T) ratios of spleen cells for 4 hours at 37C.
b) percent ^{51}Cr released into supernatant; average of 3 tests ± S.E.
c) 0.5 ml saline or saline containing 250µg poly-IC injected i.p 18 hours before assay.

NK activity was approximately twice as great with cells from rats injected with poly-IC. In the absence of ETOH or ACHO, NK activity was similar in ambient air or in chambers. However, because most ACHO (and some ETOH) is lost in ambient air (see A. Walia, these Proceedings), effects of ACHO as described below were detected at levels up to 10-fold lower when tests were conducted in chambers.

In chambers, physiologically attainable amounts of ETOH and ACHO inhibited the NK activity of NWNA spleen cells from untreated rats (Figure 1). Inhibitions by all concentrations of ETOH and ACHO tested were significant ($p<0.05$) at E:T ratios greater than 25:1. The highest concentrations of ETOH and ACHO inhibited significantly at all E:T ratios. None of the amounts tested affected the viability of spleen cells or target cells. In ambient air, 0.001% ACHO did not inhibit significantly and inhibition by 0.01% ACHO was only half that observed in the chambers.

Spleen cells from rats that were injected with poly-IC were partially resistant to the effects of ETOH and ACHO in vitro (Figure 2). There was significantly less inhibition by 0.4% ETOH or 0.05% ACHO when cells from rats injected with poly-IC were tested.

Because poly-IC is a potent IFN inducer, this prompted studies in which exogenous IFN (10^2 to 10^4 units/well) was directly added into the NK assays. It was found that recombinant rat IFN-gamma did not stimulate NK activity significantly within the 4 hour incubation period. In the absence of ETOH or ACHO, purified IFN-alpha + beta did stimulate NK activity (12%, 24% and 52% stimulation with 10^2, 10^3 and 10^4 units respectively) but had no effect on the inhibition induced by ETOH or ACHO during the incubation period. In fact, except at high amounts of IFN (10^4 units/well), no stimulation was seen when physiological amounts of ETOH or ACHO were present. Longer intervals of incubation of effector cells with IFN before assay were not tested.

Because spleen cells are a heterogenous mixture with NK cells comprising only a small percentage of the total, the effects of ETOH and ACHO on populations enriched for NK cells were tested (Table 2). Selected fractions from discontinuous Percoll gradients (LGL) exhibited approximately a 4-fold increase in NK activity compared to unfractionated spleen cells. Studies with fluorescein-labeled antibodies to rat T-cells (OX19) or surface IgM immunoglobulin and other tests (Yeralan, unpublished), showed that LGL contained 30% to 50% T-cells but less than 10% B-cells or macrophages. At all concentrations of ETOH or ACHO tested, LGL were inhibited significantly less than were unfractionated spleen cells. Similar results were observed at E:T ratios of 10:1 and 25:1.

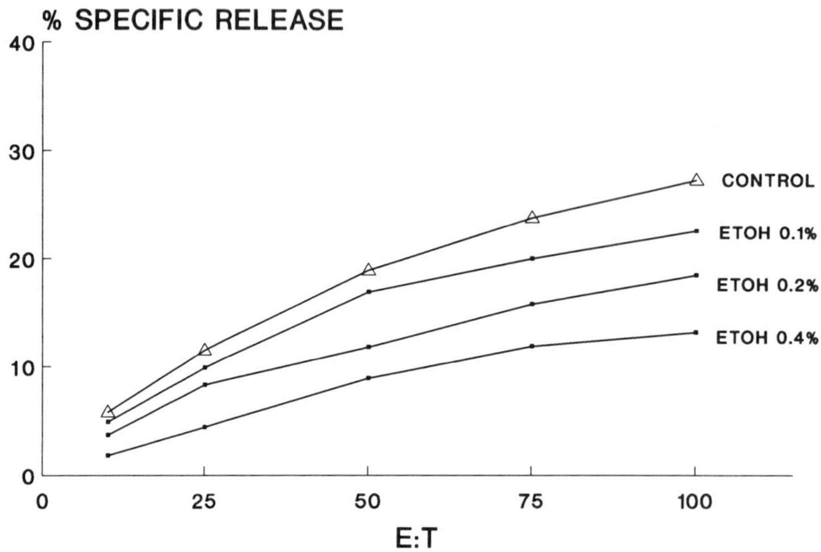

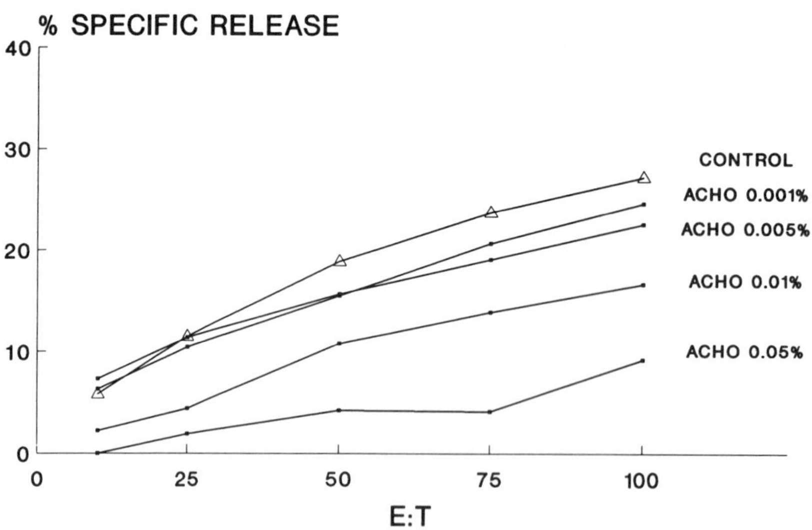

Figure 1. Effects of ETOH (upper) and ACHO (lower) on NK activity of NWNA spleen cells from untreated rats. Indicated amounts of agents (v/v) were incubated with 10^4 ^{51}Cr-YAC-1 and indicated E:T ratios of NWNA cells for 4 hours at 37C; average of 4 tests (S.E. less than 1% at all points).

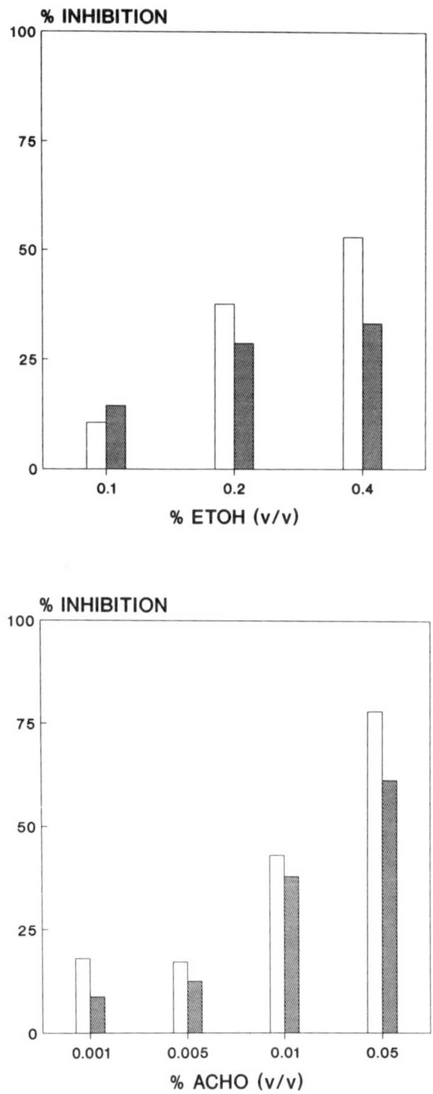

Figure 2. Inhibition by ETOH and ACHO of NK activity of NWNA spleen cells from rats injected with poly-IC. Tested as in Figure 1; E:T ratio was 50:1. Inhibition greater than 10% was significant. White bars, untreated rats; dark bars, rats injected with poly-IC.

TABLE 2. Effects of ETOH and ACHO on NK activity of unfractionated spleen cells and enriched LGL[a]

	Effectors and % specific release (% inhibition)		
Agent	Spleen	NWNA	LGL[b]
None	17.5 (0)	22.0 (0)	44.6 (0)
ETOH 0.1%	11.3 (36)	20.0 (9)	54.0 (0)
ETOH 0.2%	10.4 (41)	14.7 (32)	42.5 (4)
ETOH 0.4%	6.6 (63)	10.9 (50)	32.3 (28)
ACHO 0.0005%	15.1 (14)	21.4 (2)	53.1 (0)
ACHO 0.005%	13.2 (25)	17.4 (20)	48.0 (0)

a) Tested as in Table 1. Rats were not injected with poly-IC; E:T ratio was 50:1; average of 4 tests (S.E. less than 1% at all points). Numbers in parentheses show % inhibition; inhibition greater than 10 % was significant.
b) LGL = Percoll fraction 44.2% to 52.5% (see Methods)

DISCUSSION

The present studies confirm and extend previous reports (Saxena et al., 1982, Ristow et al., 1982, Yeralan and Jones, 1989) that alcohols can inhibit NK activity. The studies also show that amounts of ETOH and ACHO that are easily attainable in vivo will inhibit NK activity in vitro if precautions are taken to prevent the rapid evaporation of ACHO.

As expected (Djeu et al., 1979), injecting rats with the IFN inducer poly-IC, increased the NK activity but we also found that this treatment induced resistance to the inhibitory effects of ETOH and ACHO in vitro. Addition of IFN (alpha + beta) in vitro stimulated NK activity but did not provide a similar resistance to the effects of ETOH or ACHO. This could suggest that in vivo, poly-IC has effects in addition to inducing IFN. Alternatively, the differences may relate to the time intervals involved. In our tests in vitro, IFN was present for only 4 hours. Although the effects on NK activity following injection of poly-IC can be detected within 4 hours (Djeu et al., 1979), realization of the maximum effects of poly-IC in vivo or IFN in vitro may require a longer time period (Santoli et al., 1978).

Populations enriched for NK cells (LGL) were inhibited less by ETOH or ACHO than were unfractionated spleen cells. This raises the possibility that in addition to any direct effects on NK cells, these agents may act on other cells or factors in a manner that results in inhibition of NK activity. Macrophages would be a candidate for such a cell because LGL are virtually devoid of macrophages (in contrast to spleen cells) and macrophages can produce prostaglandins which are known to inhibit NK activity (Brunda et al., 1980, Koren et al., 1981). However, the LGL populations tested contained variable numbers of other cell types and tests with spleen required larger numbers of cells for a given level of activity than did LGL. Therefore, the studies must be interpreted with caution until the contribution of each cell type can be determined. Studies are in progress to establish whether indirect inhibitory effects of ETOH or ACHO on NK activity occur and if established, to identify the mechanisms involved.

REFERENCES

Brunda MJ, Herberman RB, Holden HT (1980). Inhibition of murine natural killer cell activity by prostaglandins. J Immunol 124:2682-2687.

Carpen O, Virtanen, I, Saksela, E (1981). The cytotoxic activity of human natural killer cells requires an intact secretory apparatus. Cell Immunol 58:97-106.

Djeu JY, Heinbaugh JA, Holden HT, Herberman RB (1979). Augmentation of mouse natural killer activity by interferon and interferon inducers. J Immunol 122:175-181.

Djeu JY, Heinbaugh JA, Vieira WD, Holden HT, Herberman RB (1979). The effects of immunopharmacological agents on mouse natural cell-mediated cytotoxicity and on its augmentation by poly I:C. Immunopharmacol 1:231-244.

Herberman RB (1984). Natural killer cells and their possible roles in host resistance against tumors. Transpl Proc 16: 476-480.

Hioe KM, Jones JM (1984). Effects of trimethyltin on the immune system of rats. Toxicol Lett 20:317-323.

Jerrells TR, Marietta CA, Eckardt MJ, Majchrowicz E, Weight FF (1986). Effects of ethanol administration on parameters of immunocompetency in rats. J Leuk Biol 39:499-510.

Koren HS, Anderson SJ, Fischer DG, Copeland CS, Jensen PJ (1981). Regulation of human natural killing. I. The role of monocytes, interferon, and prostaglandins. J Immunol 127:2007-2013.

Lieber CS (1988). Metabolic effects of ethanol and its interaction with other drugs, hepatotoxic agents, vitamins, and carcinogens: A 1988 update. Sem Liv Dis 8:47-68.

MacGregor RR (1986). Alcohol and immune defense. JAMA 256: 1474-1479.

Oehler JR, Lindsay LR, Nunn ME, Herberman RB (1978). Natural cell-mediated cytotoxicity in rats. I. Tissue and strain distribution and demonstration of a membrane receptor for the Fc portion of IgG. Int J Cancer 21:204-209.

Ristow SS, Starkey JR, Hass GM (1982). Inhibition of natural killer cell activity in vitro by alcohols. Biochem Biophys Res Comm 105:1315-1321.

Santoli D, Trinchieri G, Koprowski H (1978). Cell-mediated cytotoxicity against virus-infected target cells in humans. II. Interferon induction and activation of natural killer cells. J Immunol 121:532-538.

Saxena QB, Saxena RK, Adler WH (1982). Ethanol and natural killer activity. In Herberman (ed): "NK Cells and Other Natural Effector Cells," New York: Academic Press, pp 651-656.

Timonen T, Reynolds CW, Ortaldo JR, Herberman RB (1979). Isolation of human and rat natural killer cells. J Immunol Meth 51:269-277.

Watson RR, Prabhala RH, Darban HR, Yahya MD, Smith TL (1988). Changes in lymphocyte and macrophage subsets due to morphine and ethanol treatment during a retrovirus infection causing murine AIDS. Life Sci 43:5-11.

Yeralan O, Jones JM (1989). Effects of ethanol and acetaldehyde on cytotoxic lymphocytes of rats. FASEB J 3:A277.

ACKNOWLEDGEMENTS

Supported in part by UAMS GSRF. We thank Dr. David Davies for demonstrating the use of Tupperware chambers.

Alcohol, Immunomodulation, and AIDS, pages 173–180
© 1990 Alan R. Liss, Inc.

MECHANISMS OF ETHANOL-INDUCED IMMUNOSUPPRESSION*

Thomas R. Jerrells, Michael J. Eckardt and Joanne Weinberg
Dept. of Pathology, Univ. of Texas Med. Br. Galveston, TX 77550 (TRJ), Lab. of Clinical Studies, NIAAA, Bethesda, MD 20892 (MJE), and Dept. of Anatomy, Univ. of British Columbia, Vancouver, B. C. (JW)

INTRODUCTION

The ingestion of ethanol (ETOH) or administration of ETOH to experimental animals has been show to result in alterations in the immune system (Eckardt,et al. 1981, Jerrells, et al. 1986, Lauria, 1963, Macgregor, 1986, Rosell and Mendenhall, 1984). Changes have been shown to occur in both the specific immune response to a foreign antigen and in the nonspecific mechanisms of host defense including phagocytic cell function (Galante, et al. 1982) and granulocyte functions (MacGregor, et al. 1978). One of the important features of ETOH-associated changes in the immune system is the changes in cell-mediated immune functions reported by us (Jerrells, et al. 1986). The research in my laboratory has been mainly involved in the definition of the defect in the cell-mediated immunity due to ETOH and has employed the proliferative response to thymus-derived lymphocytes (T- cells) to mitogenic stimulation. It was shown by us that the administration of ETOH to rats (Jerrells, et al. 1986) or ingestion of ETOH by mice (Smith and Jerrells, in preparation) results in a broad inability to respond to mitogenic stimuli. We have also established that this proliferative defect extends to the T-cell response to recall antigen stimulation using the proliferative response to the protein antigen keyhole limpet hemocyanogen and to alloantigen stimulation as measured by the one-way mixed lymphocyte response (MLR).

*Suported In Part By Grants AA07731 (TRJ) and AA07789 (JW)

The purpose of this report is to describe the results of previously published data and preliminary studies in my laboratory that address the lymphocyte proliferative defect that results from ETOH. The results of 3 animal models will be discussed. A rat model where ETOH was administered by gastric intubation or inhalation, a mouse model where ETOH was administered in a liquid diet in a pair feeding protocol, and in a rat model of fetal alcohol exposure where the only ETOH exposure was in utero.

MATERIALS AND METHODS

Male Sprague-Dawley rats were given ETOH by gastric intubation essentially as described by Majchrowicz (1975). Briefly, animals were given 8-11 grams ETOH/Kg body weight/day in a liquid diet supplemented with vitamins. Rats were treated for 4 days with ETOH and after this treatment regime animals were allowed to with draw and during this time lab chow and water was given as libitum. Mice were given ETOH in a paired-feeding protocol using the Leiber-DeCarli diet. This protocol used diet containing ETOH as 36% of the total calories and diet calorie without ETOH. Male C57Bl/6 mice were fed ETOH or control diet for a total of 7 days and if studied after withdrawal, they were fed lab chow and water as above. The third model system was the prenatal exposure system described by Weinberg (1985). Briefly, on day 1 of gestation (determined by the presence of a vaginal plug) female Sprague-Dawley rats were randomly assigned to one of three groups: 1) liquid ETOH diet ad libitum; 2) liquid control diet, with each animal pair-fed the amount consumed (grams/kg body weight) by females in the ETOH group; 3) lab chow and water ad libitum. On day 21 of gestation experimental diets were replaced by lab chow. After birth pups and dams were left undisturbed until weaning on 22 days of age.

Immunological parameters

Animals from the above treatment groups were killed and the spleen and thymus removed aseptically as previously described (Jerrells, et al. 1986). Each organ was individually made into a single cell suspension and washed with $Ca^{++}$and Mg^{++}-free Hank's balanced salt solution

(HBSS). Cell counts were performed using an electronic cell counter (Coulter model ZM, Coulter Electronics, Hialeah, Fl). Lymphocyte proliferation assays were performed essentially as previously described. Briefly, spleen cells were adjusted to 2.5 to 5 x 10^6 per ml in RPMI 1640 supplemented with 10 mM HEPES buffer, fresh glutamine, 50 ug/ml gentamicin, 5 x 10^{-5}M 2 mercaptoethanol, and 10% heat inactivated fetal bovine serum. One hundred microliter aliquots of cells were cultured in flat bottomed microtiter plates with dilutions of concanavalin A, phytohemagglutinin, bacterial LPS or Key hole limpet hemocyanogen, or an equal number of irradiated (2500 rad) allogeneic spleen cells (MLR). After 72 to 96 hours tritiated thymidine (1 uCi/well) was added and the amount of radioactivity incorporated into the cell determined after harvesting of cells onto glass fiber filters 6 hours after addition of thymidine and liquid scintillation counting.

Production of interleukin-2 by cells stimulated with con A was determined by collecting culture supernatant 18 to 20 hours after stimulation and quantitating the level of IL-2 using the IL-2-dependent cell line CTLL as previously described. Utilization of IL-2 was measured using blast cells isolated from con A stimulated cultures after 48 hours with a ficoll-Hypaque gradient. The isolated blast cells were incubated in 2 separate 50 ml quantities of RPMI 1640 supplemented as before for 1 hour. After extensive washing the resulting cells were cultured at 5 x 10 ^{3} cells per well with various concentrations of recombinant IL-2 or a rat spleen cell supernatant. The cultures were pulsed with thymidine and harvested after 24 hours of incubation as before.

Binding of IL-2 to the IL-2 receptor was measured using ^{125}I-IL-2 as described by Robb, et al. (1984). Internalization of IL-2 was determined as described by Fujii, et al. (1986) using radiolabeled IL-2.

RESULTS AND DISCUSSION

To determine if the T-cell defect in proliferation to mitogenic stimuli extended to the secondary response to a recall antigen we immunized rats with KLH in Freund's complete adjuvant and the immune animals were given either

ETOH-containing diet or control diet by intubation. After ETOH administration the spleen cells from each group were tested for in vitro responses to KLH using the described microculture lymphocyte proliferation assay. The results of this study (Jerrells, et al. 1988) demonstrated that the response to the recall antigen KLH was suppressed similar to the suppression noted to con A stimulation. This finding indicates that the mechanism leading to suppression of the T-cell proliferation is nonspecific and not unique only to mitogens as has been suggested by others (Roselle and Mendenhall, 1984). A decreased ability to clonally expand antigen-responsive T-cells could lead to an inability to resist secondary challenges by organisms that a person has experienced before or vaccinated against. It is also possible that the impairment in T-cell-dependent antibody responses previously described (Jerrells, et al. 1986) is due to the effect of ETOH on the antigen-responsive T-cell.

We and others have shown that one effect of ETOH is a depletion of cells from the thymus and spleen (Jerrells, et al., 1986 and 1988, Tennenbaum, et al. 1969). The decreased response of spleen cells could in fact only be reflective of a lack of responding cells in the cell suspension cultured with mitogens. To test this hypothesis we cultured a cell suspension enriched for T-cells by passage of spleen cells over nylon wool columns. These isolated cells were cultured with irradiated (2500 rad) spleen cells from untreated animals and stimulated with mitogens as before. It was found that the T-cell population isolated from spleens of ETOH-treated rats still responded to con A less well than cells from control animals even though equal numbers of T- cells were in each culture (Perrit, Eckardt, and Jerrells, in preparation). These data are interpreted by us to mean that the defect in T-cell proliferation is due to some T-cell impairment and not simply to a lack of responding cells. Also, these data show that the impaired responses noted by us are not due entirely to a defect in accessory cell function because of the use in these cultures of accessory cells (irradiated spleen cells) from untreated animals. We have preliminary data (Jerrells unpublished) that shows that macrophages isolated from ETOH- treated animals produce less IL-1 than macrophages from control animals and this accessory cell defect would likely act to further decrease the ability to respond to proliferative stimuli.

Many of the characteristics associate with the effects of ETOH on the immune system are consistent with the effects of corticosteroids (Cupps and Fauchi, 1982, DelRey, et al. 1984). It has also been shown that ETOH induces relatively high levels of corticosteroids in animal models (Tabakoff, et al. 1978). To test if corticosteroids are partially or completely responsible for the observed effects we obtained adrenalectomized rats (ADX) and compared the effects of ETOH in ADX rats with rats bearing adrenal glands. The results of these studies (Jerrells, et al. Effect of adrenalectomy on ethanol-associated immunosuppression, submitted to the International Journal of Immunopharmacology) show that much of the loss of thymic cells is due to corticosteroids but the loss of spleen cells and the ability to respond to a T-cell-dependent antigen by antibody production is similarly affected in ADX and adrenal gland-bearing rats given ETOH. Again, these data are interpreted by us to mean that the effects of ETOH are not dependent on T-cell loss and also not simply due to corticosteroids.

It has been shown that the proliferative response of T-cells to antigenic and mitogenic stimuli is dependent on the production of the lymphokine IL-2 (Smith, 1988). This response is also dependent on the ability of the T-cell to bind and internalize IL-2 (Fujii, ert al., 1986, Robb, et al. 1984). It was possible that the noted effects of ETOH on T-cell responses was due to an inability to produce and/or utilize IL-2. To test these hypotheses we performed several experiments.Initially cell culture supernatant was collected and assayed for IL-2 levels using the IL-2-dependent cell line CTLL as described. In most assays performed there was no difference in the IL-2 levels produced by cells from ETOH-treated or control diet fed animals and often we noted higher levels in cultures of cells from ETOH- treated animals (Perritt, Jerrells, Eckhardt, and Marietta, Alterations in IL-2 utilization by T-cells from rats treated with an ethanol-containing diet, Submitted to Alcoholism: Clin Exp Res). In further studies it was found that the blast cells recovered from mitogen-stimulated cultures of cells from ETOH-treated rats responded significantly less to added IL-2 than cells from control rats. The addition of exogenous IL-2 to the initial cultures did not reverse the inability of T-cells to respond to con A. Taken together we interpreted these results to suggest that the T-cells from ETOH-treated animals were not able to utilize the IL-2 produced in response to con A. We have also noted a similar situation using cells from C57Bl/6 mice given ETOH in a liquid diet (Smith and Jerrells, Ethanol-induced changes in the immune system of C57Bl/6 mice, in preparation). Using ^{125}I-IL-2 we investigated the binding of IL-2 to the receptors of isolated blast cells. Surprisingly, no difference in high-affinity receptor binding of IL-2 was noted using cells isolated from ETOH-treated animals. However, there is an apparent inability to internalize IL-2 bound to the receptor. These results are preliminary and current studies using the mouse model are in progress to test this. The data generated to date would indicate that the defect in the T-cell, at least in the response to con A, is due not to an inability to produce IL-2 but to an inability to internalize and perhaps to transduce the internal signal necessary for proliferation.

Recently it has been shown that exposure to ETOH _in utero_ effects the immune response in terms of the developing thymus (Ewald and Frost, 1987) and immunological competence of the offspring (Johnson, et al., 1981, Mojan and Mandell, 1980). Using a rat model of prenatal exposure to ETOH developed in the laboratory of Joanne Weinberg (Weinberg and Gallo, 1982) the effects of prenatal exposure to ETOH was investigated. It was found in these studies that adult animals only exposed _in utero_ had a demonstrable defect in the proliferative response to con A and LPS. Interestingly this defect was noted only in the male offspring. A similar observation was recently reported by Redei (Redei, E., Mitogen-induced lymphocyte proliferation and the brain-pituitary-adrenal function in adult male rats after chronic alcohol treatment and in rats exposed to alcohol _in utero_) at this conference. As was seen in animals exposed to ETOH as adults the defect was not associated with a defect in IL-2 production but with a defect in the blast cell response to exogenous IL-2. From these preliminary studies it would seem that exposure of the developing immune system to ETOH results in defects similar to those seen in adult animals that have been treated with ETOH. It seems likely that the developing immune system is easier to alter and further it is possible that unlike the adult immune system the defect is not reversible.

In summary, a number of approaches have been taken by us to investigate the possible mechanisms of ETOH effects on the immune system. We have emphasized the T-cell and have studied extensively the effect of ETOH on the responses of T-cells to mitogenic stimulation. These defects seem to be partially due to the production of corticosteroids in response to ETOH and especially withdrawal from ETOH. It is clear, however, that other mechanisms are also responsible for some of the defects, especially antibody production in response to T-dependent antigens. The proliferative response to T-cell mitogens such as con A seems to be associated with a defect in the cells ability to utilize IL-2 rather than an inability to produce lymphokine. Similar defects were noted in animals exposed to ETOH *in utero*.

REFERENCES

Cupps, TR, Fauci, AS (1982). Corticosteroid-mediated immunoregulation in man. Immuno Rev 65:133-155.

DelRey, A, Besedovsky, H, Sorkin, E. (1984). Endogenous blood levels of corticosterone control the immunologic cell mass and B cell activity in mice. J Immunol 133:572-575.

Eckardt, MJ, Harford, TC, Kaelber, CT, Parker, ES, Rosenthal, LS, Ryback, RS, Salmoiraghi, GC, Vanderveen, E, Warren KR (1981). Health hazards associated with alcohol consumption. J Am Med Assoc 246:648-666.

Ewald, SJ, Frost, WW (1987). Effect of prenatal exposure to ethanol on development of the thymus. Thymus 9:211-215.

Fujii, M, Sugamura, K, Sano, K, Nakai, M, Sugita, K, Hinuma,Y (1986). High-affinity receptor-mediated internalization and degradation of interleukin 2 in human T cells. J Exp Med 163:550-562.

Galante, D, Andreana, A, Perna, P, Utili, R, Ruggiero,G, (1982). Decreased phagocytic and bactericidal activity of the hepatic reticuloendothelial system during chronic ethanol treatment and its restoration by levamisole. J Reticuloendol Soc 32:179-187.

Jerrells, TR, Marietta, CA, Eckardt, MJ, Majchrowicz, E, Weight, FF (1986). Effects of ethanol administration on parameters of immunocompetency in rats. J Leukocyte Biol 39:499-510.

Jerrells, TR, Marietta, CA, Bone, G, Weight, FF, Eckardt, MJ (1988). Ethanol-associated immunosuppression. In Bridge, TP, Mirsky, AF, Goodwin, FK (eds) : "Psychological, Neuropsychiatric, and Substance Abuse Aspects of
AIDS," New York: Raven Press, pp 173-185.
Johnson,S, Knight, R, Marmier, DJ, Steele, RW (1981). Immune deficiency in fetal alcohol syndrome. Pedriatic Res 15:908-922.
Lauria, DB (1963). Susceptibility to infection during experimental alcoholic intoxication. Trans Assoc Am Physicans 76:102-110.
MacGregor, RR (1986). Alcohol and immune defense. J Amer Med Assoc 256:1474-1479.
MacGrgor, RR, Gluckman, SJ, Senior, JR (1978). Granulocyte function and levels of immunoglobulins and complement in patients admitted for withdrawal from alcohol. J Infect Dis 138:747-753.
Majchrowicz, E (1975). Induction of physical dependence upon ethanol and the associated behavioral changes in rats. Psychopharmacologia 43:245-254.
Mojan, AA, Mandell, W (1980). Fetal alcohol and immunity: depression of mitogen-induced lymphocyte blastogenesis. Neurobehav Toxicol 2:213-215.
Robb, RJ, Greene, WC, Rusk, CM (1984). Low and high affinity cellular receptors for interleukin 2: implications for the level of Tac antigen. J Exp Med 160:1126-1146.
Roselle, GA, Mendenhall, CL (1984). Ethanol-induced alterations in lymphocyte function in the guinea pig. Clin Exp Res 8:62-67.
Tabakoff, B, Jaffe, RC, Ritzmann, RF (1978). Corticosterone concentrations in mice during ethanol drinking and withdrawal. J Pharm Pharmac 30:371-374.
Tennenbaum, JI, Ruppert, RD, St. Pierre, RL, Greenberger, NJ (1969). The effect of chronic alcohol administration on the immune responsiveness of rats. J Allergy 44:272-281.
Weinberg, J, (1985). Effects of ethanol and maternal nutritional status on fetal development. Alcohol & Clin Exp Res 9:49-55.

Alcohol, Immunomodulation, and AIDS, pages 181–190
© 1990 Alan R. Liss, Inc.

MODULATION OF NATURAL KILLER CELL ACTIVITY BY ALCOHOL CONSUMPTION AND NUTRITIONAL STATUS

Gary G. Meadows, Sally E. Blank and Deborah A. Duncan

College of Pharmacy and the Pharmacology/ Toxicology Graduate Program, Washington State University, Pullman, WA 99164-6510

INTRODUCTION

Agents that decrease natural killer (NK) cell function compromise important defenses against certain infectious diseases, spontaneously arising tumors, and blood-borne metastasizing tumor cells (Hanna 1982; Herberman and Holden, 1978; Herberman and Ortaldo, 1981). Alcohol is a known suppressant of both humoral and cell-mediated immune responses including NK cell activity, but the role of alcohol in immune modulation has not been systematically evaluated. Moreover, it is difficult to compare published studies because of differences in experimental design such as subject age, nutritional and health status, blood alcohol concentration, the amount and length of time that alcohol is consumed, and the NK cell assay methodology. All of these variables can influence NK cell activity. In humans, use of other drugs and tobacco, known to affect NK cell activity, further complicate evaluation of alcohol's specific modulatory role (Ferson *et al.*, 1979).

Alcoholics may have varying degrees of liver damage, and are frequently malnourished. Patients with chronic active hepatitis and cirrhosis have low NK activity (Serdengecti *et al.*, 1981; Vierling *et al.*, 1977). Starvation leading to severe malnutrition suppresses NK cell activity (Saxena *et al.*, 1980a). On the other hand, protein or specific dietary amino acid undernutrition can actually stimulate immune responses (Bounous and Kongshavn, 1978,1982; Cooper *et al.*, 1974; Jose and Good, 1973). Deficiencies in specific amino acids can either enhance (methionine) or decrease (tyrosine and phenylalanine) NK cell activity (Abdallah *et al.*, 1983), thereby further complicating the evaluation of nutritional status on NK cell activity. Thus, it is unclear whether the immunological abnormalities in alcoholics result from generalized malnutrition, malabsorption of specific nutrients, or are the consequence of direct alcohol exposure (Gross and Newberne, 1980; Neville *et al.*, 1968, Shaw and Lieber, 1978; Yew *et al.*, 1981). Given the enumerable variables that complicate evaluation of immune function in the alcohol consumer, it is not surprising that *in vivo* NK cell activity is reported to increase (Saxena *et al.*, 1980b; Saxena *et al.*, 1981), decrease (Abdallah *et al.*, 1988; Meadows *et al.*, 1989), or not change (Abdallah *et al.*, 1983; Charpentier *et al.*, 1984; Ericsson *et al.*, 1980; Mufti *et al.*, 1988) in response to alcohol consumption.

Previously, we reported that mice administered alcohol in the drinking water as the sole fluid source, maintained normal diet and fluid intake compared to non alcohol consuming mice (Abdallah *et al.*, 1983, 1988). In these studies, NK cell activity was not affected after 4 weeks and 12 weeks of continuous consumption of 10% w/v alcohol. However, when mice were given 20% w/v alcohol for 12 weeks, NK cell activity was decreased without evidence of generalized malnutrition. We report here the modulation of NK cell activity in mice after 1, 7, 14, and 30 days of exposure to 20% w/v alcohol, and specifically examine the combined effects of undernutrition and alcohol consumption on NK cell activity.

EXPERIMENTAL DESIGN AND METHODOLOGY

Treatment groups were age (8-16 weeks) and body weight matched, female, C57BL/6 mice housed singly in polycarbonate cages and fed a normal crystalline amino acid diet as previously described

(Abdallah *et al.*, 1983, 1988; Meadows *et al.*, 1989). Mice in alcohol treatment groups were given continuous access to 20% w/v alcohol in the drinking water. In the 7-day and 14-day studies, one group of mice were pair fed to alcohol consuming mice according to diet intake; however, pair feeding was unnecessary because alcohol consumption did not alter diet intake. For the undernutrition study, diet intake was restricted to 2.2 g or 1.8 g per day for 30 days. Diet restriction corresponded to approximately 75% and 60% of normal diet consumption, respectively.

Blood alcohol concentration and NK cell activity were determined as previously described (Abdallah *et al.*, 1983, 1988; Meadows *et al.*, 1989). Spleen cell number was determined in individual spleens, and then spleen cell suspensions from 3-4 mice were combined for further processing through nylon wool. Baseline NK cell activity was determined against ^{51}chromium labeled YAC-1 lymphoma cells in a standard 4-hour assay. Stimulated NK cell activity was determined after incubation of nylon wool passaged spleen cells with human recombinant interleukin-2 (rIL2) for 18-24 hours. Cytolytic activity was expressed as lytic units (L.U.) per 10^6 effector cells according to the method of Pross *et al.*, 1981. The results from 6-7 different experiments were compared using analysis of variance. Differences between two means were determined using Fisher's Protected Least Significant Difference Test and considered significant if $p<0.05$.

RESULTS AND DISCUSSION

Caloric intake and changes in body weight are presented in Table 1. Diet consumption, body weight (Table 1), and spleen weight were decreased by alcohol after one day. Diet intake in the *ad lib.* control and alcohol groups was not different at days 7, 14, and 30 (Table 1). At day 30, diet restricted mice lost considerable body weight. However, mice given alcohol lost significantly less body weight than their respective control

Table 1. Caloric Intake and Body Weight Change During Various Alcohol Feeding Regimens[a]

Day	Group	Body Weight Change(g)	Calories Per Day Diet	Calories Per Day Alcohol
1	C *ad lib.*	-0.6±0.1	10.5±3.4	
	A *ad lib.*	-1.6±0.2[b]	6.8±1.6[b]	3.0±0.8
7	C Pair fed	0.5±0.6	10.7±1.0	
	A *ad lib.*	0.1±0.6	12.1±1.8	4.4±0.7
14	C Pair fed	0.7±1.3	10.5±0.9	
	A *ad lib.*	0.3±1.1	12.8±2.0	4.8±0.4
30	C *ad lib.*	1.9±1.4	12.5±1.0	
	C 2.2 g	-4.2±1.2[b]	8.5±0.1[b]	
	C 1.8 g	-4.9±0.5[b]	7.0±0.1[b,c]	
	A *ad lib.*	1.7±1.5	11.0±1.4	4.7±0.5
	A 2.2 g	0.4±0.8[b,d]	8.5±0.2[b,d]	4.9±0.3
	A 1.8 g	-1.8±1.4[b,d]	7.0±0.2[b,d,e]	4.6±0.4

[a] Mean±S.D.; C = control; A = alcohol; C or A 2.2g and 1.8g = diet restricted groups. Each group contained 18-21 mice.
[b] Different from C *ad lib.* group.
[c] Different from C 2.2 g group.
[d] Different from A *ad lib.* group.
[e] Different from A 2.2 g group.

group. Alcohol intake was maintained independently of changes in body weight or diet intake (Table 1). The mean alcohol derived calories ranged from 27.1 to 30.9±6% in the *ad lib.* groups to as high as 39.5±2.2% in the "A 1.8 g" group. Blood alcohol concentrations at the time of NK assay varied from 0-<75 mg/dl even though mice consumed a large proportion of their calories as alcohol.

Alcohol consumption did not influence spleen weight in the *ad lib.* groups. No differences in the number of spleen cells were observed except at

14 days when the mean cell number per spleen in the alcohol *ad lib.* group was 33.1±0.2% lower compared to the control *ad lib.* and pair-fed groups. Significant spleen cell loss was observed in the diet restricted animals in the 30-day experiment as indicated in Table 2. Decrease in spleen weight and in the total numbers of cells per spleen paralleled losses in body weight. However, the degree of loss was more pronounced in the dietary restricted control groups than in the alcohol consuming groups. Food restricted alcohol consuming groups maintained higher body weight throughout the 30-day treatment than their control counterparts (Table 1).

Table 2. Effect of Diet Restriction on Spleen Weight and Cell Number at Day 30[a]

Group	Spleen Weight (mg)	Spleen Cell No. ($\times 10^7$)	Spleen Cell No. / Spleen Weight ($\times 10^5$)
C *ad lib.*	56.4±10.6	3.3±0.9	5.9±1.4
C 2.2 g	30.1± 8.1[b]	1.5±0.5[b]	4.9±1.5
C 1.8 g	21.9± 5.8[b]	1.1±0.5[b]	5.4±2.6
A *ad lib.*	52.2±13.3	2.5±1.1	4.9±1.9
A 2.2 g	38.4± 9.8[b]	2.1±0.6[b]	5.8±2.5
A 1.8 g	30.5± 5.9[b]	1.7±0.1[b]	5.5±2.9

[a] Mean±S.D. C = control; A = alcohol; C or A 2.2 g and 1.8 g = diet restricted groups.
[b] Different from all other groups.

Consumption of 20% w/v alcohol significantly decreased baseline NK cell activity at 7, 14, and 30 days, but no significant difference in activity was observed after one day of alcohol consumption (Table 3). The suppression of NK cell activity was greatest at 7 days. rIL2 stimulated NK cell activity in *ad lib.* groups at all time periods. Alcohol and control *ad lib.* groups were augmented to the same degree at day 1 and day 14; however, NK cells were more responsive to rIL2 stimulation at 7 and 30 days.

Table 3. NK Cell Activity in *ad lib.* Alcohol Consuming Groups Compared to Control Groups at Different Time Periods

	NK Cell Activity (% of Control)[a]		Degree of Augmentation[b]	
Days	Baseline	Stimulated	Control	Alcohol
1	79.3	84.5	2.6	2.7
7	38.2[c]	70.3[c]	2.0	3.6
14	66.9[c]	55.8[c]	2.2	1.8
30	51.3[c]	82.2	2.7	4.3

[a] $\% \text{ of Control} = \dfrac{\text{L.U. Alcohol group}}{\text{L.U. Control group}} \times 100;$

At 7 and 14 days the L.U. for the control group represent combined values from *ad lib.* and pair fed groups since NK cell activity did not differ between these groups.

[b] $\text{Degree of Augmentation} = \dfrac{\text{L.U. Stimulated}}{\text{L.U. Baseline}}$

[c] NK cell activity significantly lower in alcohol group compared to control group.

Diet restriction consistently decreased baseline NK cell activity independently of alcohol consumption (Figure 1). We observed no differences between the diet restricted groups and alcohol consuming mice given free access to diet. Although there was a tendency in the diet restricted groups for alcohol consuming mice to have higher rIL2 stimulated activity than the non alcohol consuming diet restricted groups, the values were not significantly different. Stimulated NK cell activity was lower in all diet restricted groups relative to the stimulated activity of control and alcohol *ad lib.* groups.

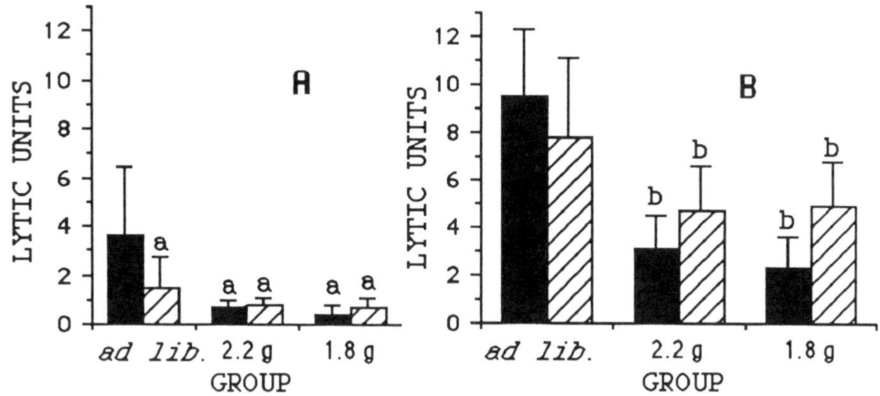

Figure 1. Baseline (A) and rIL2 stimulated (B) NK cell activity in control (filled bars) and alcohol consuming (cross-hatched bars) mice as a function of undernutrition. *ad lib.* = unrestricted diet intake; 2.2g and 1.8 g = diet restricted groups; a = different from control *ad lib.* group; b = different from control and alcohol *ad lib.* groups.

Alcohol consuming mice given free access to diet were not undernourished; therefore, poor nutritional status did not contribute to the decrease in baseline NK cell activity. These data confirm previous work indicating suppression of baseline NK cell activity after 12 weeks of treatment (Abdallah *et al.*, 1988). Some possible explanations for the suppression of NK cell activity include decreased effector to target binding, interference with the signal transduction mechanisms involved in the cytolytic event, decreased production of cytotoxic factors, or decreased proportion of NK to other T lymphocytes in the nylon wool enriched spleen cell preparation used for determination of cytolytic activity.

Diet restriction dramatically decreased NK cell activity in both control and alcohol consuming groups. In undernourished mice, alcohol did not significantly contribute to the overall decrease in NK cell activity. Alcohol actually inhibited the loss of body weight, spleen weight, and splenocyte number. The most consistent indicator of undernutrition was spleen weight. These data suggest that alcohol derived calories play an important metabolic role in the undernourished animal. NK cell activity was not further suppressed by alcohol consumption in the undernourished mice, which suggests that alcohol or its metabolites may not have a direct role in modulating NK activity *in vivo*. NK cell activity can be modulated directly by alcohol-associated release of corticosteroids, prostaglandins, or immune regulatory factors produced by other lymphocytes, and these could impact NK cell activity *in situ* (Bagasra *et al.*, 1987; Jerrells *et al.*, 1986; Kaplan 1986; Roselle and Mendenhall, 1984). Additional work is necessary to identify the specific mechanism(s) responsible for the suppressive effect of alcohol on NK cell activity.

ACKNOWLEDGEMENT

This work was funded by grant number AA07293 from the National Institute for Alcohol Abuse and Alcoholism.

REFERENCES

Abdallah RM, Starkey JR, Meadows GG (1983). Alcohol and related dietary effects on mouse natural killer-cell activity. Immunology 50:131-137.

Abdallah RM, Starkey JR, Meadows GG (1988). Toxicity of chronic high alcohol intake on mouse natural killer cell activity. Res Commun Chem Pathol Pharmacol 59:245-258.

Bagasra O, Howeedy A, Dorio R, Kajdacsy-Balla A 1987. Functional analysis of T-cell subsets in chronic experimental alcoholism. Immunology 61:63-69, 1987.

Bounous G, Kongshavn PAL (1978). The effect of dietary amino acids on immune reactivity. Immunology 35:257-266.

Bounous G, Kongshavn PAL (1982). Influence of dietary proteins on the immune system of mice. J Nutr 112:1747-1755.

Charpentier, B, Franco D, Paci L, Charra M, Martin B, Vuitton D, Fries D (1984). Deficient natural killer cell activity in alcoholic cirrhosis. Clin Exp Immunol 58:107-105.
Cooper, WC, Good RA, Mariani T (1974). Effects of protein insufficiency on immune responsiveness. Am J Clin Nutr 27:647-664.
Ericsson CD, Kohl S, Pickering LK, Davis J, Glass GS, Faillace LA (1980). Mechanisms of host defense in well nourished patients with chronic alcoholism. Alcoholism: Clin Exp Res 4:261-265.
Ferson M, Edwards A, Lind A, Milton GW, Hersey P (1979). Low natural killer-cell activity and immunoglobulin levels associated with smoking in human subjects. Int J Cancer 23:603-609.
Gross RL, Newberne PM (1980). Role of nutrition in immunologic function. Physiol Rev 60:188-302.
Hanna N (1982). Role of natural killer cells in control of cancer metastasis. Cancer Met Rev 1:45-64.
Herberman RB, Holden HT (1978). Natural cell-mediated immunity. Adv Cancer Res 27:305-377.
Herberman RB, Ortaldo JR (1981). Natural-killer cells: Their role in defense against disease. Science 214:24-30.
Jerrells TR, Marietta CA, Eckardt MJ, Majchrowicz E, Weight FF (1986). Effects of ethanol administration on parameters of immunocompetency in rats. J Leukocyte Biol 29:499-510.
Jose DG, Good RA (1973). Quantitative effects of nutritional protein and calorie deficiency upon immune responses to tumors in mice. Cancer Res 33:807-811.
Kaplan DR (1986). A novel mechanism of immunosuppression mediated by ethanol. Cell Immunol 102:1-9.
Meadows GG, Blank SE, Duncan DA (1989). Influence of ethanol consumption on natural killer cell activity in mice. Alcoholism: Clin Exp Res 13: (in press).
Mufti SI, Prabhala, R, Moriguchi S, Sipes IG, Watson RR (1988). Functional and numerical alterations induced by ethanol in the cellular immune system. Immunopharmacology 15:85-93.

Neville JN, Eagles JA, Samson G, Olson RE (1968). Nutrition status of alcoholics. Am J Clin Nutr 21:1329-1340.
Pross HF, Baines MG, Rubin P, Shragge P, Patterson MS (1981). Spontaneous human lymphocyte-mediated cytotoxicity against tumor target cells. IX: The quantitation of natural killer cell activity. J Clin Immunol 1:51-63.
Roselle GA, Mendenhall CL (1984). Ethanol-induced alterations in lymphocyte function in the guinea pig. Alcoholism: Clin Exp Res 8:62-67.
Saxena QB, Mezey E, Adler WH (1980b). Regulation of natural killer activity *in vivo*. II. The effect of alcohol consumption on human peripheral blood natural killer activity. Int J Cancer 28:413-417.
Saxena QB, Saxena RK, Adler WH (1981). Regulation of natural killer activity *in vivo*: Part IV--High natural killer activity in alcohol drinking mice. Ind J Exp Biol 19:1001-1006.
Saxena RK, Saxena QB, Adler WH (1980a). Regulation of natural killer activity *in vivo*: Part I--Loss of natural killer activity during starvation. Indian J Exp Biol 18:1383-1386.
Shaw S, Lieber CS (1978). Plasma amino acid abnormalities in the alcoholic: respective role of alcohol, nutrition and liver injury. Gastroenterology 74:677-682.
Serdengecti S, Jones DB, Holdstock G, Wright R (1981). Natural killer activity in patients with biopsy proven liver disease. Clin Exp Immunol 45:361-364.
Vierling JM, Nelson DL, Strober W, Bundy BM, Jones EA (1977). *In vitro* cell-mediated cytotoxicity in primary biliary cirrhosis and chronic hepatitis. Dysfunction of spontaneous cell-mediated cytotoxicity in primary biliary cirrhosis. J Clin Invest 60:1116-1128.
Yew MS, Moore S, Biesele MM (1981). Effects of chronic "moderate" alcohol consumption on vitamins A and C status of male Sprague-Dawley rats. Nutr Rep Int 23:427-436.

Alcohol, Immunomodulation, and AIDS, pages 191–200
© 1990 Alan R. Liss, Inc.

LYMPHOCYTE POPULATIONS AND IMMUNE RESPONSES IN MICE PRENATALLY EXPOSED TO ETHANOL

Sandra J. Ewald and Ching Huang

Department of Microbiology, Montana

State University, Bozeman, Montana 59717

INTRODUCTION

Prenatal exposure to ethanol is known to be teratogenic for many organ systems, in both humans and experimental animals (for review, see Abel, 1984). The effect of in utero alcohol exposure on the developing immune system, however, has received relatively little attention. In humans there are reports from two different groups (Johnson et al., 1981; Calvani et al., 1985) of long-lasting immune deficiency involving both T- and B-cell populations in children of alcoholic mothers. Yet another report (Ammann et al., 1982) shows an association of DiGeorge syndrome (a complex of disorders including thymic aplasia, heart anomalies, and parathyroid insufficiency) with maternal alcoholism. In experimental animals, Monjan and Mandell (1980) reported long-term reduction of T-cell responses in a limited study of rats born to alcohol-treated dams.

More recently, we (Ewald and Frost, 1987; Ewald and Walden, 1988) have undertaken studies to examine the effect of prenatal exposure to ethanol on development of the thymus in mice. Normal fetal thymus development has been particularly well characterized in this species (for a recent review, see Adkins et al., 1987). The epithelial thymus anlage forms at gestational day (g.d.) 9-10 mainly from third pharyngeal pouch endoderm with possible contribution from pharyngeal cleft ectoderm (reviewed in Owen and Jenkinson, 1984) and neural crest (Bockman and Kirby, 1984). Between g.d. 10.5 and 13 the thymus is colonized by lymphoid stem cells (Jotereau et al., 1987). The Thy-1 antigen typical of all murine T-cells is expressed at high levels on fetal murine thymocytes by g.d. 15 (Itoh, 1987). The Lyt-2 (CD8) antigen is expressed at g.d. 16, and the L3T4 (CD4) antigen at day 17 (Ceredig et al., 1983). Double-positive ($CD4^+CD8^+$) thymocytes give rise to single-positive thymocytes ($CD4^+CD8^-$ helper cells and $CD4^-CD8^+$ cytotoxic/suppressor cells) which do not appear in adult proportions until about g.d. 19, just before birth.

Our studies have shown impaired development of the thymus, in terms of both cell number and maturation, in late-term mouse fetuses examined immediately after chronic prenatal ethanol exposure. We were further interested to determine if exposure to alcohol at extremely high doses during critical periods of prenatal development might completely arrest formation of the epithelial thymus, thus producing one characteristic feature of DiGeorge syndrome in mice. Others have shown that very high maternal blood alcohol levels at critical developmental periods are teratogenic for a number of organ systems (Webster et al., 1983), and may produce heart defects similar to those seen in the human DiGeorge syndrome (Daft et al., 1986).

METHODS AND RESULTS

Effect of chronic prenatal exposure to ethanol on development of the thymus in late-term fetuses.

Age- and weight-matched C57BL/6 female mice were assigned to one of three diet groups: (1) 25% EDC (ethanol-derived calories): fed a liquid diet (Bio-Serv, Inc.) containing ethanol in a concentration that contributed 25% of the total calories; (2) pair-fed: fed isocaloric control diet (identical to the 25% EDC diet except that maltose-dextrin replaced ethanol) in quantities equal to the amount consumed by 25% EDC mice at the same day of pregnancy; or (3) ad-lib: fed isocaloric control diet ad-libitum.

The females in the 25% EDC diet group were fed that diet from day 1 to day 18 of gestation (before mating, these mice were on a 10% EDC diet followed by one more week on 20% EDC to accustom them to ethanol in the diet). Pair-fed mice were paired against 10% EDC and 20% EDC before mating, and against 25% EDC mice after a plug was detected.

Blood alcohol concentrations in mice receiving the 25% EDC diet averaged about 150 mg/100 ml. In all three diet groups, fetuses were obtained at 18 days' gestation. For each litter, all the fetuses were weighed, and the thymus was obtained from the smallest, the largest, and the fetus closest in weight to the average. Cell counts were individually determined for each of the three thymuses, and the cells were then pooled for staining with reagents for FACS analysis. Results from these analyses are shown below (Figure 1).

As can be seen from Fig. 1, fetuses from the 25% EDC group were smaller (by about 22%) than fetuses from the control diet groups. The thymus was even more reduced in size (by about 74%) in fetuses from the alcohol-fed dams. Prenatal alcohol exposure also led to reduced proportions of thymocytes positive for the CD4 and CD8 differentiation antigens. All these differences were statistically significant ($p < 0.01$), when EDC mice were compared with either control group.

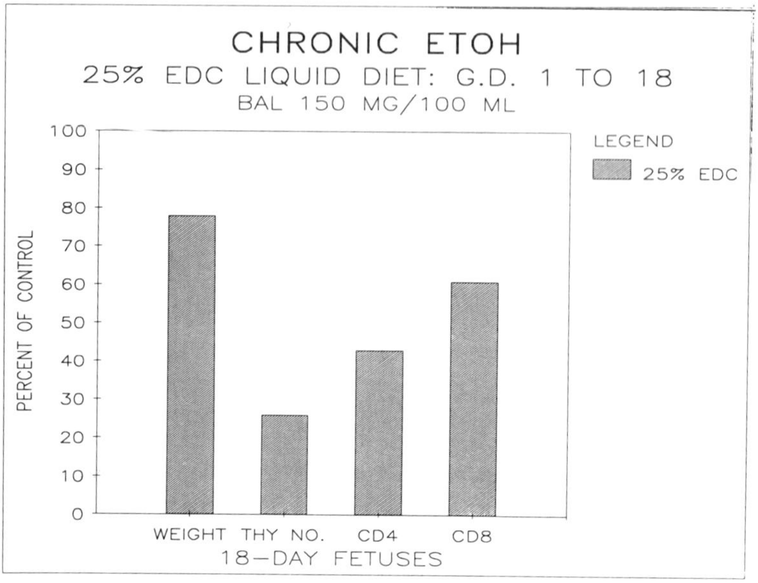

Fig. 1. Effect of chronic ethanol exposure on fetal weight and thymus development. In this figure, values for fetal weight, thymus cell number, proportion of thymocytes expressing CD4 or CD8 antigens are expressed for fetuses from the 25% EDC diet group as a percentage of those values for the pair-fed fetuses (which are set at 100%). Values for these parameters were not significantly different between pair-fed and ad-lib diet groups. (From data published in Ewald and Walden, 1988).

Effect of acute prenatal exposure to teratogenic concentrations of ethanol on development of the thymus in late-term fetuses.

DiGeorge syndrome in humans is a complex of disorders involving heart, face, parathyroids and thymus. These structures have in common contributions from the neural crest, at least in the chicken (Bockman and Kirby, 1984). There is one report in mice that acute prenatal exposure to ethanol during the time that neural crest cells are migrating can lead to heart defects similar to those seen in DiGeorge syndrome (Daft et al., 1986). Certainly, very high blood alcohol concentrations at critical periods of organogenesis can produce malformations of a number of organs and structures, including face, heart and limbs (Webster et al., 1983).

Because of the known teratogenic effects of ethanol on a variety of organs, and the report of an association between DiGeorge syndrome and maternal alcoholism in humans (Ammann et al., 1982), we wondered whether high doses of alcohol <u>in utero</u> might produce "athymia" in mice. Pregnant C57BL/6 mice received 2 intraperitoneal injections, spaced 4 hr apart, of 25% (v/v) alcohol (2.9 g/kg) or saline on one of several days of gestation. This regimen of alcohol injection produced maternal blood alcohol levels (BAL) of 400 to 600 mg/100 ml, as previously reported by others (Webster et al., 1983). Ethanol-injected mice were comatose for several hours following each injection; mice injected with saline were deprived of food and water for 8 hr following the first injection to control for this variable. With this exception, all dams were fed standard lab chow and water <u>ad-libitum</u> throughout gestation.

Fetuses were removed at g.d. 18, weighed, examined for external malformations, and thymus dissected and analyzed. We arbitrarily chose 0.8 g as the cut-off point for intrauterine growth retardation (IUG) (control pups weighed on average more than 0.9 g). As shown in Table 1, when dams were injected on g.d. (plus 12 hr and 16 hr) 7, 8, 9, 10, or 11, some of the pups in each group showed IUG (the most consistent feature of fetal alcohol syndrome). Furthermore, fetuses from dams injected with ethanol on g.d. 9, 12 hr and 16 hr, included a high proportion of pups with forelimb abnormalities (missing fifth, or fourth and fifth, digits). These results are very similar to those of Webster, who reported a high percentage of such forelimb defects in fetuses exposed to ethanol at g.d. 9 or 10. On the other hand, in no group did we find fetuses missing a thymus.

Table 1. Effect of acute prenatal exposure to ethanol on 18-day fetuses

Gestational day (+ 12 hr and 16 hr)	n	Fetuses Weighing <0.8 g	Fetuses with limb defects	Fetuses with athymia
Injection with EtOH (2.9 g/kg):				
day 7	31[4][a]	3[2][a]	0	0
day 8	73[8]	16[5]	0	0
day 9	47[5]	14[4]	14[3]	0
day 10	4[2][b]	4[2]	0	0
day 11	12[2][b]	10[2]	0	0
Injection with saline:				
day 8	29[3]	1[1]	0	0
day 9	20[2]	0	0	0
day 10	10[1]	0	0	0

[a] n = total fetuses [number of litters]
[b] Ethanol injection at days 10 and 11 resulted in a high rate of resorption.

Despite the fact that none of the ethanol-exposed fetuses were completely lacking a thymus (the murine equivalent of DiGeorge syndrome), it was possible that the thymus in some of these animals was abnormal in cell number or antigenic phenotype. Thymuses from all the viable fetuses were dissected, counted, and a pool from 3 fetuses in each litter was analyzed by FACS. Only the data for mice from the 8 day, 12 hr and 16 hr injection group are shown below in Fig. 2. Because data from others (Webster et al., 1983) demonstrate that fetuses with structural malformations are usually lighter in weight than normal fetuses from the same litter, in Fig. 2 we also show data for only those fetuses weighing less than 0.8 g.

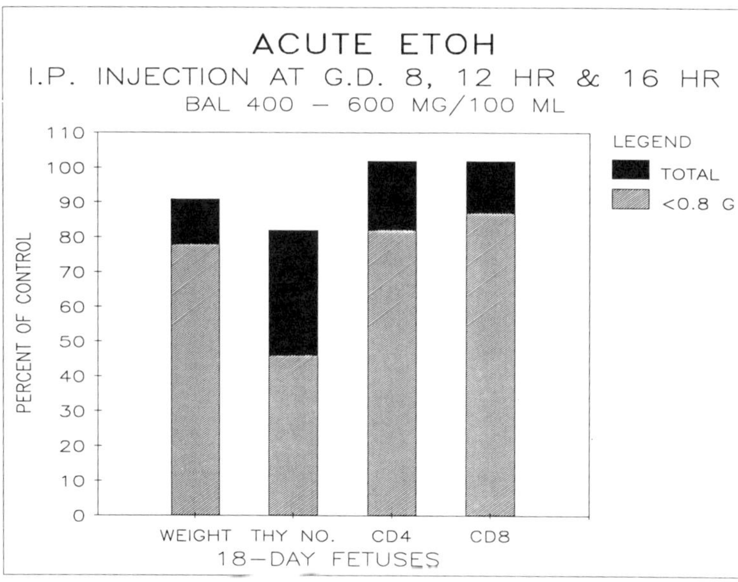

Fig. 2. Effect of acute ethanol exposure at gestational age 8 days, 12 hr and 16 hr, on fetal weight and thymus development. In this figure, values for fetal weight, thymus cell number, and proportion of thymocytes expressing CD4 and CD8 antigens from ethanol-exposed fetuses are expressed as a percentage of those values for fetuses from saline-injected (control) dams. Hatched bars represent the values for only those fetuses weighing less than 0.8 g. The black bars are the values for all fetuses from the alcohol-injected dams.

The results of these analyses indicate that the average weight of fetuses from dams injected with ethanol on g.d. 8, 12 hr and 16 hr is 91% ($p < 0.05$) of the value for saline-injected fetuses (Fig. 2). Thymus size for all litters in the ethanol-injected fetuses is 82% ($p > 0.10$) that of the controls, while CD4 and CD8 expression are normal. If only the fetuses weighing less than 0.8 g are considered, thymus number is 46% of the control value compared to fetal weight 78% of the control. CD4 and CD8 expression are reduced to about the same extent as fetal weight (82% and 87% of controls, respectively).

DISCUSSION

Results from these studies in mice demonstrate that chronic prenatal exposure to ethanol at levels yielding maternal BAL typical of human alcoholics (BAL >100 mg/100 ml) caused retardation of thymus development. Both thymus cell number and expression of CD4 and CD8 differentiation antigens were reduced in thymuses of 18-day fetuses from dams fed a 25% EDC diet throughout gestation.

One obvious question is whether effects of prenatal alcohol exposure on the immune system persist after birth. Preliminary data (Huang, Reed, and Ewald, manuscript in preparation) indicate that _in utero_ exposure to ethanol (23% EDC) in mice leads to changes in immune responses such as delayed-type hypersensitivity and spleen plaque-forming cell numbers, when pups are tested 4-7 weeks after birth.

In utero exposure of mice to extremely high doses of ethanol (maternal BAL >400 mg/100 ml) during developmental stages when the thymus was forming did not lead to athymia. However, some of the mice in our experimental groups demonstrated limb defects and intrauterine growth retardation (as previously described by Webster et al., 1983, as well as others); therefore, our experimental regimen did reproduce some of the teratogenic effects of alcohol previously described. It may be that alcohol contributes to DiGeorge syndrome (including absent thymus), but must interact with other cofactors such as genetic predisposition or other drugs. Certainly, human alcoholics have been reported with blood alcohol levels in the range of those attained in mice in these studies (e.g., Lindblad and Olsson, 1976), so that a human fetus might be exposed to such teratogenic ethanol concentrations.

In summary, our studies show that chronic maternal consumption of ethanol during pregnancy led to impaired thymus development in late-term fetal mice. Acute exposure to high maternal blood alcohol levels during gestational periods critical for thymus development did not result in failure of epithelial thymus formation, though these same alcohol treatments were teratogenic to other systems. Work is in progress to determine longer-term consequences of chronic prenatal alcohol exposure to immune system development.

Acknowledgments. This work was supported by research grant #AA07010 and by a Research Scientist Development Award #K02 AA00105, both from the ADAMHA awarding Institute NIAAA.

REFERENCES

Abel ER (1984). "Fetal Alcohol Syndrome and Fetal Alcohol Effects." New York: Plenum Press.

Adkins B, Mueller C, Okada C, Reichert R, Weissman IL, Spangrude GJ (1987). Early events in T-cell maturation. Ann Rev Immunol 5:325-365.

Ammann AJ, Wara D, Cowan MJ, Barrett DJ, Stiehm ER (1982). The DiGeorge syndrome and the fetal alcohol syndrome. Am J Dis Child 136:906-908.

Bockman DE, Kirby ML (1984). Dependence of thymus development on derivatives of the neural crest. Science 223:498-500.

Calvani M, Ghirelli D, Calvani M, Fortuna C, Lalli F, Marcolini P (1985). Fetal alcohol syndrome: Clinical, metabolic, and immunologic follow-up in 14 cases. Minerva Pediatr 37:77-88.

Ceredig R, Dialynas DP, Fitch F, MacDonald HR (1983). Precursors of T cell growth factor producing cells in the thymus: Ontogeny, frequency, and quantitative recovery in a subpopulation of phenotypically mature thymocytes defined by monoclonal antibody GK-1.5. J Exp Med 158:1654-1671.

Daft PA, Johnston MC, Sulik KK (1986). Abnormal heart and great vessel development following acute ethanol exposure in mice. Teratology 33:93-104.

Ewald SJ, Frost WW (1987). Effect of prenatal exposure to ethanol on development of the thymus. Thymus 9:211-215.

Ewald SJ, Walden SM (1988). Flow cytometric and histological analysis of mouse thymus in fetal alcohol syndrome. J Leuk Biol 44:434-440.

Itoh T (1987). Development of Thy 1 positive mouse thymocytes. Analysis of early fetal thymocytes by flow microfluorometry. Thymus 9:217-223.

Johnson S, Knight R, Marmier DJ, Steele RW (1981). Immune deficiency in fetal alcohol syndrome. Pediatr Res 15:908-911.

Jotereau F, Heuze F, Salomon-Vie V, Gascan H (1987). Cell kinetics in the fetal mouse thymus: Precursor cell input, proliferation, and emigration. J Immunol 138:1026-1030.

Lindblad B, Olsson R (1976). Unusually high levels of blood alcohol? JAMA 236:1600-1602.

Monjan AA, Mandell W (1980). Fetal alcohol and immunity: Depression of mitogen-induced lymphocyte blasto- genesis. Neurobehavioral Toxicology 2:213-215.

Owen JJT, Jenkinson EJ (1984). Early events in T lymphocyte genesis in the fetal thymus. Am J Anat 170:301-310.

Webster WS, Walsh DA, McEwen SE, Lipson AH (1983). Some teratogenic properties of ethanol and acetaldehyde in C57BL/6J mice: Implications for the study of the fetal alcohol syndrome. Teratology 27:231-243.

Alcohol, Immunomodulation, and AIDS, pages 201–209
© 1990 Alan R. Liss, Inc.

EFFECTS OF CHRONIC ALCOHOL INTAKE ON PLACENTAL TRANSPORT OF IgG

William P. Jollie and Hamdy M. Aly

Department of Anatomy, Medical College of Virginia, Virginia Commonwealth University, Richmond, VA 23298

INTRODUCTION

Alcohol abuse during pregnancy is known to produce intrauterine growth retardation (Stein and Susser, 1984; Lin, 1985; Halmesmaki et al., 1986; Synder, Singh and Pullen, 1986). Moreover, in new-born infants associated with intrauterine growth retardation immunoglobulin concentrations are known to be suppressed (Yang, et al., 1983). Although it has been found that serum levels of immunoglobulins in alcoholics are abnormal, however, it is the level of IgA that increases; the IgG level is unaltered (Drew et al., 1984). If indeed the concentration of IgG remains unaffected by alcohol, then a failure in the acquisition of neonatal immunity is likely the result of failure in mechanisms for maternofetal exchange of this immunoglobulin class, since it is the transport of IgG across the placental membrane that provides humans with neonatal immunocompetence before birth (Burnett, 1968). Moreover, alcohol consumption has been shown to have an acute deleterious effect on the fine structure of the human placenta (Amankwah and Kaufman, 1984). The controlling cellular mechanisms for placental transport of IgG during pregnancy are very poorly understood; the effects of chronic alcohol intake on such mechanisms are unknown.

Placentas from chronically alcoholic women rarely are available. Moreover, ethical restraint prevents the use of pregnant women in any investigation of placental transport mechanisms. Furthermore, use of human tissues would introduce too many variables for meaningful data-assessment of results of alcohol intake in such a study. Only by using a suitable animal model is it possible to examine the effects of alcohol on placental transport without interference from such compounding variables as nutritional status, multidrug abuse, prior exposure to alcohol and other drugs, and resultant organ damage. The laboratory rat has been the animal model of choice for such studies for several reasons. After the human, it is the species whose reproductive biology is most completely understood. Furthermore, alcohol can be self-administered in pharmacologically significant amounts from a completely liquid, nutritionally adequate diet that contains ethanol as a fixed percentage of total daily caloric intake. A suitable pair-feeding system can be used to insure the absence of other variables, even circadian variables in feeding patterns. Maintenance on such a system over time assures that any variations in transfer of immunity to the fetus are a result of alcohol, not of malnutrition. Moreover, it has been been known for more than 30 years that in rats, like in humans, neonatal immunity is acquired by transfer of antibody as IgG from maternal to fetal blood compartments just before term (Bramble, 1958; Mayersbach, 1958). Although the membranes responsible for such placental transport are not homologous in the two species, uptake of the antibody by receptor-mediated endocytosis, its intracellular sorting either for ultimate hydrolysis or for translocation and exocytosis, and its final deposition into a peripheral fetal placental capillary network are by similar, if not identical cellular mechanisms (Jollie, 1985; 1986).

The purpose of the present study was to determine the effects of drinking alcohol during pregnancy on the development of immunocompetency in the fetus. Specifically the protocol was designed to assess the effects of ethanol consumption in rats on the controlling mechanisms for cellular translocation of antibody through placental membranes during antepartum acquisition of neonatal immunity. For this investigation a model system was developed for studying immunity-transporting placental membranes in an in-vitro system. The long-term objective of such studies is to ascertain and characterize the pernicious effects of maternal alcohol consumption on the cellular mechanisms for placental transfer by means of which, at the end of pregnancy, an individual acquires immunologic protection until, following birth, it develops its own immunologic competence.

EXPERIMENTAL PROCEDURES

Care and Breeding of Animals: Ten 200-250 gm Sprague Dawley rats were maintained on a high protein liquid diet (Liquid Rat Diet for Pregnant Animals: BioServ, Inc.) in which 36% of the total calories were provided by ethanol; 10 females similarly were maintained on a liquid diet (ibid.) made isocaloric with maltose and dextrose (Lieber and DeCarli, 1982); the animals were simultaneously pair-fed (Israel, Oporto and Macdonald, 1984) to insure both equal daily caloric intake and identical feeding patterns. After a minimum of six weeks on such a feeding system, vaginal lavages were taken daily to identify proestrus. The animals were caged (fasting) overnight with breeder males, and a second lavage was made the following morning. The day when sperm were identified in the second lavage was designated as the first day of pregnancy. Placental tissues were taken by surgical removal, and the animals were subsequently euthanized on either the 12th, 17th or 22nd days of pregnancy (term = 23 days).

Tissue Culture Techniques: By uterine incision the visceral yolk sacs of 4 fetuses from each animal were exposed; and, in 12- and 17- day pregnancies the entire membrane together with both the attached chorioallantois and enclosed fetus was removed and transferred immediately to sterile Dulbecco's minimum essential medium (MEM) at 37°C that contained either 2 mg horseradish perioxidase-conjugated-rat immunoglobulin G (HRP-IgG) per ml MEM, 1 mg HRP alone /ml MEM, or 1 mg rat IgG alone/ml MEM. At autopsy for 22-day pregnancies the visceral yolk sac was removed from opened gestation sacs and cultured similarly. Tissues were cultured in the three media at 37°C in a humidified (95.5%) CO_2 incubator for 1 hr.

Tissue Preparation for Electron Microscopic Immunocytochemistry: After a quick wash in MEM alone at room temperature, cultured visceral yolk-sac membranes were fixed in 2% paraformaldehyde, 1% glutaraldehyde and 0.1 M phosphate buffer with 0.01% $CaCl_2$ at pH 7.4 and at room temperature for 1 hour. They were washed briefly in 0.1 M phosphate buffer plus 5% sucrose at pH 7.4, then in 0.05 M Tris-HCl buffer at pH 7.5. Subsequently each membrance was incubated in 3 mg diaminobenzidime tetrahydrochloride in 10 ml 0.05 M Tris-HCl buffer at pH 7.5 with 0.01% H_2O_2 for 30 minutes, washed briefly in first 0.05M Tris-Hcl, then 0.1 M phosphate buffer, and post fixed in 2% OsO_4 in 0.1 M phosphate buffer at pH 7.4 and at 4° C for 2 hours. Finally they were dehydrated through a graded series of ethanols, passed through propylene oxide and embedded in Durcupan. Thin sections were cut on a LKB Ultratome-II and mounted on copper grids; the grids were examined and photographed at 75 kV in a Zeiss EM 10C electron microscope without contrast enhancement with heavy metal salts.

An additional yolk-sac membrane upon surgical removal from each of the 20 animals was fixed directly in the paraformaldehyde/glutaraldehyde mixture and processed for routine electron microscopy and with heavy metal salt contrast enhancement to characterize the effects of prolonged alcohol intake on the fine structure of the yolk-sac placental membrane at each of the 3 stages of pregnancy.

RESULTS

Yolk-sac epithelial tissues that have been exposed to chronic alcoholism show alterations in the fine structure of the visceral endodermal absorptive epithelium. Golgi elements are hypertrophied and often appear organized in a GERL configuration in which several flattened cisterns are separated off the concave side of the Golgi stack and are straightened (Fig.1). Primary lysosomes are markedly abundant (Figs. 1 and 2). Cisterns of granular endoplasmic reticulum are constricted and often appear beaded; and mitochondria reveal an internal organization in which cristae are in tubular and/or vesicular forms (Fig. 2).

Compared to cultured tissues from control liquid-diet-fed animals (Fig. 3), cultured tissues from alcohol-diet fed animals showed a marked reduction in stored reaction product of HRP-IgG localization in the subapical cytoplasm of the absorptive epithelium (Fig. 4); binding of HRP-IgG to specific receptor sites on the exposed cell membrane of these cells and its internalization into the apical cytoplasm, however, appeared unaffected by alcohol.

Cultured tissues from control-fed animals, however, contained an absorptive epithelium in which the reaction product of HRP-IgG localization could be identified in an infranuclear position within individual epithelial cells, even adjacent to the basal plasmalemma; furthermore, reaction product occasionally was localized both in the endothelium of subepithelial fetal capillaries and in fetal red blood cells (Fig. 5).

CONCLUSIONS

1. Ingestion of a nutritionally complete high protein liquid diet in which ethanol provides 36% of the caloric intake both for 6 weeks and a subsequent pregnancy, produces ultrastructural differences in the cells of the absorptive epithelium of the visceral yolk-sac placentas of rats; among them: hypertrophy of Golgi elements; a narrowing of cisterns of granular endoplasmic reticulum; increased production of primary lysosomes; and conversion of mitochondrial cristae to tubular and vesicular forms. Such changes denote increased production of lysosomes from Golgi elements and augmented acid hydrolase activity as a result of exposure to alcohol.

2. By immunocytochemical localization, such an alcohol diet appears not to affect binding of HRP-conjugated rat IgG to specific receptor sites on the exposed surface of the epithelium and its endocytosis in membranes cultured *in vitro*, but to impede sorting of antibody and translocation across the epithelium for exocytosis and transfer into the vitelline circulation.

3. Although in the *in-vivo* system receptor-mediated endocytosis of antibody, its translocation for basal exocytosis and transfer to vitelline capillaries previously has been identified only in visceral yolk-sac membranes near term (at 22 days of a 23 day gestation period), in tissues from animals on an isocaloric, but alcohol-free, liquid diet, such maternofetal transfer has been demonstrated immunocytochemically as well in 12- and 17-day yolk-sac placentas that are maintained for an hour *in vitro*.

This last observation calls into question the efficacy of the *in-vitro* method for studying cellular mechanisms for placental transfer and strongly suggests the need for an *in-vivo* model.

Supported by the Franklin Fund of the Medical College of Virginia Foundation.

FIGURES

Figure 1. Alcohol-exposed 22-day yolk-sac epithelial cell cytoplasm. Note the hypertrophied Golgi stacks (GS), the associated flattened GERL cisterns (GERL), and the abundance of primary lysosomes (*). X 75,000

Figure 2, Alcohol-exposed 22-day yolk-sac epithelial cell. Primary lysosomes (arrows), constricted, beaded cisterns of granular endoplasmic reticulum (C), and mitochondria with tubular and/or vesicular cristae (M) are abundant. X 1,500

Figure 3. Control yolk-sac placental membrane cultured 1 hr on MEM with HRP-IgG. Note the abundance of reaction product in the subapical cytoplasm of the absorptive epithelium. L-lipid droplet; YSC = yolk-sac cavity; RBC = fetal erythrocyte. X 12,500

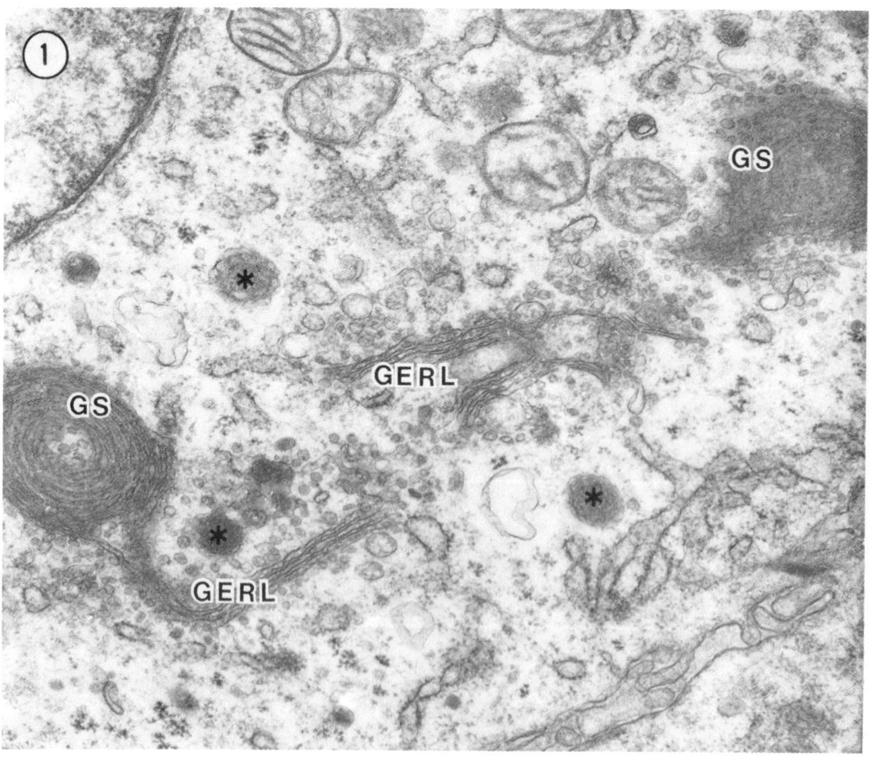

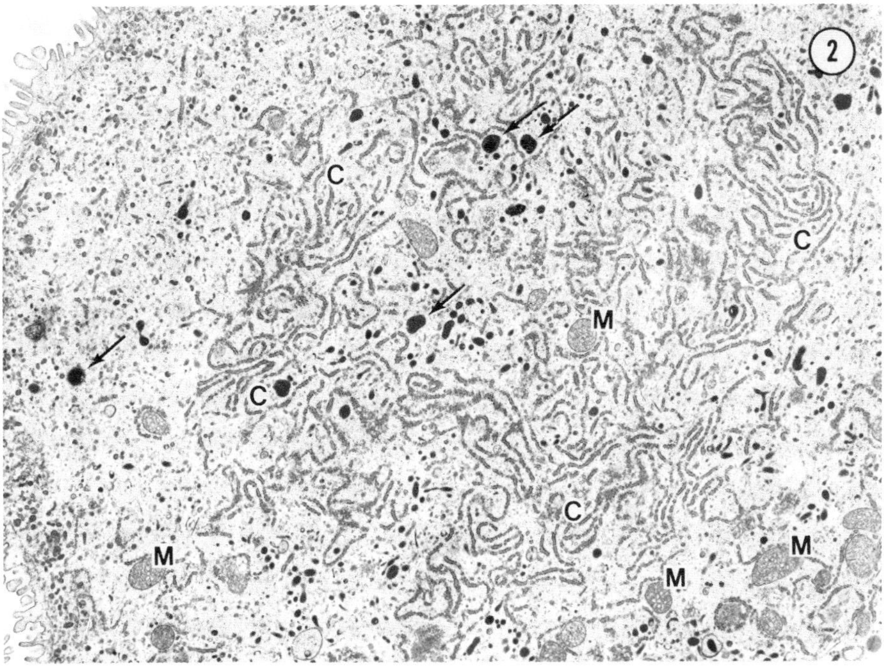
2
C
C
M
C
C
M
M
M

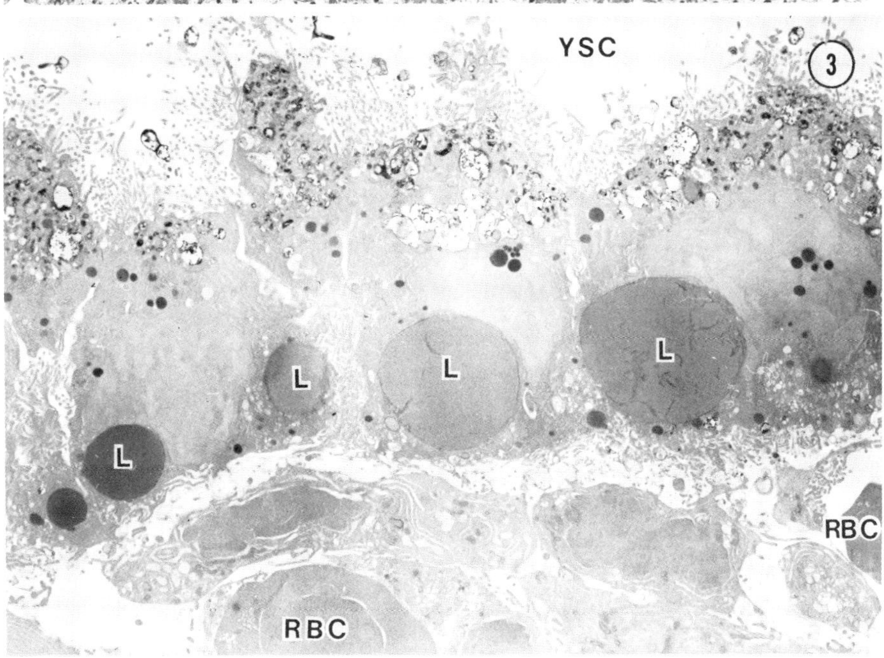
YSC
3
L
L
L
L
RBC
RBC

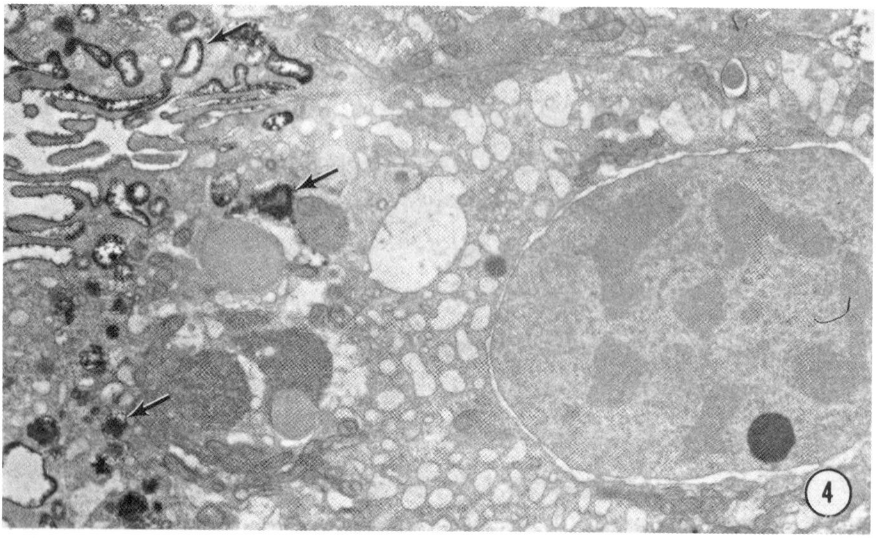

Figure 4. Alcohol-exposed placental membrane cultured as above. Note binding of reaction product to the apical membrane and evidence of endocytosis (arrows). X 20,000

Figure 5. Basal aspect of the absorptive epithelium and subjacent connective tissue compartment in a 12-day cultured control yolk sac. Note the presence of reaction product in epithelial cells, in the endothelium of a capillary (EN), and in a fetal erythrocyte (RBC). X 75,000

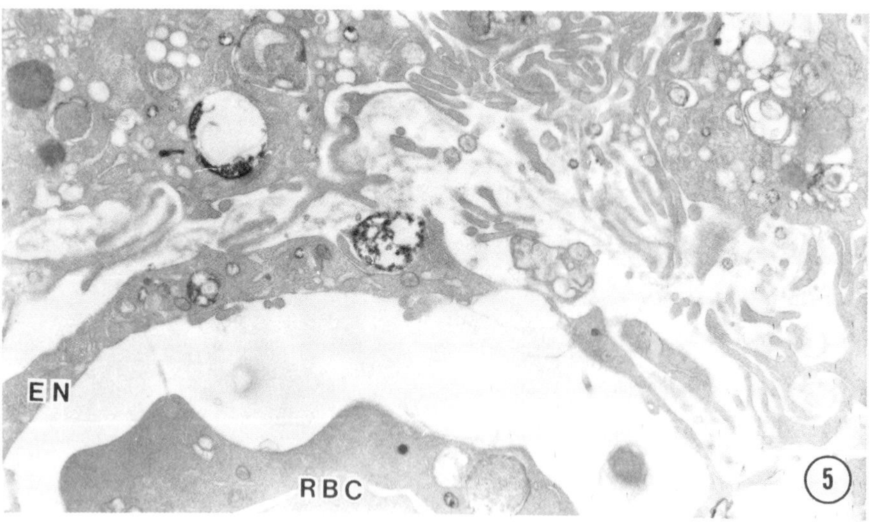

REFERENCES

Amanakwah KS, Kaufman RC (1984). Ultrastructure of human placenta: effects of maternal drinking. Gynecol Obstet Invest 18:311-316.

Brambell FWR (1958). The passive immunity of the young mammal. Biol Rev 33:485-531.

Burnett LS (1968). Development of the immune process. In: Intrauterine Development. Barnes AC, ed. Lea & Febiger (Philadelphia).

Drew PA, Clifton PM, LaBroog JT, Shearman DJ (1984). Polyclonal B cell activation in alcoholic patients with no evidence of liver dysfunction. Clin Exp Immunol 57:479-486.

Halmesmaki E, Autti I, Granstom ML, Heikenheimo M, Raivio KL, Ylikorkala (1986). Alpha-fetoprotein, human placental lactogen and pregnancy-specific beta 1-glycoprotein in pregnant women who drink:relation to fetal alcohol syndrome. Am J Obstet Gynecol 155:598-602.

Israel Y, Oporto B, Macdonald, A (1984). Simultaneous pair-feeding system for the administration of alcohol-containing liquid diets. Alcohol Clin Exp Res 8:1-9.

Jollie WP (1985). Immunocytochemical localization of antibody during placental transmission of immunity in rats. J Reprod Immunol 7:261-274.

Jollie WP (1986). Ultrastructural studies of protein transfer across the rodent yolk sac. Placenta 7:263-281.

Lieber CS, DeCarli LM (1982). The feeding of alcohol in liquid diets: two decades of application and 1982 update. Alc Clin Exp Res 6:2-10.

Lin CC (1985). Intrauterine growth retardation. Obstet Gynecol Annu 14:127-221.

Mayersbach HV (1958). Zur Frage des Proteinüberganges von der Mutter zum Föten. I. Befunde an Ratten am Ende der Schwangerschaft. Zeit für Zellforsch Mikrosk Anat 48:479-504.

Snyder AK, Singh SP, Pullen GL (1986). Ethanol-induced intrauterine growth retardation: correlation with placental glucose transfer. Alcoholism 10:167-170.

Stein ZA, Susser M (1984). Intrauterine growth retardation: epidemiological issues and public health significance. Semin Perinatol pp 5-14.

Yang SL, Lin CC, River P, Moawad AH (1983). Immunoglobulin concentrations in newborn infants associated with intra-uterine growth retardation. Obstet Gynecol 62:561-564.

Alcohol, Immunomodulation, and AIDS, pages 211–220
© 1990 Alan R. Liss, Inc.

ALCOHOL-INDUCED SUPPRESSION OF TUMOR NECROSIS FACTOR-A POTENTIAL RISK FACTOR FOR SECONDARY INFECTION IN THE ACQUIRED IMMUNODEFICIENCY SYNDROME.

Steve Nelson, Gregory J. Bagby, and Warren R. Summer

Departments of Pulmonary/Critical Care Medicine and Physiology, Louisiana State University Medical Center, New Orleans, LA 70112

INTRODUCTION

The immunoregulatory function of macrophages is of primary importance in normal host defenses against invasive microorganisms (Toews, 1986). The alveolar macrophage (AM) represents the first-line of defense for the respiratory membranes. In addition to its potent phagocytic capabilities, the AM is an active secretory cell and can markedly influence the immune response of the host to potential pathogens from the initial breech of the lower respiratory tract to its eventual repair (Nathan, 1987).

Ethanol has been shown to suppress selected functions of the immune system thereby compromising host defenses (MacGregor, 1986). Pneumonia is among the most common of these infections affecting the alcoholic host (MacGregor, 1986). Patients with the acquired immunodeficiency syndrome (AIDS) also typically manifest their disease with recurrent pulmonary opportunistic infections (Murray et al., 1987). Defective monocyte and macrophage function is an integral part of the immunopathology of alcoholism and AIDS, leading to the failure of the host to control these pathogens (Bender et al., 1988). It is possible that alcohol may pharmacologically modify the interaction of the human immunodeficiency virus (HIV) with the host resulting in a depression of the immune mechanisms which functionally serve to limit its clinical expression.

Although not widely appreciated, it has become increasingly clear that in addition to opportunistic infections, patients infected with HIV are at an increased risk for bacterial pneumonias and have a higher incidence of these infections when compared to the general population (Polsky et al., 1986; Schlamm and Yancovitz, 1989). Indeed, the development of bacterial pneumonia in HIV-infected patients may be a harbinger of their underlying disease and identify patients at risk for AIDS (Witt et al., 1987). In these immunocompromised patients, any factor that further compromises the remaining, intact antimicrobial systems, such as alcohol,might abrogate the protective redundancy of the host defense system and lead to an increased incidence of bacterial infection.

Tumor necrosis factor-alpha (TNF), a macrophage-derived cytokine, is a potent mediator of the inflammatory cascade and plays a central role in mobilizing host defenses against invasive microorganisms (Beutler and Cerami, 1987). We propose that one mechanism by which alcohol impairs host defenses is by suppressing macrophage synthesis and release of TNF. In order to determine this, we studied the effect of acute alcohol administration on bronchoalveolar lavage (BAL) fluid TNF, cellular response, and intrapulmonary bactericidal activity in animals intratracheally challenged with Staphylococcus aureus or Klebsiella pneumoniae, two common pathogens in bacterial pneumonia.

METHODS

Saline or ethanol (5.5 g/kg as a 20% solution) was administered intraperitoneally to 200-225 gm Sprague-Dawley male rats followed 30 min later by intratracheal saline, Klebsiella pneumoniae or Staphylococcus aureus.

Staphylococcus aureus 209 P, Phage type 42D (American Type Culture Collection, Rockville, MD) or Klebsiella pneumoniae (laboratory strain) was incubated in 125 ml of tryptic soy broth (TSB) at 37^{0} C in a rotating shaker water bath. After 18 h, the culture was centrifuged (3,000 x g for 10 min), washed twice with phosphate-buffered saline solution (PBS), and resuspended in 10 ml of TSB. Intratracheally challenged rats were placed under mild anesthesia with ether, and a midline incision was performed above the sternum exposing the trachea by blunt dissection.

A 28-gauge needle was then inserted into the trachea above the carina, and 0.5 ml of the bacterial suspension was instilled.

Following intratracheal challenge, rats were killed immediately (zero hour) and at 4 h. The lungs were aseptically removed and cultured quantitatively by standard pour plate techniques in 5% NaCl-tryptic soy agar for S. aureus and in MacConkey agar for K. pneumoniae. Quantitation of bacterial colony-forming units (CFU) was determined after 48 h of incubation at 37° C. Pulmonary bactericidal activity was quantitated as the percentage of the number of viable bacteria in the lungs at 4 h post-intratracheal challenge compared to the mean bacterial count deposited in the lungs at 0 h.

Total and differential counts of free pulmonary cells obtained by bronchoalveolar lavage were quantified prior to and at 240 min post-intratracheal bacterial challenge. The rats were euthanized with ether and each pair of lungs were surgically removed in toto and lavaged with PBS containing 3 mM ethylenediaminetetraacetic acid at room temperature.

The recovered lavage fluid was centrifuged (200 x g for 5 min), and the cell pellet resuspended in 1.0 ml of Hank's balanced salt solution. Direct cell counts were performed with a hemacytometer. Morphologic differentiation was performed on cell monlayers prepared by cytocentrifugation and stained with Wright-Giemsa solution. TNF activity was measured in lavage fluid in a separate group of rats 2 h after intratracheal bacterial challenge and expressed as units per ml of recovered lavage fluid.

TNF-alpha activity in BAL specimens was determined with a cytotoxicity assay utilizing L929 cells obtained from American Type Culture Collection, Rockville, MD. Briefly, 2 x 10^4 L929 cells were planted in the wells of microtiter plates and allowed to adhere overnight. The next day wells were treated with serial dilutions of the specimens followed by addition of actinomycin D (1.0 ug/ml, final conc.). After an 18 h incubation at 37° C in 5% CO_2, the wells were washed and surviving cells indexed with a chromogenic assay for hexosaminidase (Landegren, 1984). A unit of TNF activity was defined as the reciprocal of the dilution required to kill 50% of the cells which was normalized against murine recombinant TNF-alpha. Cell lytic activity in BAL samples was completely neutralized by the addition of rabbit antibody against murine recombinant TNF-alpha (Genentech, Inc., San Francisco, CA) indicating that cell killing was due specifically to TNF-alpha.

Blood alcohol levels were quantitated by an enzymatic assay (Kit #332-UV, Sigma) which spectrophotmetrically detects reduction of nicotinamide adenosine dinucleotide during oxidation by alcohol dehydrogenase. All data are reported as mean ± standard error. Data were analyzed using analysis of variance and a Student's two tailed t-test where indicated.

RESULTS

TNF was not detected in the BAL fluid from normal rats challenged with saline. In contrast, intratracheal challenge with S. aureus or K. pneumoniae in normal rats resulted in the appearance of significant TNF activity in BAL fluid at 2 h post-challenge (Table 1). Acute alcohol administration markedly attenuated (>75%) S. aureus or K. pneumoniae induced TNF activity in lung lavage specimens. In these animals, blood ethanol levels were in the range of 300-350 mg/dl during the 4 h observation period.

TABLE 1. Tumor Necrosis Factor in Control and Ethanol-Treated Rats Two Hours Following Intratracheal Bacterial Challenge.

Bacterial Challenge	Group	BAL TNF units/ml
S. aureus	Control	1537±199
	Ethanol	239±86*
K. pneumoniae	Control	3012±356
	Ethanol	678±114*

Data expressed as mean ± SEM, n=6-8
*Statistical difference from matched control ($p \leq 0.01$)

Intratracheal inoculation of S. aureus deposited $6.1 \pm 0.4 \times 10^7$ CFU in the lungs of the control animals at zero hour. By 4 h, 58±3% of the initial bacterial challenge remained viable. In marked contrast, in alcohol-treated rats the bacteria proliferated to 126±4%, indicating a significant failure of pulmonary antibacterial defenses in these animals against S. aureus (Table 2). At zero hour, 6.5±0.2 x 10^7 CFU of K. pneumoniae were deposited in the lungs of intratracheally challenged rats. In control animals, 72±5% of their initial challenge was viable at 4 h. However, in alcohol intoxicated rats, 282±7% of the initial bacterial challenge remained viable within the lung (Table 2). These differences in pulmonary bactericidal activities between control and alcohol-treated rats in response to intratracheal S. aureus or K pneumoniae were highly significant ($p \leq 0.01$).

TABLE 2. Pulmonary Bactericidal Activity and Total and Differential Cell Counts in BAL Fluid Four Hours Following Bacterial Challenge.

Bacterial Challenge	Group	CELL COUNTS Total ($\times 10^6$)	% AM	% PMN	% Bacteria Viable
S. aureus	Control	12.2±0.9	57.2±2.6	42.8±2.6	58±3
	Ethanol	6.3±0.6*	97.8±1.0*	2.2±1.0*	126±4*
K. pneumoniae	Control	57.9±3.0	17.8±1.7	82.2±1.7	72±5
	Ethanol	10.1±0.9*	72.4±2.0*	27.6±2.0*	282±7*

Data expressed as mean ± SEM, n=6-8
*Statistical difference from matched control ($p \leq 0.01$)

The total cell counts and percentage of polymorphonuclear leukocytes (PMN) and AM recovered by lung lavage from control and alcohol-treated rats in response to intratracheal S. aureus or K. pneumoniae are shown in Table 2. Bronchoalveolar lavage in rats prior to intratracheal challenge recovered approximately 5.5 ±0.6 x 10^6 cells of which 99% were alveolar macrophages and 1% were PMN. Acute alcohol administration did not significantly affect the number of cells recovered prior to bacterial challenge. Intrapulmonary instillation of S. aureus or K. pneumoniae elicited large increases in the number of PMN recovered by bronchoalveolar lavage. In contrast, acute alcohol administration markedly suppressed this intrapulmonary inflammatory response to the challenge organism.

DISCUSSION

These data show that acute alcohol intoxication markedly suppresses BAL fluid TNF, PMN recruitment, and the antibacterial defenses of the lung against both S. aureus and K. pneumoniae. Our laboratory has recently reported that ethanol similarly suppresses serum and lung TNF elicited in response to challenges with intravenous or intratracheal lipopolysaccharide (LPS) (Nelson et al., 1989). We propose that alcohol-induced inhibition of TNF may be a potential pathway increasing host susceptibility to invasive bacterial infections.

The predominant pathophysiologic effects of TNF are largely unknown. TNF is a 17-kd polypeptide produced by the macrophage in response to multiple stimuli including viruses and bacteria and their products, such as LPS (Beutler and Cerami, 1987). TNF is a potent activator of phagocyte functions and a proximal mediator of the inflammatory cascade. As such, much of the recent literature has implicated excessive, systemic levels of TNF in the pathogenesis of endotoxemia and septic shock (Tracey et al., 1988). However, the role of TNF locally produced and released within the lung may have entirely different consequences to the host. We have previously reported that intratracheal LPS-induced TNF is compartmentalized and does not spillover into the vascular space (Nelson et al., 1989). In these normal animals, the increase in BAL fluid TNF, from non-detectable levels in the unchallenged lung, precedes the development of an inflammatory response within the lung. Similar findings have been reported with intratracheal challenges of Legionella pneumophilia (Blanchard et al., 1987). Aerosol administration of TNF to animals also does not result in significant serum levels and, furthermore, primes the alveolar macrophage for enhanced secretory activity (Debs et al., 1988). Finally, administration of recombinant TNF has been reported by others to enhance the bactericidal capacity of the lung against L. pneumophilia and by our group against S. aureus (Blanchard et al., 1988; Nelson et al., 1989). Therefore, like most other inflammatory mediators, TNF, depending upon the specific stimulus, underlying host status, and the magnitude of the response, may be either beneficial or potentially harmful to the host.

Recently, TNF has been detected in sera from patients infected with HIV suggesting a possible correlation between TNF concentration and the severity of their disease (Lahdevirta et al., 1988). Asymptomatic carriers of HIV had the lowest levels of TNF while actively infected patients with manifest AIDS had the highest levels. An alternative explanation for these observations is that the higher TNF levels in the patients with AIDS was directly a consequence of an active secondary infection in these patients. In the majority of the patients studied, TNF levels were highest in those patients with an active secondary infection and were lower in these individuals during periods of less secondary infection. It is known that normal, healthy individuals produce TNF in response to an infectious stimulus (Michie et al., 1988). Therefore, it is possible that the TNF detected in these HIV-infected patients was an appropriate and beneficial response to their secondary infection. Indeed, given their propensity for relapse and re-infections, patients infected with HIV may be, in fact, hypo-responders and this may be one of the underlying mechanisms of their immunosuppressed status. Furthermore, recent studies suggest that TNF does have an antiviral effect <u>in vitro</u>, and thus, conceivably, could offer protection from HIV itself in addition to other invading pathogens (Wong and Goeddel, 1986).

Considerable evidence exists for the suppression of multiple facets of PMN function by alcohol (MacGregor, 1986; MacGregor et al., 1988). At present, there is no evidence to suggest that PMN play a role in the host response to primary infection with HIV. However, the PMN does play a pivotal role in the host's response to many bacterial pathogens affecting HIV-infected patients, and a defect in the inflammatory response would significantly decrease host resistance in these individuals. It is clear that HIV is capable of infecting mononuclear phagocytic cells and macrophages may comprise a major tissue target for the virus. Macrophages of patients with AIDS demonstrate a wide variety of <u>in vitro</u> and <u>in vivo</u> abnormalities (Bender et al., 1988). Since many of the microorganisms causing infections in AIDS are intracellular pathogens that are normally held in check by these cells, it is likely that defective macrophage function contributes to the multiple occurrence of infections in AIDS. To date, the effect of HIV infection on alveolar macrophage TNF activity is unknown. However, it is at this site of action, that alcohol may act as a co-factor in the pathogenesis of infections in these patients.

These studies demonstrate that alcohol intoxication markedly suppresses AM-derived TNF within the alveolar space produced in response to intratracheal challenges with either a gram-positive or a gram-negative bacterium. This impaired response was associated with a significant inhibition of PMN recruitment and resulted in the proliferation of the pathogens within the lung. TNF has been shown to have opposing effects on PMN chemotaxis that appear to be dose-dependent (Yonemaru et al., 1988). At low concentrations it stimulates chemotaxis while at higher concentrations it inhibits chemotaxis. This dual effect may serve to both initiate and then localize the inflammatory response of the host to an invading pathogen. This would provide an effective mechanism of "stand and fight" by which these cells combat invading microorganisms.

Infection is the clinical manifestation of multiple interactions involving immunologic defenses, metabolism, and nutrition. Clearly, the multiple diverse effects of alcohol on these factors renders the otherwise normal host more susceptible to infections. It is likely that in patients infected with HIV, whose host defenses are operational at a tenuous level at best, alcohol consumption may be an important co-factor in the pathogenesis and clinical manifestations of their disease.

ACKNOWLEDGMENTS

This work was supported by grant #AA07710 from the National Institute on Alcoholism and Alcohol Abuse. We thank Amy Weinberg, Rhonda R. Martinez and Amad Jawda for their technical support and Debbie McNamara for her secretarial assistance.

REFERENCES

Bender BS, Davidson BL, Kline R, Brown C, Quinn TC (1988). Role of the mononuclear phagocyte system in the immunopathogenesis of human immunodeficiency virus infection and the acquired immunodeficiency syndrome. Rev Infect Dis 10:1142-1154.

Beutler B, Cerami A (1987). Cachectin: more than a tumor necrosis factor. N Engl J Med 316:379-385.

Blanchard DK, Djeu JY, Klein TW, Friedman H, Stewart WE (1987). Induction of tumor necrosis factor by Legionella pneumophila. Infect Immun 55:433-437.

Blanchard DK, Djeu JY, Klein TW, Friedman H, Stewart WE (1988). Protective effects of tumor necrosis factor in experimental Legionella pneumophila infections of mice via activation of PMN function. J Leukocyte Biol 43:429-435.

Debs RJ, Fuchs HJ, Philip R, Montgomery AB, Brunette EN, Liggitt D, Patton JS, Shellito JE (1988). Lung-specific delivery of cytokines induces sustained pulmonary and systemic immunomodulation in rats. J Immunol 140:3482-3488.

Lahdevirta J, Maury CPJ, Teppo AM, Repo H (1988). Elevated levels of circulating cachectin/tumor necrosis factor in patients with acquired immunodeficiency syndrome. Am J Med 85:289-291.

Landegren U (1984). Measurement of cell numbers by means of the endogenous enzyme hexosaminidase. Applications to detection of lymphokines and cell surface antigens. J Immunol Methods 67:379-388.

MacGregor RR (1986). Alcohol and immune defense. JAMA 256:1474-1479.

MacGregor RR, Safford M, Shalit M (1988). Effect of ethanol on functions required for the delivery of neutrophils to sites of inflammation. J Infect Dis 157:682-689.

Michie HR, Manogue KR, Spriggs DR, Revhaug A, O'Dwyer S, Dinarello CA, Cerami A, Wolff SM, Wilmore DW (1988). Detection of circulating tumor necrosis factor after endotoxin administration. N Engl J Med 318:1481-1486.

Murray JF, Garay SM, Hopewell PC, Mills J, Snider GL, Stover DE (1987). Pulmonary complications of the acquired immunodeficiency syndrome: an update. Am Rev Respir Dis 135:504-509.

Nathan CF (1987). Secretory products of macrophages. J Clin Invest 79:319-326.

Nelson S, Bagby G, Summer WR (1989). Alcohol suppresses lipopolysaccharide-induced tumor necrosis factor activity

in serum and lung. Life Sciences 44:673-676.
Nelson S, Bagby GJ, Bainton BG, Wilson LA, Thompson JJ, Summer WR (1989). Compartmentalization of intraalveolar and systemic lipopolysaccharide-induced tumor necrosis factor and the pulmonary inflammatory response. J Infect Dis 159:189-194.
Nelson S, Noel P, Bokulic R, Bagby G, Summer WR (1989). Murine recombinant tumor necrosis factor enhances host defenses against Staphylococcus aureus. Am Rev Respir Dis 139S:357.
Polsky B, Gold JWM, Whimbey E, Dryjanski J, Brown AE, Schiffman G, Armstrong D (1986). Bacterial pneumonia in patients with the acquired immunodeficiency syndrome. Ann Int Med 104:38-41.
Schlamm HT, Yancovitz SR (1989). Haemophilus influenzae pneumonia in young adults with AIDS, ARC, or risk of AIDS. Am J Med 86:11-14.
Toews GB (1986). Determinants of bacterial clearance from the lower respiratory tract. Semin Respir Infect 1:68-78.
Tracey KJ, Lowry SF, Cerami A (1988). Cachectin/TNF-alpha in septic shock and septic adult respiratory distress syndrome. Am Rev Respir Dis 138:1377-1379.
Witt DJ, Craven DE, McCabe WR (1987). Bacterial infections in adult patients with the acquired immune deficiency syndrome (AIDS) and AIDS-related complex. Am J Med 82:900-906.
Wong GHW, Goeddel DV (1986). Tumor necrosis factors alpha and beta inhibit virus replication and synergize with interferons. Nature 323:819-822.
Yonemaru M, Zheng H, Stephens KE, Ishizaka A, Sandhu JS, Hatherill JR, Hogue RS, Raffin TA (1988). Biphasic effect of tumor necrosis factor on polymorphonuclear leukocyte chemotaxis. Am Rev Respir Dis 137S:42.

Alcohol, Immunomodulation, and AIDS, pages 221–230
© 1990 Alan R. Liss, Inc.

IMMUNOREGULATORY EFFECTS OF ALCOHOL ON LYMPHOCYTE RESPONSES TO HUMAN IMMUNODEFICIENCY VIRUS PROTEINS

Madhavan P. N. Nair, Stanley A. Schwartz, Ziad A. Kronfol, Edgar P. Heimer, Raveendran Pottathil and John F. Greden

Departments of Pediatrics, Epidemiology (M.P.N.N. and S.A.S.), Psychiatry (M.P.N.N., Z.A.K. and J.F.G.) and the Alcohol Research Center (M.P.N.N., S.A.S., Z.A.K. and J.F.G.), The University of Michigan, Ann Arbor, Michigan 48109 and Hoffman LaRoche, Inc., (E.P.H. and R.P.), Nutley, New Jersey

INTRODUCTION

High intake of recreational drugs such as alcohol is associated with an increased risk of infections and malignancies (Pollack et al., 1984). Previous studies have shown that chronic alcohol consumption is also associated with abnormalities of humoral and cellular immunity including dysfunction of suppressor, helper and cytotoxic lymphocyte activities (Mutchnick and Lee, 1988; Drew et al., 1984; Watson et al., 1984). Because of these inhibitory effects of alcohol on various immunologic mechanisms, it is reasonable to speculate that alcohol may compromise host immune reactions to HIV infections. This investigation examines the effect of alcohol on various lymphocyte responses to different peptides derived from HIV.

RESULTS

Effect of Alcohol on Natural and Lymphokine Activated Killer Cell Activity

In view of the findings that natural killer (NK) and lymphokine activated killer (LAK) cell activities are important defense mechanisms against tumors and virus infections (Herberman, 1984; Rosenberg et al., 1986; Nair and Schwartz, 1988; Nair et al., 1986) we examined the effect of alcohol on NK and LAK cell activities of lymphocytes from normal donors. Data presented in Figure 1 demonstrate that isolated large granular lymphocytes (LGL) from normal subjects precultured for 72 hr with 0.4% ethanol (EtOH) demonstrated significant suppression (P<.05) of NK activity.

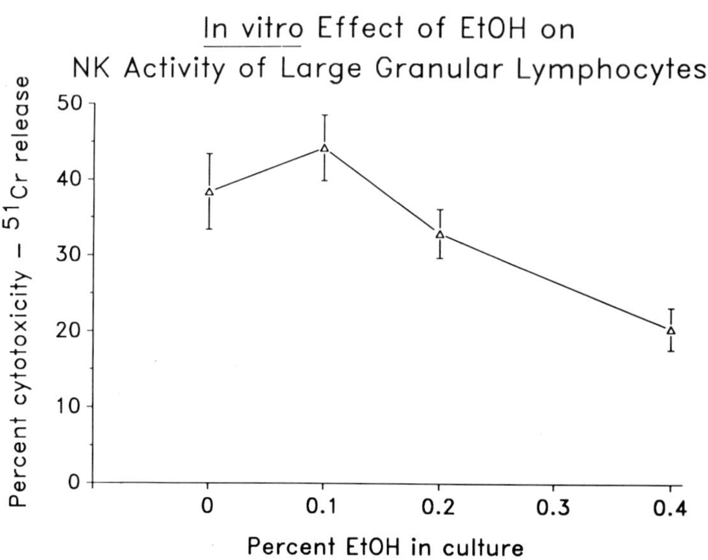

Figure 1. Effect of EtOH on the NK activity of LGL. LGL precultured with different concentrations of EtOH for 72 hr were washed and tested for NK activity against ^{51}Cr-labeled K562 target cells at a 5:1 effector-to-target (E:T) ratio. LGL were prepared on a discontinuous density gradient of Percoll as described. The least dense fraction of lymphocytes banding at the 37.5% Percoll interface consistently showed the

highest NK activity and was used as LGL. Approximately 7 to 10% of the input cells were recovered at the 37.5% Percoll interface and 75 to 80% of this fraction were stained with a monoclonal antibody specific for NKH-1. Values are the mean ± SD of 4 experiments performed in triplicate.

Figure 2 shows the cytotoxic activity of LAK cells generated in the presence of EtOH against the NK nonsensitive and NK sensitive target cells, SB and HSB respectively. PBL precultured in media containing 0.4% alcohol demonstrated significant inhibition of LAK cell activities against both HSB (P<.025) and SB targets (P<.05).

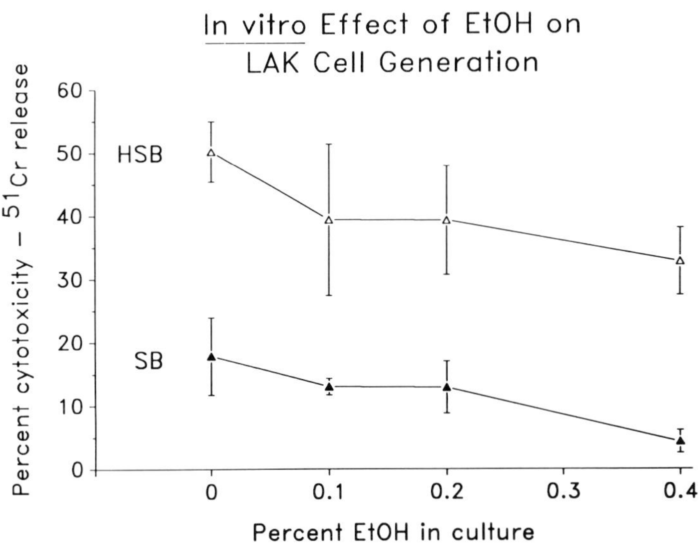

Figure 2. Lymphocytes (1 x 10^6/ml) were precultured with 5 to 10 U/ml of recombinant IL2 with or without different concentrations of EtOH for 5 to 6 days, washed and tested against NK resistant (SB) and NK sensitive (HSB) targets at a 10:1 E:T cell ratio.

Effect of Alcohol on Lymphocyte Proliferative Responses to T Cell and B Cell Mitogens

Alcoholic patients have also been shown to have impaired T and B cell functions (Mutchnick et al., 1988; Drew et al., 1984; Watson et al., 1984). Studies were carried out to investigate the effect of alcohol on T and B cell proliferative responses as measured by ^3H thymidine incorporation. Data presented in Figures 3 and 4 demonstrate that alcohol at a final concentration of 0.4% significantly suppressed T cell proliferative responses to PHA ($P<.025$) and B cell proliferative responses to killed Staphylococcus aureus cells (SAC) ($P<.01$). The suppressive effects of alcohol were not observed at higher concentrations of either PHA, or SAC and the suppression was more effective when the mononuclear cells were in an increased proliferative state.

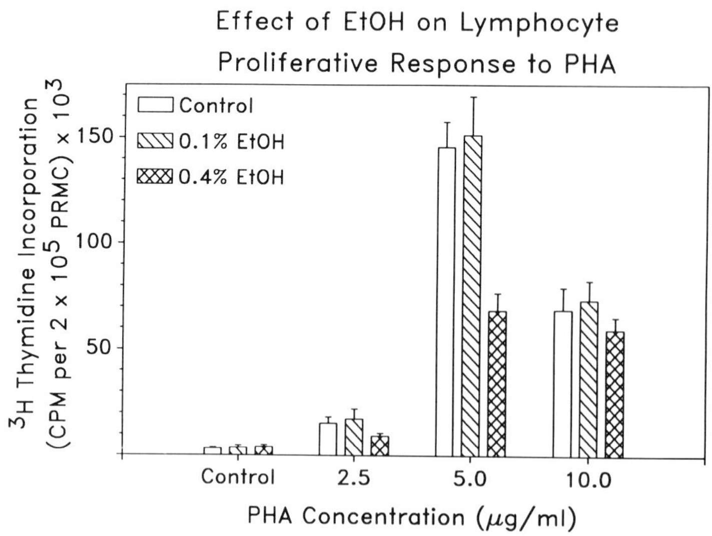

Figure 3. Mononuclear leukocytes (2×10^5 cells) were cultured with different concentrations of

PHA, to which alcohol at 0.1 or 0.4% final concentrations were added and proliferative responses were measured as a function of incorporation of ^{3}H thymidine. Values represent the mean ± SEM of 3 separate experiments performed in triplicate.

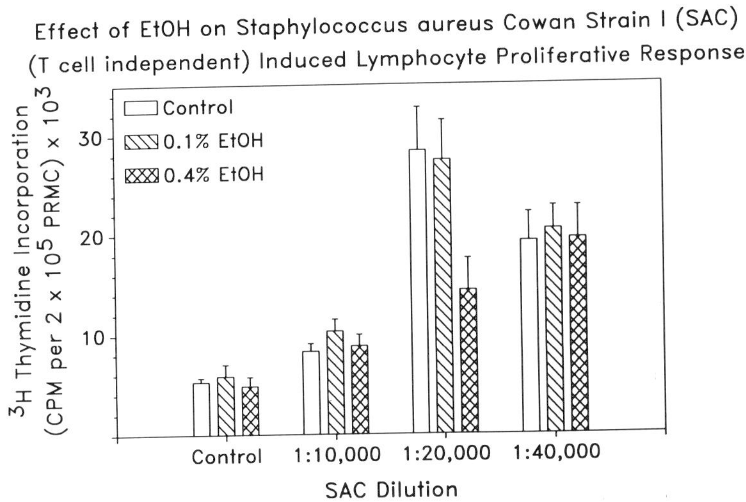

Figure 4. Mononuclear leukocytes (2 x 10^5 cells) were cultured with different concentrations of SAC, to which alcohol at 0.1 or 0.4% final concentrations was added and proliferative responses were measured as a function of incorporation of ^{3}H thymidine. Values represent the mean ± SEM of 3 separate experiments performed in triplicate.

NK Cell Activities of Lymphocytes from Alcoholic Patients

Lymphocytes from 2 alcoholic patients who presented with DSM-III R criteria for alcohol abuse or dependence and with a Michigan Alcohol

Screening Test score of ≥5 without coexisting illnesses including affective disorders as determined by SADS-L, liver disease or infections, were examined for NK activity in comparison with age and sex matched normal controls (Table 1). Both patients demonstrated decreased NK activity against K562 targets at various E:T cell ratios compared to control lymphocytes. This reduced NK activity is consistent with the reported increased susceptibility to various infections and malignancies in alcoholic patients (Pollack et al., 1984).

TABLE 1. NK Activity of Lymphocytes from Alcoholic Patients and Sex and Age Matched Controls at Various Effector to Target (E:T) Cell Ratios[a]

	Lymphocyte Source	E:T Cell Ratios 25:1	12.5:1	6.25:1
Exp#1	Patient	28.7(50.8)	21.9(54.6)	12.7(65.3)
	Control	58.4	48.3	36.7
Exp#2	Patient	35.4(49.0)	24.9(54.9)	11.4(72.4)
	Control	69.5	55.3	39.9

a. Effector cells were depleted of adherent cells by passage through a Sephadex G10 column. K562 target cells were labeled with ^{51}Cr and mixed with effector cells at varying E:T cell ratios. Values represent mean % cytotoxicity from triplicate determinations of each subject. Data in parentheses indicate percent suppression of NK activity compared to control.

Effect of Alcohol on Lymphocyte Proliferative Responses to HIV Peptides

Alcohol may be a cofactor in reducing the immune response to HIV infection potentially enhancing progression to clinical AIDS (MacGregor, 1987; Stall 1987; Siegal, 1986). Our previous studies demonstrated that both recombinant and synthetic HIV peptides can stimulate lymphocyte proliferative responses and suppress polyclonal immunoglobulin production by normal lymphocytes (Nair et al., 1988). In the present investigation, we examined the effect of alcohol on proliferative responses of peripheral blood mononuclear cells (PBMC) to specific HIV-specific peptides. Env-gag, a recombinant HIV fusion peptide, at 5 and 50 ng/ml produced significant proliferation as determined by ^3H thymidine incorporation. PBMC precultured with env-gag plus 0.1% alcohol produced a slight increase in their proliferative responses, while alcohol at an increased concentration of 0.4% produced significant suppression (P<.05) of env-gag induced proliferation.

Effect of EtOH on HIV Peptide, env-gag, Induced Lymphocyte Proliferation

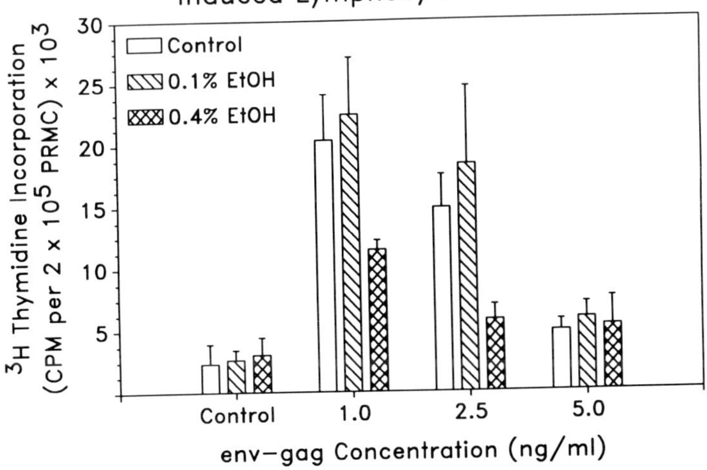

Figure 5. Mononuclear leukocytes (2 x 10^5 cells) were cultured with different concentrations of the

(continued overleaf)

Fig. 5 (continued)

HIV peptide, env-gag, to which alcohol at 0.1 and 0.4% concentrations was added and proliferative responses were measured as in the legend for Figure 3. Values represent mean ± SEM of 3 separate experiments performed in triplicate.

PBMC precultured with 10 ng/ml of env 80-DHFR, another HIV recombinant peptide which corresponds to the superconserved region of gp 41, showed significant proliferative responses, which were significantly inhibited by alcohol at a concentration of 0.4% ($P<.05$).

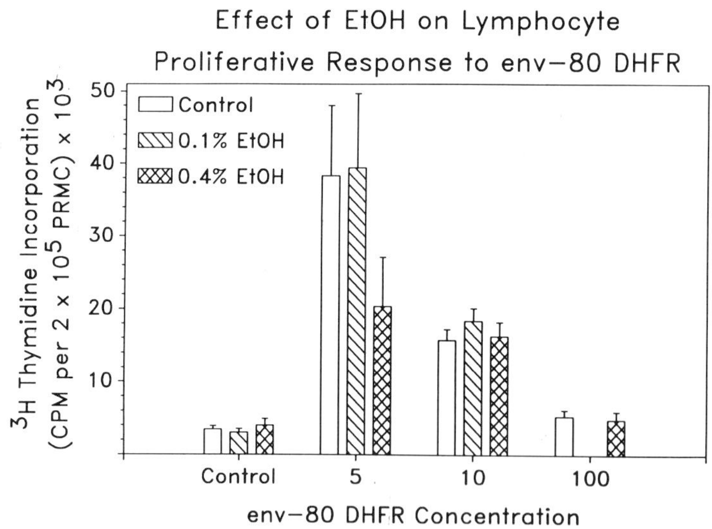

Figure 6. Mononuclear leukocytes (2×10^5 cells) were cultured with different concentrations of the HIV peptide, env 80-DHFR, to which alcohol at 0.1 and 0.4% concentrations was added and proliferative responses were measured as in the legend for Figure 3.

CONCLUDING REMARKS

Because of the inhibitory effects of alcohol on various immunologic functions of normal lymphocytes as well as the observed depressed immune status of both alcoholic and AIDS patients, alcohol may be considered as a potential cofactor in reducing the host's immune responses to HIV infections and potentially leading to progression to clinical AIDS. Our studies have demonstrated that alcohol can suppress NK and LAK cell activities, which are considered to be a primary host defense mechanism against tumors and viral infections. Further, we have demonstrated that alcohol can inhibit both T and B cell responses and suppress lymphocyte proliferative responses to recombinant HIV peptides. The mechanisms underlying the proliferative responses of lymphocytes from uninfected, healthy donors to HIV peptides and alcohol mediated suppression of HIV induced lymphocyte response are not clearly understood. Nonetheless, these studies present evidence that alcohol can suppress the host's immune response to HIV antigens thus supporting the premise that alcohol may act as a cofactor in HIV infections and progression of disease.

REFERENCES

Drew PA, Clifton PM, Labrooy JT, Shearman DJC (1984). Polyclonal B cell activation in alcoholic patients with no evidence of livers dysfunction. Clin Exp Immunol 51:479-486.

Herberman RB (1984). "NK and Other Effector Cells." New York: Academic Press.

MacGregor RR (1987). Alcohol and drugs as cofactors for AIDS. Advan Alcohol Sub Abuse 7(2):47-71.

Mutchnick MG, Lee HH (1988). Impaired lymphocytes proliferative response to mitogen in alcoholic patients. Absence of a relation to liver disease activity. Alcoholism Clin Exp Res 12:155-158.

Nair MPN, Laing TJ, Schwartz SA (1986). Decreased natural and antibody-dependent cellular cytotoxic activities in intravenous drug abusers. Clin. Immunol Immunopathol 38:68-78.

Nair MPN, Schwartz SA (1988). Immunoregulation of lymphokine activated killer cells. Clin Immunol Immunopathol 49:28-40.

Nair MPN, Pottathil R, Heimer EP, Schwartz SA (1988). Immunoregulatory activities of human immunodeficiency virus proteins. I. Effect of HIV recombinant and synthetic peptides on immunoglobulin synthesis and proliferative responses by normal lymphocytes. Proc Natl Acad Sci USA 85:6498-6502.

Pollack ES, Nomura AMY, Helburn LK, Stemmerman GN, Green SB (1984). Prospective study of alcohol consumption and cancer. N Eng J Med 310:617-621.

Rosenberg SA, Spiess P, LaFreniere R (1986). A new approach to the adoptive immuntherapy of cancer with tumor infiltrating lymphocytes. Science 233:1318-1321.

Siegal L (1986). AIDS: Relationship to alcohol and other drugs. J Sub Abuse Treat 3:271-274.

Stall R (1987). The prevention of HIV infection associated with drug and alcohol use during sexual activity. Adv Alcohol Abuse 7:73-89.

Watson RR, Eskelson C, Hartman BR (1984). Severe alcohol abuse and cellular immune functions. Arizona Med 41:665-668.

Alcohol, Immunomodulation, and AIDS, pages 231–238
© 1990 Alan R. Liss, Inc.

BIOCHEMICAL CHANGES IN ETHANOL-TREATED HL-60 CELLS

Lester K. Leung, Peter Kinkade and Joseph M. Wu

Department of Biochemistry and Molecular Biology, New York Medical College, Valhalla, New York 10595

INTRODUCTION

Acquired immune deficiency syndrome (AIDS) is a debilating and consequentially fatal disease with no known cure. It exhibits multilevel symptoms spanning from central nervous disorders to immune dysfunctions and is recognized as the one single detrimental disease facing mankind. Concerted international research efforts led to the isolation of the human immunodeficiency virus (HIV) in 1983 from patients with AIDS and the AIDS-related complex thereby establishing HIV as the etiologic agent of this newly recognized human disease (1). Although it was initially thought to be restrictive in its infectivity to peripheral blood mononuclear cells, particularly T helper lymphocytes, HIV is now known to attack a number of other cells including monocytes/macrophages, other hematopoietic, brain, skin and colon cells (2).

Several casually observed correlations existing in the literature have guided the research focus of this laboratory and have provided the impetus for the preliminary studies described in this communication. First, the incidence of AIDS is known to be more prevalent among certain social groups among which are intravenous drug users (1). Second, the relative risk for drug abuse is about four times higher among those with alcoholism than for non-alcholics (3,4). Third, prolonged and excessive alcohol intake alters the host defense mechanism as evidenced by an increased susceptibility to pathogenic and opportunistic infections (5).

POSING THE QUESTIONS

Because of the considerations described in the last section, we have posed the following questions: Does excessive alcohol intake reduce the effectiveness of therapeutically efficacious drugs such as AZT? Is alcoholism a risk factor and possibly a link to the development and progression of AIDS? (Contributions of other abused substances are recognized but are omitted.)

WORKING HYPOTHESIS

The salient features of our working hypothesis are:
(1) Prolonged and sustained exposure to physiologically achievable chronic concentrations of ethanol (0.2-0.3%) elicits membrane, cytoplasmic and nuclear changes in responsive target cells. The magnitude of the responses may be inversely proportional to the ability of the target cells to metabolize ethanol.
(2) Transient exposure to acute potentially lethal doses of ethanol elicits changes which may be irreversible or often slowly "repaired" in the target cells.
(3) Ethanol-induced (acute or chronic) cellular perturbations significantly alter the ability of these cells to interact with biological immunomodulators, e.g. interferon.
(4) The ethanol-elicited changes contribute in part to the progression and establishment of AIDS.

TESTING THE HYPOTHESIS: EXPERIMENTAL DESIGN

As a first step in testing this hypothesis, we have investigated the effects of ethanol treatment on the HL-60 promyelocytic leukemic cells. Cells were simultaneously exposed to or previous treated with various ethanol concentrations (0.3-1.5%) for different periods of time and the experimental parameters illustrated in Table 1 were determined.

MATERIALS AND METHODS

(1) HL-60 Cell Culture methods were as described in previous publications from this laboratory (6,7). Cells between passages 30-40 were used. To initiate ethanol treatment, HL-60 cells were seeded at an initial density of 3-4 x 10^5 cells/ml. Fourteen hours later, ethanol at

Table 1. Biochemical parameters measured in ethanol-treated HL-60 cells.

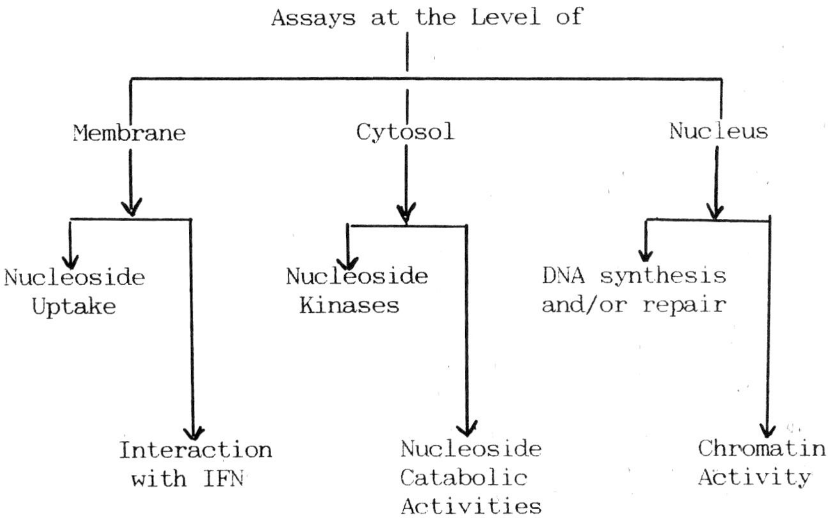

various concentrations were added. After an additional 24 or 48 hours in culture, cells were used for pulse labeling studies. Alternatively, after the 48 hour incubation period with ethanol, cells were washed free of ethanol and then incubated for an additional 24 or 72 hours in the absence of ethanol, followed by pulse labeling or enzymatic studies.

(2) Uptake Studies. Control or treated cells were incubated with 5uCi/ml [^{3}H] thymidine (ICN Radiochemicals, 70 Ci/mmol) or [^{3}H] AZT (Moravek Radiochemicals, 15 Ci/mmol) for 60 min, 37°C at the end of which cells were pelleted, washed once with phosphate buffered saline. The acid-soluble molecules were prepared by extraction with Freon as described by Pogolotti et al. (8) and their composition analyzed by HPLC. The acid-insoluble material was suspended in 0.5M KOH, precipitated with 5% trichloroacetic acid (TCA) for 15 min at 4°C, and filtered on a Millipore filter manifold. The filter-bound radioactivity was quantitated by scintillation counting.

(3) Treatment with Interferon and Assay of 2',5' Oligoadenylate Synthetase. Control or ethanol treated HL-60 cells were further treated with 200 IU/ml human

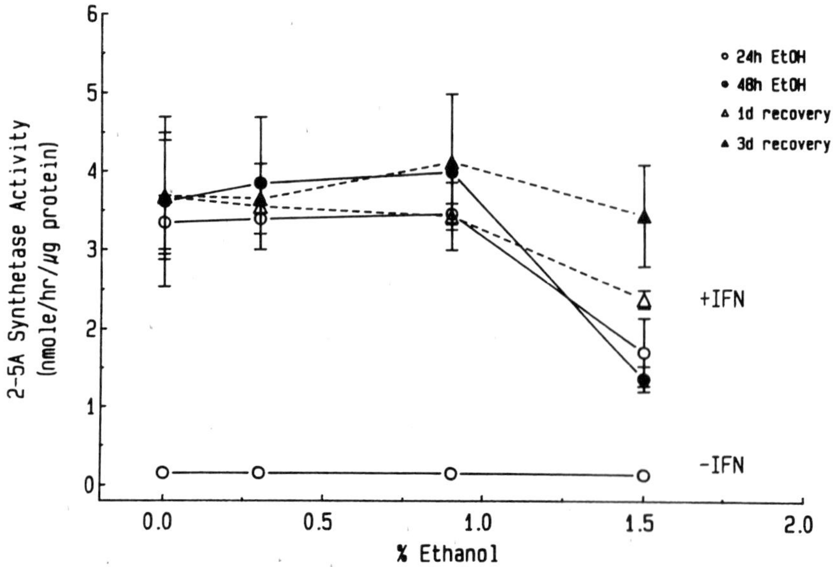

Figure 1. Varying times of ethanol treatment on 2-5A synthetase activity. (A) 24 hour ethanol treatment, 24 hour IFN treatment; (B) 48 hour ethanol treatment, 24 hour IFN treatment; (C) 48 hour ethanol treatment, wash, 1 day recovery, 24 hour IFN treatment; (D) 48 hour ethanol treatment, wash, 3 day recovery, 24 hour IFN treatment.

observation). The difference in the metabolism of the naturally occuring thymidine in comparison to the analog AZT may be related to the substrate specificity and kinetic properties of the intracellular kinases. Extrapolating this laboratory observation to clinical studies would imply that the therapeutic value of AZT in treating AIDS may be of less significance. Continuous treatment shows thymidine and AZT uptake to be affected only by 1.5% ethanol, with the harmful effects of ethanol amplified after the cells were allowed to recover in ethanol free media for 1 day (fig 2). Studies are currently in progress to determine whether a similar effect of ethanol can be shown with cultured human monocytes/macrophages.

(2) Incorporation of thymidine and AZT into DNA. Thymidine and AZT are incorporated into DNA, although the latter is incorporated at 1% efficiency compared to thymidine. This is expected since AZT 5'-triphosphate is known to act as a DNA chain terminator. When cells were treated with 1.5% ethanol, we consistently observe a 2-3 fold increase in the incorporation of AZT into DNA. While the exact mechanism for this apparent stimulation remains to be determined, it should be noted that we have observed significant DNA fragmentation and breakage at the high ethanol concentration. (Fraioli and Wu, unpublished data) It may be surmised that the ethanol-induced DNA breaks create additional sites for AZT incorporation into DNA. The disproportionate decrease in the incorporation of thymidine into DNA compared to the suppression in thymidine uptake is also consistent with the notion that ethanol has another role in inhibiting DNA synthesis/repair.

(3) Status of receptor structure/function. Our studies on 2-5A synthetase as an indirect assessment of receptor structure/function show that high levels of ethanol adversely affected the cellular response to IFN. In contrast to our uptake studies, the recovery of receptor function and affinity appears to be more efficient; suggesting that membrane component involved in interaction with interferon is distinctly different than that in deoxynucleoside uptake.

ACKNOWLEDGEMENTS

Supported in part by a grant from Lederle Laboratories and a grant from the Smokeless Tobacco Research Council, Inc. (STRC 0186-01).

REFERENCES

1. Broder, S., and Gallo, R.C. (1984). A pathogenic retrovirus (HTLV-III) linked to AIDS. N. Engl. J. Med. 311:1292-1297.
2. Levy, J.A. (1988). The human immunodeficiency virus and its pathogenesis. In Sande, M.A. and Volberding, P.A. (eds.): "The medical management of AIDS," Philadelphia: W.B. Saunders Co., pp. 1-17.

3. Rose, R.M. and Barrett, J.E. (eds.): "Alcoholism: Origins and Outcome," New York: Raven Press (1988).
4. Weiss, R.D., Mirin, S.M., Griffin, M.L., and Michael, J.L. (1988). A comparison of alcoholic and non-alcoholic drug abusers. J. of Studies on Alcohol. 49:510-515.
5. Jerrels, T.R., Marietta, E.A., Bone, G., Weight, F.F., and Eckardt, M.J. (1988) Ethanol associated immunosuppression. In Bridge, T.P., et al. (eds.): "Psychological, neuropsychiatric and substance abuse aspects of AIDS," New York: Raven Press.
6. Konno, S., Borelli, T.J., and Wu, J.M. (1986). Partial purification and characterization of phorbol ester-regulated translational inhibitor(s) in human HL-60 leukemic cells. J. Biol. Chem. 261:5010-5017.
7. Konno, S., Chiao, J.W. and Wu, J.M. (1986). Effects of nicotine on cellular proliferation, cell cycle phase distribution and macromolecular synthesis in human promyelocytic HL-60 leukemic cells. Canc. Letters 33:91-97.
8. Pogolotti, A.L., Jr., and Santi, D.V. (1982). High-pressure liquid chromatography-ultraviolet analysis of intracellular nucleotides. Anal. Biochem. 126:335-345.
9. Wu, J.M., Semproni, A.R., Wang, C.H., Borelli, T.J., and Alessandroni, R. (1986). The effect of ammonium ion on the induction of (2'-5')-$(A)_n$ synthetase and (2'-5')-$(A)_n$-dependent endoribonuclease activity by interferon in mouse BALB/C 3T3 cells. J. Interferon Research 6:297-303.

Alcohol, Immunomodulation, and AIDS, pages 239–254
© 1990 Alan R. Liss, Inc.

AN OBSERVED MECHANISM FOR DECREASING BLOOD ALCOHOL LEVELS IN RATS BY USING SODIUM ACETATE

C.D. Eskelson, Ph.D., L. Meeks, L. Myers,
R. MacDonald, P. Thut, Ph.D. E. Tucker, M.D.

Department of Surgery and Pharmacology and Toxicology, University of Arizona Health Sciences Center, Tucson, Arizona 85724, The College of Pharmacy, Community Resources Specialist in Additions, University of Arizona Health Sciences Center, Tucson, Arizona 85721 and The Veterans Administration Hospital, Tucson, Arizona 85723

INTRODUCTION

The rate of ethanol* metabolism is determined by the availability of the oxidized nucleotides (NAD) for alcohol dehydrogenase (ADH) (Hawkins and Kalant, 1972). During the metabolism of ethanol to acetate, NAD is rapidly converted to NADH and the amount of NAD available for ADH utilization is significantly reduced. It has been proposed that by increasing the availability of NAD in animals would increase the rate of alcohol metabolism.

Acetate is a product of ethanol's metabolism and is compound which should increase NAD levels during ethanol metabolism since it can be converted to various lipids (fatty acids, cholesterol, triacylglycerols) by utilizing the reduced nucleotides (NADPH). Therefore, would acetate facilitate the metabolism of ethanol by increasing ethanol's metabolic rate due to increased conversion of NADH to NAD? Rats given acetate and ethanol intraperitoneally (I.P.) do not significantly increase the ethanolic metabolic rate (Table 1), but rats given ethanol orally (P.O.) and acetate I.P. or P.O. have decreased blood alcohol levels (Table 2) and an apparent decreased rate of ethanol metabolism.

* Ethanol and alcohol as used here are equivalent.

TABLE 1. Some Effects of Sodium Acetate on Alcohol Metabolism when Alcohol and Sodium Acetate are Given Intraperitoneally (2.25 g alcohol I.P. per kg body weight)

Treatment	No.of Rats	I Hour	2 Hours	3 Hours	4 Hours
Control	5	.216	.145	.076	.025
Std. Dev.		.020	.025	.029	.025
Acetate I.P.					
1.6 g/kg	5	.201	.152	.111	.038
Std. Dev.		.057	.048	.055	.028

The five rats in each of the two groups were intraperitoneally given 2.25 g of alcohol per kg body weight. Sodium acetate was given to the experimental rats in the administered alcohol solution.

TABLE 2. Some Effects of Sodium Acetate on the Gastrointestinal Tract Ethanol Content and Plasma Alcohol Levels in Rats 5 Hours after Administering 3.4 g of Alcohol Orally per kg Body Weight (Values expressed in g of alcohol per 100 ml of plasma)

Treatment	No.of Rats	I Hour	2 Hours	3 Hours	4 Hours	5 Hours	Stomach mg	Gut mg
Saline, I.P.	4	.150	.099	.045	.011	.0002	228	3
Std Dev.		.011	.013	.010	.010	.0004	74	6
Acetate, I.P.								
I.6 g/kg	5	.075*	.023*	.003	.003	.002*	409*	5
Std. Dev.		.016	.017	.005	.006	.004	128	6

* Significant from saline at P values equal to or less than .05 level. The rats in each group were orally given 3.4 g of alcohol per kg body weight. Immediately following alcohol administration each group of rats was intraperitoneally given the same volume of solution on a weight basis. The control group was given intraperitoneally a saline solution and the experimental group was given intraperitoneally a sodium acetate solution.

The purposes of this research are to determine whether acetate influences the metabolism of alcohol and whether acetate plays a homeostatic role during alcohol metabolism. Previous studies show that large doses of alcohol inhibit gastric emptying both in rats (Barboriak and Meade, 1969) and man (Barboriak and Meade, 1970). Additionally, Lalyre et al (Lalyre et al, 1974) reported that prostaglandin E_1 increases the release of alcohol from rat stomach. These reports indicate that ethanol or a metabolite of ethanol may inhibit gastric emptying during alcohol metabolism, thus controlling alcohol release from the stomach.

The observation that there is a suppression of food intake in ruminants following the infusion of sodium acetate into the ruminoreticulum (Simkins et al, 1965; Baile et al, 1969) may be related to the inhibition of gastric emptying following alcohol administration to rats and man. Baile et al (Baile and Mayer, 1969; Baile, 1968) suggested a receptor site mechanism for acetate which causes decreased food intake in animals given sodium acetate. These observations concerning alcohol and acetate suggest that the suppression of appetite produced by sodium acetate administration to ruminants and the inhibition of gastric emptying following alcohol intake in man and animals may be related since alcohol metabolism produces free acetate resulting in increased blood acetate levels (Lundquist et al, 1962).

MATERIALS AND METHODS

Non-fasted male Sprague-Dawley rats (150-330 g) were used. The weight range in any given study was less than 65 g. Basically the experiments consisted of rats given either I.P. or P.O. doses of alcohol with or without the administration of acetate or other anions. Controls received a volume of saline equivalent to those of alcohol, acetate or anions given to the experimental animals.

The I.P. alcohol was given as a 22.5% (w/v) solution and the alcohol given P.O., in a 33.7% (w/v) solution. Sodium acetate was given as an 8% solution with pH adjusted to 7.4. The doses of alcohol were given at the level of either 2.25 g per kg body weight or 3.37 g per kg body weight (P.O.). The sodium acetate dose was 1.6 g per kg body weight and that of potassium butyrate was given at various doses.

Acetate determinations were done by the enzymatic methods of

Ballard (Ballard, 1972 A, 1972). The rats were guillotined at various times after the alcohol dose and the bloods collected. Serum was obtained by centrifugation and was stored frozen until analyzed.

Bloods for alcohol analysis were obtained by cutting off the tip of the rat's tail and collecting it in heparinized capillary tubes, usually on an hourly basis, for up to 5 hours. The capillary tubes were then centrifuged, the red blood cell layer broken away and the tube containing plasma sealed and stored up to 48 hours at 4°C. Plasma alcohol levels (PAL) were determined by a gas chromatographic method described by Palo and Ilkova, 1970. The data obtained from the various groups of rats in the study were averaged and the standard deviations were determined on the average values. Statistical significance between experimental groups of animals was determined, using the Student "t" test. Significance was accepted at the 95% level, or greater. Linear regression analysis was performed on some of the lines in the graphs with the lines standard error of the estimate and correlation coefficient.

In studies in which decreased alcohol absorption was suspected, the level of alcohol in the gastrointestinal tract (GIT) of each animal was determined by removing the GIT and homogenizing it with its contents in 100 ml of ice-cold saline. At times the stomachs with its contents were separated from the rest of the GIT and their ethanol contents determined by homogenizing both with 100 ml of ice-cold saline. A polytron homogenizer was used for the homogenization procedure. The homogenates were centrifuged for 30 minutes at 9000 x g at 0°C. The supernatants were stored, frozen (-30°) in sealed tubes until analyzed for alcohol content. The alcohol contents of the supernatant fluid from the homogenates of the stomach, GIT and gut with their contents were analyzed as described earlier (Palo and Ilkova, 1970).

RESULTS

FIGURE I

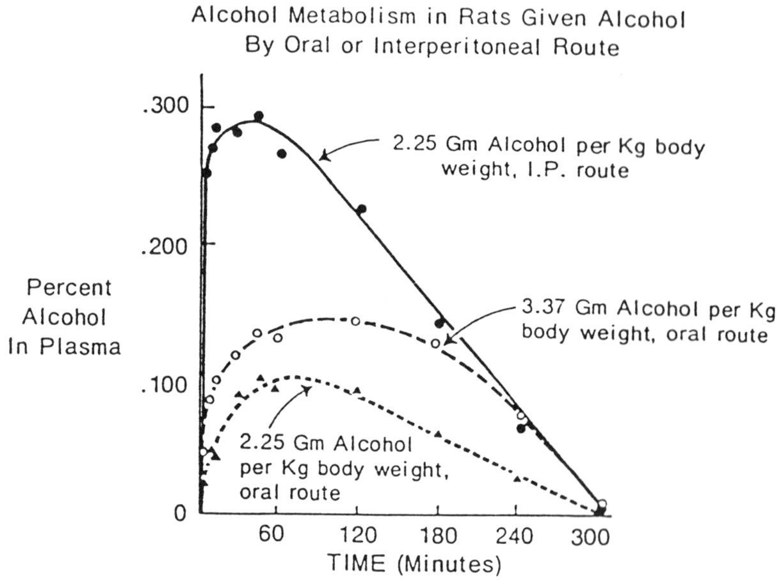

Legend

Percent alcohol in plasma is expressed as g of alcohol per 100 ml of plasma.
Each point in the graph represents the average level of alcohol in plasma of 5 rats.
Figure 1 graphically demonstrates the clearance of alcohol from rat plasma when 2.25 g of alcohol per kg body weight is administered P.O. or I.P.

The PAL of rats given alcohol I.P. is greater than that of rats given the same amount of alcohol P.O. Even after the oral administration of a larger dose of alcohol, the PAL is greater in the rats given the lesser amount of alcohol I.P. In addition, the PAL in all groups of rats are near zero levels within 5 hours regardless of administration route.

The alcohol clearance rate from plasma appears 2 times greater in rats given alcohol I.P. compared with the apparent rate of alcohol clearance from plasma in rats given alcohol P.O. (Equations 1, 2 and 3 in Table 3). When the alcohol content of the GIT of these rats was determined, only 2% of the original alcohol load was recoverable in rats given alcohol I.P.; however, approximately 20% of the alcohol load was recoverable in the GIT of rats given P.O. 2.25 g of alcohol per kg body weight and approximately 27% of the alcohol load was recovered in the GIT of rats P.O. given 3.37 g of alcohol per kg body weight (Table 4).

Rats given acetate I.P. 60 minutes following an oral dose of the ethanol had an ethanol removal rate approaching that equal to those rats given ethanol I.P. Rats P.O. given (3.4 g of ethanol per kg body weight) an ethanol solution followed immediately by giving them an I.P. dose (1.6 g of sodium acetate per kg body weight) of sodium acetate contained 1.8 times more alcohol in their stomachs than stomachs from rats not given sodium acetate (Table 2). The PAL of rats given sodium acetate were 2-12 times less than rats not given acetate (Table 2) up to 3 hours post alcohol treatment.

To determine whether acetate was the only organic anion that inhibited gastric emptying, differing amounts of potassium butyrate was given to rats I.P. immediately following an oral alcohol load. The PAL was reduced at 1 and 2 hours post ethanol administration but only at the highest levels of butyrate given. However, 3 and 4 hours post treatment, the PAL returned near to the level of rats given ethanol but not potassium butyrate (Table 5).

Increased acetate levels occurred in blood of rats metabolizing ethanol (Figure 2). When acetate was given to rats I.P. and ethanol given P.O., the acetate levels in plasma were greater than the acetate levels in plasma of rats given no alcohol and only sodium acetate. The valley in acetate plasma levels at 3 hours in both groups of rats given ethanol is followed by a plasma acetate rise at 4 hours. This valley was not detected in rats given only acetate (Figure 2).

TABLE 3. Equations for Ethanol Removal from Plasma in Rats given Ethanol Orally or Intraperitoneally and in Rats given Ethanol Orally and given Sodium Acetate 60 minutes after the Ethanol Dose

Group No.	Treatment	Number of Samples/Line	Equation for the Line[1]	Corr[2] Coeff.	Std.Error of Est.[3]
1	2.25 g of alcohol I.P.	31	y[4] = - .00113 X[5] + 0.353	0.915[6]	0.025
2	2.25 g of alcohol P.O.	30	y = - .000525 X + 0.145	0.677	0.028
3	3.4 g of alcohol P.O.	15	y = - .000565 X + 0.230	0.678	0.030
4	3.4 g of alcohol P.O. plus 1.6 g of sodium acetate 1 hour after alcohol administration	20	y = - .000956 X + 0.250	0.811	0.031

1. The data for the equations for the lines were taken at 120, 180 and 240 minutes after the alcohol dose (see Figure 1) for treatments numbers 1-3 and at 60, 120, 180 and 240 minutes for treatment number 4.
2. Corr. Coeff. = Correlation coefficient
3. Standard Error of Est. = Standard error of the estimate
4. y = g of alcohol per 100 ml of plasma
5. X = time in minutes
6. All Corr. Coeff. have P-values less than the 1% level

FIGURE 2

Plasma Acetate Levels in Rats After Acetate; Acetate and Alcohol; and Alcohol Treatment

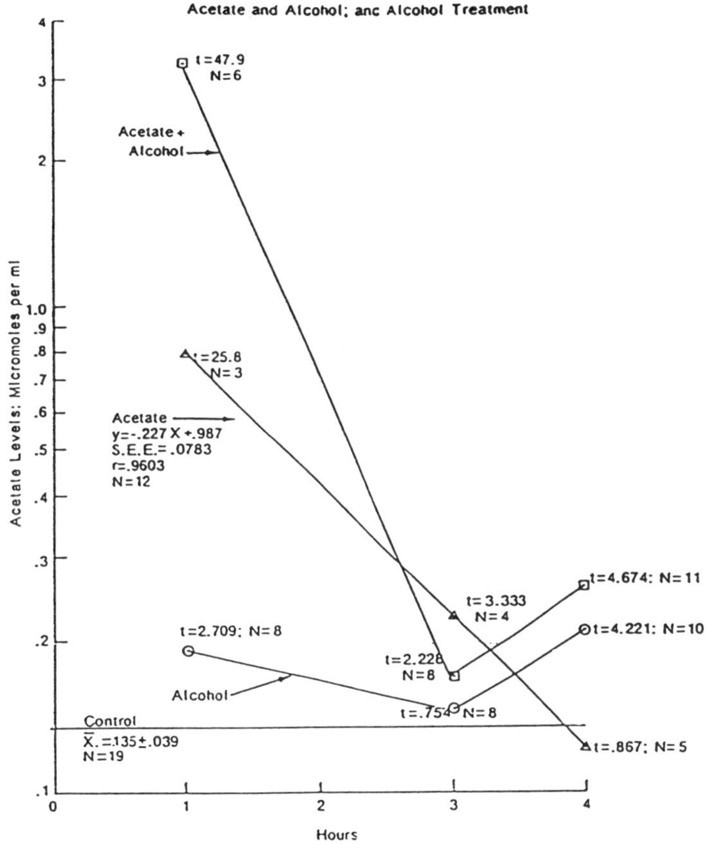

"N" is the number of animals used to determine the average level of acetate per ml of serum for each point in the graph. "t" was determined by the Student "t" test and compares the control level of acetate with the experimental values. All "t" values are significant at less than the 0.05 level of probability except for "t" values 0.754 and 0.867 which are not significant.
Each rat given alcohol was given P.O. 3.4 g of alcohol per kg body weight.

Each rat given acetate was given, I.P., 1.6 g of sodium acetate per kg body weight.
The correlation coefficients are significant at 1>p>.1

TABLE 4. Alcohol Content in Rat Gastrointestinal Tract 5 Hours after Receiving Differing Amounts of Alcohol Orally or Intraperitoneally

Group No.	Amount of Alcohol Given Each Rat	No. of Rats	Average Amount of Alcohol in Gastrointestinal Tract and Contents		Rat Weight Range
			mg	Std.Dev.	
1	2.25 g/kg I.P.	5	10	1	210-245
2	2.25 g/kg P.O.	5	100	60	225-240
3	3.37 g/kg P.O.	5	231	70	235-275

Rats treated as in Figure 1.
Rats in Group 1 were intraperitoneally given 2.25 g of alcohol per kg body weight.
Rats in Group 2 were orally given 2.25 g of alcohol per kg body weight.
Rats in Group 3 were orally given 3.37 g of alcohol per kg body weight.
The alcohol contents of the gastrointestinal tracts of the rats were determined 5 hours after alcohol administration. The data are recorded as the average value and standard deviation of the 5 rats in each group.

TABLE 5. Effects of Potassium Butyrate on Plasma Alcohol Levels[1]

Group No.	Treatment	No. of Rats	1 Hour	2 Hours	3 Hours	4 Hours
1	Control[2]	10	.131	.137	.122	.098
	Std. Dev.		.049	.055	.047	.047
2	Butyrate(100mg/kg)[3]	5	.089	.117	.115	.081
	Std. Dev.		.044	.082	.089	.093
3	Butyrate(500mg/kg)[3]	5	.083	.069	.103	.083
	Std. Dev.		.036	.035*	.090	.083
4	Butyrate(1 g/kg)[4]	5	.043*	.055*	.083	.050
	Std. Dev.		.021	.026	.067	.052
	Student "t" value		3.789	3.12	N.S.	N.S.
			1>P>.5	1>P>.5		

* Student "t" value = 2.265; 5>P>2.5

1. All plasma alcohol levels are expressed as g per 100 ml.
2. Control rats received intraperitoneally equivalent volume of saline as rats in Groups 2 and 3.
3. The potassium butyrate was given intraperitoneally after the oral alcohol dose.
4. The potassium butyrate was given orally with the alcohol dose.

Since ethanol is metabolized more slowly when rats are fasted, (Vitale et al, 1953) they were fasted for 17 hours before they were given ethanol. This should reduce their ability to form acetate from ethanol. These animals at 5 hours did not retain as much ethanol in the stomach as non-fasting rats (Table 6). Five hours after the dose of ethanol, the alcohol content of the gut was 5 times greater in fasted rats than that of the non-fasted rats. The PAL at 5 hours of fasted rats was 7 times greater than the PAL of non-fasted rats. The removal rate of ethanol from non-fasted rats is 1.25 times greater than the alcohol metabolic rate of fasted rats. The alcohol metabolic rate in rats weighing 271 $\pm$ 16 g and normally fed is 398 mg of ethanol per kg body weight or 40 mg per 100 g body weight (Table 6). The ethanolic metabolic rate for alcohol metabolism in fasted rats is 307 mg of ethanol per kg body weight or 30.7 mg per 100 g per hour. The alcohol removal rate from plasma of non-fasted rats equal 42.5 mg per dL per hour and fasted rats equal 32.7 mg per dL per hour.

DISCUSSION

Since the rate of alcohol metabolism is fairly constant at blood alcohol levels above 10-20 mg per 100 ml (Hawkins and Kalant, 1972), the alcohol removal rate from plasma in rats given alcohol P.O. should equal that of rats given alcohol I.P. The apparent differences that are observed here may be explained by the fact that alcohol is also added to serum by being absorbed from the GIT of animals given alcohol P.O. Alcohol absorption from the GIT into the plasma may account for the apparent decreased alcohol removal rate from plasma (compare Equations 1 with Equations 2 and 3 in Table 3). If this were true, then, using the equations in Table 1, the calculated absorption rate of alcohol from the GIT of these rats is 6 ug into 1 ml of blood plasma per minute on the descending limb of the plasma alcohol curve. Note that after 1 hour the slope of the plasma alcohol curve in Figure 1 of the P.O. treated rats is negative, thus the rate of alcohol absorption from the GIT must be less than the alcohol removal rate from plasma. We concluded, therefore, that 5 hours after giving the alcohol load P.O., when the PAL is essentially zero, that the GIT must contain significant amounts of alcohol.

Table 6. Alcohol Metabolism in Fasted and Non-fasted Rats 5 Hours After an Oral Alcohol Load

Treatment	No.of Rats	Alcohol in Stomach	Alcohol in Gut	Plasma(1) Alcohol Level	Average Amount of Alcohol Administered	Alcohol(2) in Carcass and GIT (calculated)	Alcohol Metabo-lized in 5 Hours	Rate(3) of Alcohol Metabolized per hour	Average Rat Weight in grams
		mg	mg		mg	mg	mg	mg/hour	
Non-fasting	8	319(4)	5	.025	905	365	539	108	271
Std. Dev.(5)		134	7	.036	55	91	88	18	16
Fasting	8	114*	25*	.183*	949	491*	440*	87*	283
Std. Dev.		52	6	.061	60	71	84	16	19

* Significant from non-fasting rats at P values equal to or less than .05 level.

The experimental rats were fasted for 17 hours while the control rats were allowed food ad libitum. The two groups of rats were given 3.37 g of alcohol per kg body weight orally. The alcohol content of the stomach and gut was determined 5 hours after alcohol administration. Plasma alcohol levels were also obtained 5 hours after alcohol administration.

1. Grams of alcohol per 100 ml of plasma.
2. The amount of alcohol in the rat carcass was determined by assuming a water content of 65% and assuming the alcohol level in the water of plasma is representative of total body water.
3. The amount of alcohol given the rats is known, therefore the amount of alcohol removed primarily by metabolism could be obtained by subtracting the total alcohol content remaining in the carcass and gastrointestinal tract from the amount of alcohol given each rat. Assuming that all of the alcohol removed was metabolized then an estimate of alcohol metabolism per hour was obtained.
4. All values are expressed as the average value of 8 rats.
5. Std. Dev. = Standard Deviation.

Analysis of the GIT and/or the gut and stomach for alcohol content revealed that at 5 hours the stomach may retain greater than 30% of the original ethanol burden even though PAL is near zero in the rats (Table 6). However, stomachs from fasted rats which have a reduced ethanolic metabolic rate contained less ethanol. This implies that gastric release of ethanol was not as controlled in fasted rats and that an "ethanol metabolite" was not synthesized at a rate rapid enough to elicit the inhibition of gastric emptying. That an alcohol-metabolite was involved or controlling alcohol removal from the stomach is supported by studies in which acetate was P.O. given to rats immediately following the oral ethanol burden. The acetate treated rats contained 18 times more ethanol in their stomachs 5 hours after the alcohol burden than did rats not dosed with sodium acetate. The data indicate that acetate inhibits the loss of alcohol from the stomach (Table 2, Table 6). Interestingly, some of our preliminary data indicate that gastric tissue has the capacity for concentrating acetate above that found in the plasma, suggesting that the anion, acetate, is actively concentrated by gastric tissue similarly as chloride.

The valley at 3 hours post ethanol treatment observed in the plasma acetate levels of rats metabolizing ethanol or ethanol and acetate may be caused by plasma acetate levels becoming decreased enough that acetate no longer affects gastric emptying. The rise in plasma acetate levels at 4 hours then could be explained by the release of ethanol from the stomach and its metabolic conversion to acetate so that the level of acetate in plasma reaches some "critical level" which again inhibits gastric emptying. PAL at 3 hours in rats given ethanol P.O. are approaching the PAL where the ADH is not saturated with ethanol, thus acetate levels may fall. However this concept is at variance with others.

Additionally that acetate does not influence the rate of alcohol metabolism is illustrated by data in Table 1 where alcohol and acetate were given in a single dose I.P. to rats. There was no increase in ethanol removal from the plasma of rats given the dose of acetate and ethanol. The data in Figure 2 indicate that plasma acetate levels are greater in rats metabolizing ethanol and in rats metabolizing ethanol and given acetate. The apparent rate (slope) of acetate removal from plasma seems stimulated in rats metabolizing ethanol. This could suggest that acetate is being utilized by increased fatty acid synthesis which probably is caused by the increased levels of the reduced NADH associated with alcohol metabolism.

When potassium butyrate was studied to determine whether the butyrate anion would also inhibit gastric emptying, the data indicated that butyrate inhibited gastric emptying but was not as effective as acetate (Table 5). A mixture of anions containing fumarate pyruvate glycerate, citrate oxaloacetate was not significantly effective at inhibiting gastric emptying of rats given ethanol (data not shown).

In summary, fed rats given alcohol P.O. have a control mechanism for alcohol absorption. The mechanism depends upon the alcohol metabolite, acetate, and operates through a feedback mechanism as follows: 1) alcohol is absorbed from the GIT and transported to the liver where it is metabolized to acetate; 2) some of the acetate formed in the liver is released to the blood and transported to the stomach or some other location (CNS) resulting in an inhibition of gastric emptying. Alcohol is absorbed more slowly from the stomach than the gut; thus ethanol's release to the plasma is slowed. The reason for the greater alcohol levels in plasma of fasting rats compared to non-fasting rats is that alcohol is not retained in the stomach since the alcohol metabolite, acetate, is not synthesized at a rate sufficient to inhibit gastric emptying. Because sodium acetate administration accentuates the inhibition of gastric emptying in rats metabolizing alcohol, it is postulated that a feedback mechanism involving acetate occurs in fed-rats metabolizing alcohol which causes an inhibition of gastric emptying. This mechanism prevents rapid alcohol absorption from the GIT and significantly controls blood alcohol levels in fed rats.

REFERENCES

Baile, C.A. (1968) Regulation of feed intake in ruminants. Fed. Proc. 27:1361-1366.

Baile, C.A. and Mayer, J. (1969) Depression of feed intake of goats by metabolites injected during meals. Am. J. Physiology 217:1830-1836.

Ballard, F.J. (1972) Supply and utilization of acetate in mammals. Am. J. Clin. Nutrition. 25:773-779.

Ballard, F.J., Filsell, O.H. and Jarrett, C.G. (1972 A) Effects of carbohydrate availability on lipogenesis in sheep. Biochem. J. 126:193.

Barboriak, J.J. and Meade, R.C. (1969) Ethanol and gastrointestinal processing of food abst no 2050, Fed. Proc. 28:626.
Barboriak, J.J. and Meade, R.C. (1970) Effect of alcohol on gastric emptying in man. Am.J. Clin. Nutr. 23:1151-1153.
Hawkins, R.D. and Kalant, H. (1972) The metabolism of ethanol and its metabolic effects. Pharmacology Reviews 24:67-157.
Lalyre, Y. Scruggs, W. and Wilson, D.E. (1974) Prostaglandin E, effects on ethanol metabolism in the rat. Prostaglandins 6:489-494.
Lundquist, F., Tygstrup, N., Winkler, K. Mellemgaard K., and Munck-Petersen S. (1962) Ethanol metabolism and production of free acetate in the human liver. J. Clin. Invest. 41:955-961.
Palo, V., likova H. (1970) Direct gas chromatographic estimation of lower alcohols, acetaldehyde, acetone and discetyl in milk products. J. Chorm. 53:363-387.
Simkins, K.L., Jr., Suttie, J.W. and Baumgardt, B.R. (1965) Regulation of food intake in ruminants. Effect of acetate, propionate, butyrate and glucose on voluntary food intake in dairy cattle. J. Dairy Sci. 48:1635-1642.
Vitale, J.J., DiGiobgoio, J., McGrath, H., Nay, J. and Hegsted, D.M. (1953) Alcohol oxidation in relation to alcohol dosage and the effect of fasting. J. Biol. Chem. 204:254-264.

Alcohol, Immunomodulation, and AIDS, pages 255–265
© 1990 Alan R. Liss, Inc.

ETHANOL, ACETALDEHYDE AND KUPFFER CELL FUNCTION: POTENTIAL ROLE FOR KUPFFER CELLS IN ALCOHOL INDUCED LIVER INJURY

David L. Earnest, M.D., Winnie W. Sim, Ph.D., Thomas L. Smith, Ph.D., and Cleamond D. Eskelson, Ph.D.

Departments of Medicine (DLE, WWS), Surgery (CDE) and Pharmacology (TLS), University of Arizona College of Medicine, Tucson, AZ 85724

INTRODUCTION:

Hepatic Kupffer cells constitute about 80-90% of fixed tissue macrophages in humans and are responsible for clearing most circulating foreign particles especially bacteria from the blood (Biozzi, 1965). It is well recognized clinically that alcoholics have a high incidence of bacterial infections, and studies in humans as well as experimental animals suggest that chronic ethanol consumption depresses immune defense and Kupffer cell function (MagGregor, 1986). Alcohol induces liver injury by mechanisms which remain incompletely defined. Clearly, it causes a direct toxic effect on hepatic parenchymal cell metabolism (Lieber, 1988). It also potentiates the hepatotoxic effect of a variety of drugs and chemicals (Sato, 1981). Most work on the pathogenesis of ethanol-induced liver injury has focused on alterations in the parenchymal cell since metabolism of ethanol and of hepatotoxic xenobiotics potentiated by ethanol occur in this cell type. However, it was recently reported that macrophages including liver Kupffer cells metabolize large amounts of ethanol (Wickramasinghe, 1987). Moreover, there is increasing evidence that these phagocytic cells also secrete a large variety of important mediators which play key roles in regulatory mechanisms for both the immune system as well as liver parenchymal cell homeostasis (Nathan, 1987). The possibility that metabolism of, or simply exposure to alcohol may enhance or suppress the secretory function of macrophages, in addition to its effect on phagocytosis, has not been adequately considered. We have found that activated Kupffer cells potentiate carbon tetrachloride liver injury by secretion of excess amounts of reactive oxygen associated with enhanced phagocytosis (El Sisi, 1987). Thus, it is conceivable that Kupffer cells may play a significant role in alcohol-induced liver injury through induced changes in phagocytosis and mediator secretion.

Kupffer cells are located within the hepatic sinusoids, are bathed directly by portal blood and thus are exposed to similar concentrations of alcohol as the parenchymal cells. It is recognized that ethanol can induce hepatic abnormalities and modify liver function when ingested either in large quantities consumed at a single time or when taken in smaller amounts chronically over months to years. In this report, we present <u>in vitro</u> and <u>in vivo</u> data which demonstrate that acute and repeated doses of ethanol significantly effect Kupffer cell function and that the type of response to ethanol is both dose and time dependant.

METHODS

In order to determine the concentrations of ethanol to which Kupffer cells are exposed in portal blood after acute ethanol ingestion, non-fasting male Sprague Dawley rats were gavaged with ethanol (4 g/kg) and blood samples obtained from the portal vein and inferior vena cava simultaneously. Different groups of rats were used in order to develop a six hour dose response curve. Blood ethanol content was quantitated by gas liquid chromatography using a porpak Q column (Palo, 1970).

The effects of ethanol and its metabolite acetaldehyde on Kupffer cell function <u>in vitro</u> were evaluated using Kupffer cells prepared from the liver of normal two month old Sprague Dawley rats. Kupffer cells were isolated by standard methods which utilized initial liver perfusion with collagenase and pronase followed by sinusoidal cell separation by metrizamide gradient centrifugation. Finally, Kupffer cells were purified and isolated by centrifugal elutriation (Knook, 1976) and placed in culture in IMDM medium (1.0 X 10^6 cells/ml) for twenty four hours prior to study. Varying concentrations of ethanol (0-1000 mg/dl), and in separate experiments acetaldehyde

(0–0.5 mg/dl), were then added in fresh media to the Kupffer cell cultures which were maintained at 37°C in 95% O_2, 5% CO_2. After twenty four hours, the effects of ethanol and acetaldehyde on Kupffer cell phagocytosis of opsonized ^{51}chromium-labelled sheep erythrocytes were measured (Tachibana, 1984).

We also evaluated the effects of varying concentrations (0–1840 mg/dl) of ethanol in vitro on Kupffer cell plasma membrane microviscosity. For this, 10 ml of freshly prepared Kupffer cells (1 X 10^6 cells/ml) suspended in phosphate buffer were incubated for 30 minutes at 25°C with 10ul of a 2mM solution of the fluorescent probe diphenylhexatriene (DPH). Fluorescence polarization was determined using a T-format spectrofluorometer and microviscosity (P) calculated with an on line microcomputer (Shinitzky, 1971).

To determine the effects on Kupffer cell function in vivo of either acute or repeated exposure to concentrations of ethanol similar to those studied in vitro, we administered the same oral dose of ethanol (4g/kg) used to assess portal blood ethanol concentration and measured clearance of colloidal carbon. We later evaluated the effects of three lower ethanol doses: 0.5, 1.0, and 2.0 g/kg given by gavage. Carbon clearance was quantitated one hour after the single oral dose of alcohol or one hour after the last of three repeated doses (given every eight hours over a twenty four hour period). The colloidal carbon suspension was injected in the jugular vein and serial blood samples obtained from the tail vein over thirty minutes. The concentration of carbon in blood was determined by a spectrophotometer (OD = 670nm). The half life ($t_{1/2}$) for carbon clearance was calculated from the slope of the plasma carbon concentration curve ($K = t_{1/2}/0.301$).

Statistical comparisons of data in this study were made between individual treatment groups of animals and cell cultures. The significance of observed differences was judged by using a non-paired student's t-test.

RESULTS

Table 1 shows the concentrations of ethanol in blood obtained simultaneously from the portal vein and inferior vena cava (IVC) after a single oral dose (4g/kg) of ethanol.

TABLE 1. Ethanol Concentration in Portal and Systemic Blood During the Six Hours After a Single Oral Dose (4g/kg) of Ethanol in Non-Fasting Rats.

	Blood Ethanol Concentration (mg/dl; mean + SEM)				
	0.5 hr.	1.0 hr.	2.0 hr.	4.0 hr.	6.0 hr.
Systemic*	233±11.3	212±19.9	184±18.3	139±22.9	26±6.9
Portal	406±39.9	400±64.2	293±42.3	225±42.9	123±11.6

*Systemic blood obtained from inferior vena cava simultaneously with blood from portal vein.

The concentration of ethanol in IVC blood is assumed to be similar to that which would be measured in systemic peripheral veins. Alcohol concentration in portal blood was highest at thirty and sixty minutes after oral dosing and fell progressively thereafter. Of note, the concentration of ethanol bathing Kupffer cells was approximately 400mg/dl at one hour. Moreover, ethanol content of portal blood was almost twice that present in the peripheral venous system at all time points tested.

Kupffer cells were cultured in concentrations of ethanol both below and above the amounts measured in vivo in portal blood. Table 2 shows the effects of such ethanol concentrations on Kupffer cell phagocytosis of opsonized ^{51}chromium-labelled sheep erythrocytes.

TABLE 2. Phagocytosis of Opsonized ^{51}Cr-labelled Sheep Erythrocytes by Rat Kupffer Cells Cultured in Varying Concentrations of Ethanol

	Ethanol Concentration (mg/dl)				
	200	300	500	800	1000
Phagocytosis % control (Mean ± SEM)	111±2.8	117±3.1*	119±2.2*	87±2.9*	52±3.8*

*p ≤ 0.05 compared to control

Concentrations of ethanol between 300-500 mg/dl caused significant stimulation of phagocytosis while concentrations greater than 800 mg/dl suppressed this function. Thus, ethanol induced a biphasic response in Kupffer cell phagocytic function *in vitro*, causing cell activation at ethanol concentrations found in portal blood after acute oral dosing and depression of activity at higher concentrations. A different pattern of response was seen with acetaldehyde (Table 3). All concentrations of acetaldehyde tested suppressed Kupffer cell phagocytosis, with significant impairment in function occuring at acetaldehyde concentrations above 0.15 mg/dl.

TABLE 3. Phagocytosis of Opsonized ^{51}Cr-labelled Sheep Erythrocytes by Rat Kupffer Cells Cultured in Varying Concentrations of Acetaldehyde

	Acetaldehyde Concentration (mg/dl)				
	0.05	0.10	0.15	0.30	0.50
Phagocytosis % control (Mean ± SEM)	83±9.4	84±8.5	61±5.1*	66±4.2*	62±4.5*

* p ≤ 0.05

Incubation of Kupffer cells in ethanol at concentrations from 0-1840 mg/dl caused marked changes in membrane microviscosity (Figure 1). Ethanol induced a fluidizing effect which became significantly different from control at concentrations above 260 mg/dl. We observed no plateau or decrease in the fluidizing effect of ethanol at any of the concentrations tested.

Figure 1. Plasma membrane microviscosity (P) of rat Kupffer cells exposed to varying concentrations of ethanol.

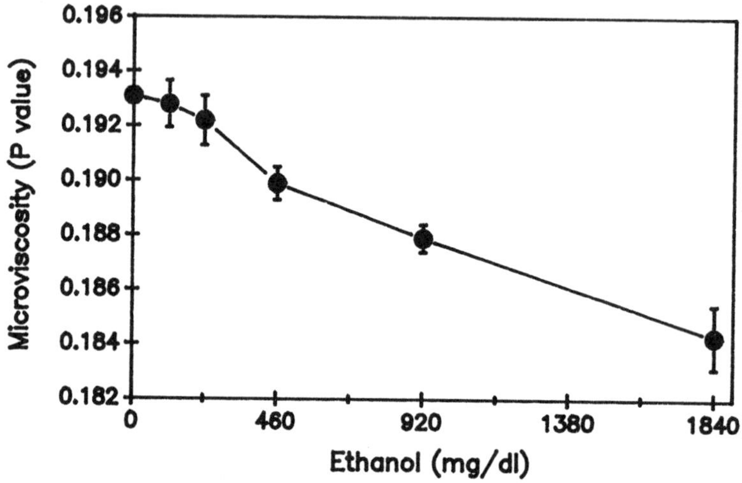

The effects of varying acute and also repeated doses of ethanol on blood clearance of colloidial carbon is shown in Table 4. A single oral doses of ethanol (1-4 g/kg) led to activated macrophage (Kupffer cell) function as reflected by enhanced carbon clearance, i.e. a shorter blood carbon half life ($t_{1/2}$). In contrast, when the same dose of ethanol was given three times (8 hour intervals) over twenty four hours there was significant prolongation of carbon clearance by all four ethanol doses, reflecting significant suppression of macrophage and Kupffer cell function.

TABLE 4. Effects of Varying Oral Doses of Ethanol on Half Life ($t_{1/2}$) of Colloidal Carbon in the Rat**

ETHANOL DOSE	CONTROL	1 DOSE OF ETHANOL	3 DOSES OF ETHANOL
0	16.1±0.5	-	-
0.5g/kg	-	17.3±0.4	20.3±0.7*
1.0g/kg	-	13.6±0.6*	19.1±0.6*
2.0g/kg	-	12.5±0.9*	20.0±0.3*
4.0g/kg	-	12.0±0.2*	25.3±1.8*

* $p \leq 0.05$ from control

** Clearance test started 1 hour after last dose of ethanol.

DISCUSSION

The results of these studies clearly demonstrate that ethanol can modify Kupffer cell phagocytosis in vitro and in vivo. Concentrations of ethanol similar to that observed in portal blood of rats given a single large oral dose of ethanol stimulated Kupffer cell phagocytic function. In contrast, higher concentrations of ethanol, which might have been reached in portal blood at larger or repeated doses of ethanol produced significant suppression of Kupffer cell function. Of interest, the ethanol metabolite acetaldehyde, which is not normally measureable in peripheral blood but during alcohol metabolism is likely present in hepatic sinusoidal blood bathing Kupffer cells, caused significant suppression of phagocytosis at all concentrations tested. Our observations support the possibility that acetaldehyde produced from ethanol metabolism in hepatic parenchymal cells or within the Kupffer cell itself might be responsible for causing the impairment of Kupffer cell function described with chronic alcohol consumption (MacGregor, 1986).

It is well recognized that ethanol fluidizes the bulk lipid of membranes of a variety of cells and that this effect can alter cell function (Wood and Schroeder, 1988). In the liver, previous studies have shown that ethanol has a fluidizing effect and causes an alteration in function of parenchymal cells (Schacter, 1984). We observed that ethanol also causes a dose related fluidizing effect on the Kupffer cell plasma membrane. A decrease in membrane microviscosity might be anticipated to augment phagocytosis whereas development of a rigid membrane structure would conceivably impair phagocytosis. It is of interest to note that enhanced phagocytosis occurred at concentrations of ethanol which reduced membrane microviscosity (see Table 2 and Figure 1). However, higher doses of ethanol, which were associated with depression in phagocytosis, caused an even greater increase in membrane fluidity. Therefore, it seems unlikely that alterations in Kupffer cell phagocytosis induced by ethanol result solely from an effect of ethanol on physical properties of the cell plasma membrane.

Single oral doses of ethanol (1-4 g/kg) activated macrophage function in vivo as reflected by enhanced blood clearance of colloidal carbon. However, repeated application of the same dose of ethanol over a twenty four hour period led to significant impairment of macrophage clearance of the injected particles. Thus, individuals acutely consuming a variety of large doses of alcohol could theoretically experience consequences of activated Kupffer cell function such as enhanced phagocytosis and possibly increased secretion of mediators (Adams, 1984). In contrast, repeated ethanol consumption would likely cause impairment of this cellular response. One consequence of the latter situation which has been recognized clinically is impaired clearance of foreign particles and bacteria from the blood leading to increased risk of infection (Rimola, 1984). Conceivably, repeated doses of ethanol would also impair release of important macrophage derived cytokines, the consequences of which are less clear.

The results of these studies do not directly assign a role for the Kupffer cell in pathogenesis of alcoholic liver disease. However, the fact that ethanol can both stimulate as well as depress Kupffer cell function suggests a number of possibilities which merit further consideration. For example, activated Kupffer cells not only exhibit enhanced phagocytosis, they also secrete increased amounts of cytokines and mediators including reactive oxygen species, products of arachidonic acid metabolism, interleukins, tumor necrosis factor and a variety of other substances which could augment toxic effects of ethanol on the liver (Adams, 1984). Some Kupffer cell secretory products are also chemotactic and recruit leukocytes as well as activated mononuclear cells into liver tissue, a consequence which could further augment or promote liver damage (Adams, 1984, Nathan, 1987). Conversely, depression of macrophage function by repeated exposure to ethanol might contribute to liver injury by reducing Kupffer cell degredation of endotoxin in portal blood and by suppressing Kupffer cell synthesis and release of those cytokines or mediators which are cytoprotective and promote normal liver homeostasis (Rimola, 1984, Nathan, 1987). For example, Kupffer cells synthesize and secrete both prostaglandin E_1 and E_2 (Decker, 1989). PGE_1 has an inhibitory effect on cell mediated cytotoxicity of effector spleen cells against hepatocytes in experimental autoimmune hepatitis (Ogawa, 1988). PGE_2 has been shown to have a cytoprotective effect on liver parenchymal cells exposed to carbon tetrachloride and to galactosamine (Stachura, 1980, Stachura, 1981). In addition, PGE_2 decreases the release of extracellular collagen from fibroblasts (Steinman, 1982). In other experiments, rats fed a lipotrope deficient, liver fibrosis-inducing diet had less increase in hepatic synthesis of hydroxyproline and collagen when given exogenous PGE_2 than did control rats fed the same diet (Ruwart, 1988). Thus, suppression of Kupffer cell secretion of at least PGE_1 and PGE_2 conceivably could increase the susceptibility of hepatic parenchymal cells to damage by ethanol or other hepatotoxins and also promote synthesis and deposition of collagen in liver in response to minimal injury.

Lastly, when chronic ethanol consumption is discontinued, recovery of Kupffer cell function may lead to rebound secretion of various mediator substances that could promote or enhance liver injury. One candidate cytokine might be leukotriene B_4 (LTB-4), a potent chemotactic agent secreted by Kupffer cells (Nathan, 1987, McCuskey, 1987). Recruitment of large numbers of polymorphonuclear leukocytes into liver tissue by LTB-4 could result in increased injury from these cells to parenchymal cells which were only minimally damaged by the ethanol itself. Indeed, a common clinical finding is the unexplained worsening of alcoholic hepatitis some 5-7 days after acute alcohol ingestion has been discontinued.

In view of the large number of cytokines and mediator substances secreted by Kupffer cells and the biphasic effects of ethanol on Kupffer cell function observed in these studies, we postulate that ethanol-induced alterations in Kupffer cell function may play a significant contributory role in the pathogenesis of alcohol-induced liver injury. Further investigation of this possibility is clearly indicated.

REFERENCES

Adams DO, Hamilton TA (1984). The Cell biology of macrophage activation. Ann Rev Immunol 2:283-318.

Biozzi G, Stiffel C, (1965). The physiopathology of the reticuloendothelial cells of the liver and spleen. Prog Liver Dis 2:166-191.

Decker T, Lohmann-Matthes ML, Karck U, Peters T, Decker K (1989). Comparative study of cytotoxicity, tumor necrosis factor and prostaglandin release after stimulation of rat Kupffer cells, murine Kupffer cells and murine inflammatory liver macrophages. J Leukocyt Biol 45:139-146.

El Sisi, AE, Earnest DK, Sipes IG (1987). Potentiation of carbon tetrachloride hepatotoxicity by hypervitaminosis A is mediatred in part by reactive oxygen species secreted by Kupffer cells. Gastroenterol 92:894.

Fox ES, Thomas P, Broitman SA (1989). Clearance of gut-derived endotoxins by the liver. Release and modification of ^3H, ^{14}C-lipopolysaccharide by isolated rat Kupffer cells. Gastroenterol 96:456-461.

Knook DL, Sleyster ECH (1976). Separation of Kupffer and endothelial cells of the rat liver by centrifugal elutriation. Experim Cell Res 99:444-456

Lieber CS (1988). Biochemical and molecular basis of alcohol-induced injury to liver and other tissues. N Eng J Med 319:1639-1650.

MacGregor RR (1986). Alcohol and immune defense. JAMA 256:1474-1479.

McCuskey RS, McCuskey PA, Urbaschek R, Urbaschek B (1987). Kupffer cell function in host defense. Rev Infect Dis 9:(supp 15):S616-619.

Nathan CF (1987). Secretory products of macrophages. J Clin Invest 79:319-326.

Ogawa M, Mori T, Mori Y, Ueda S, Yoshida H, Kato T, Iesato K, Wakashin Y, Wakashin M, Okuda K (1988). Inhibitory effects of prostaglandin E_1 on T-cell mediated cytotoxicity against isolated mouse liver cells. Gastroenterol 94:1024-1030.

Palo V, Likova H (1970). Direct gas chromatographic estimation of lower alcohols, acetaldehyde, acetone and diacotyl in milk products. J Chrom 53:363-367.

Rimola A, Soto R, Bory F, Arryoy V, Piera C, Rodes J (1984). Reticuloendothelial system phagocytic activity and cirrhosis and its relation to bacterial infections and prognosis. Hepatology 4:53-58.

Ruwart MJ, Rush BD, Syder KF, Peters RM, Appelman HD, Henley KS (1988). 16,16-dimethyl prostaglandin E-2 delays collagen formation in nutritional injury in rat liver. Hepatology 8:61-64.

Sato C, Matsuda Y, Lieber CS (1981). Increased hepatotoxicity of acetominophen after chronic ethanol consumption in the rat. Gastroenterol 80:140-148.

Schacter D (1984). Fluidity and function of hepatocyte plasma membranes. Hepatol 4:140-151.

Scott WA, Pawlowski NA, Murry HW, Andreach M, Zrike J, Cohn ZA (1982). The regulation of arachidonic acid metabolism by macrophage activation. J Exp Med 155:1148-1161.

Shinitzky M, Dianoux A, Gitler C (1971). Microviscosity and order in the hydorcarbon region of micelles and membranes determined with fluroescent probes. Biochem 10:2106-2113.

Stachura J, Tarnawski A, Ivey KJ, Mach T, Bogdad J, Szczudrawa J, Klimczyk B (1981). Prostaglandin protection of carbon tetrachloride-induced liver necrosis in the rat. Gastroenterol 81:211-217.

Stachura J, Tarnawski A, Szuzudrawa J, (1980). Cytoprotective effects of 16, 16-dimethyl prostaglandin E_2 and some drugs on acute galactosamine induced liver damage in the rat. Folia Histochem Cytochem 9:311-318.

Steinman BU, Abe S, Martin GR (1982). Modulation of type I and type II collagen production in normal and mutant human skin fibroblasts by cell density, prostaglandin E_2 and epidermal growth factor. Collagen Rel Res 2:185-195.

Tachibana K, Sone S, Tsubura E, Kishino Y (1984). Stimulatory effects of vitamin A on tumoricidal activity of rat alveolar macrophages. Brit J Cancer 49:343.

Wickramasinghe SN, Barden G, Levy L (1987). The capacity of macrophages from different murine tissues to metabolize ethanol and generate an ethanol-dependent nondialysable cytotoxic activity in vitro. Alcohol and Alcoholism 22:31-39.

ACKNOWLEDGEMENT

The study was supported in part by NIAAA Grant No. AA08037. The excellent secretarial assistance of Debbie Markley is gratefully recognized.

Alcohol, Immunomodulation, and AIDS, pages 267–271
© 1990 Alan R. Liss, Inc.

THE EFFECT OF ALCOHOL ON HIV INFECTION IN VITRO

Louis D. Saravolatz, Robert F. Cerra, Donald J. Pohlod and Susan Smereck

Infectious Disease and Surgical Research Laboratories, Henry Ford Hospital, Detroit, Michigan 48202

INTRODUCTION

Alcohol may serve as a potential risk factor for HIV infection through either a behavioral or physiological mechanism. Consumption of alcohol may result in behavioral disinhibition leading to increased high risk behavior. In addition, alcohol may produce an immune dysregulation directly or indirectly. One direct effect alcohol may have on cell physiology is to increase the susceptibility to HIV infection through modulation of CD4 (+) cell surface receptors, the known binding site of the gp120 viral coat protein (2,5). Ethanol treatment of cells has previously been shown to produce alteration in membrane fluidity, lipid content, and modulation of HLA antigens (1,3,4,6). We have attempted to determine whether alcohol does increase infectivity of CD4 (+) cells by exposing the CEM cell line to various ethanol concentrations and measuring the amount of viral antigen produced. Although no difference in cell growth or viability was observed, a marked dose dependent increase in HIV production was found with increasing ethanol concentrations, suggesting alcohol does alter the susceptibility of a lymphocyte to HIV infection.

METHODS

CELLS/VIRUS

The CEM cells and the HIV isolates were obtained from Dr. L. Guskey at the Michigan Department of Public Health and the cells were maintained in RPMI-1640 containing L-glutamine, penicillin-streptomycin-neomycin supplemented with 10% heat inactivated fetal bovine serum. Virus was propagated by co-culture of HIV(+) CEM cells with an equal number of uninfected CEM cells in fresh culture media. Cell viability was determined by trypan blue exclusion.

ALCOHOL TREATMENT/INFECTION OF CELLS

CEM cells were incubated in tissue culture media containing 0, 50, 100, 150 and 250 mM ethanol. After 24 hours, the cells were washed free of the alcohol and 1 x 10^6 cells in 5 ml media were inoculated with a 1:1000 dilution of HIV(+) media. Twenty-four hours later, 5 ml of fresh media was added to the culture (day 1) and at the indicated times an aliquot was removed and assayed as described below. Data is presented as the amount of p24 antigen produced by ethanol treated cells normalized to the amount produced by cells not pretreated with alcohol.

p24 ANTIGEN ASSAY

The Abbott HIV antigen EIA detection kit was used for p24 analysis according to manufactures directions. Briefly, the aliquot of cells and media was solubilized in 0.1% Triton X-100 and incubated with antibody to p24 immobilized on polystyrene beads. After washing, the beads are inoculated with rabbit antibody to p24 followed by peroxidase conjugated goat anti-rabbit IgG. The amount of antigen is detected using OPD substrate.

RESULTS

The viability of the CEM cells after 24 hour ethanol exposure is shown in Figure 1. Following the incubation in 50 and 250 mM ethanol, no significant difference was observed between the alcohol treated cells and untreated controls. The CEM cells maintained greater than 80% viability immediately after removal of the ethanol and continued to survive over prolonged culture.

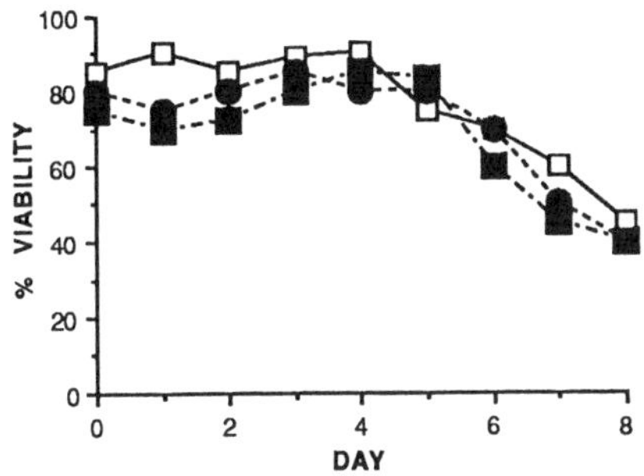

Figure 1 - Viability of CEM cells following Ethanol Exposure. CEM cells were exposed to 0(□), 50 (●), or 250 (■) mM ethanol for 24 hours. Viability was determined by trypan blue exclusion.

Cells exposed to ethanol for 24 hours were then examined for susceptibility to infection by HIV (Figure 2). Treated cells were washed free of ethanol and inoculated with HIV(+) cell free conditioned media. A marked dose-dependent rise in amounts of p24 antigen production is observed for cells treated with increasing ethanol concentrations indicating increased virus production. The p24 antigen levels increase from control levels on day 1 to 3 times control levels by day 8 for the 250 mM ethanol exposure. A similar increase is also seen with the 150 mM level. However, at 50 and 100 mM ethanol only, a minimal increase of p24 antigen was seen compared to the controls.

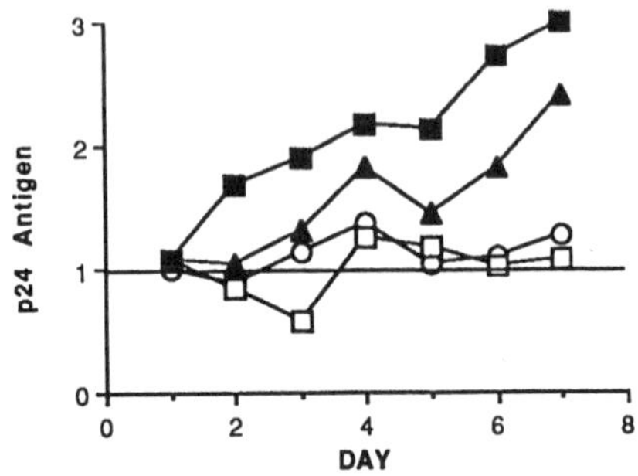

Figure 2 - Production of p24 antigen by cells exposed to ethanol. CEM cells were exposed to 50 (□), 100 (○), 150 (▲), or 250 (■) mM ethanol for 24 hours and inoculated with HIV(+) conditioned media.

DISCUSSION

We have attempted to evaluate the susceptibility to infection by HIV of CD4(+) cells which have been exposed to ethanol. High concentrations of ethanol, which do not affect the viability of the CEM cells, induce a marked rise in HIV core antigen production in a dose dependent fashion. Whether the increased production of HIV - p24 antigen results from a greater number of cells being infected or induction and replication of HIV in a few cells which are infected is not known. We would postulate that a modulation of cell surface molecules has led to increased number of cells being infected. Ethanol is a known immunomodulator that affects cellular physiology and cell surface biochemistry. After ethanol exposure, the number of CD4 receptors may be increased which would facilitate a more productive infection. Alternatively, receptor affinities may be increased or cell surface rearrangements may occur also resulting in a greater likelihood of infection. We are currently attempting to elucidate the mechanism of the increased infection that is observed.

REFERENCES

1. Dalgleish AG, Beverly PCL, Clapham PR, Crawford DH, Greaves MF, Weiss RA. (1984) Nature 312:763.
2. Maddon PH, Dalgleish AG, MCDougal JS, Clapham PR, Weiss RA, Axel R. (1986) Cell 47:333.
3. Vanderkooi, JM. (1979) Alcoholism 3:60.
4. Chin JH, Goldstein DB, Parsons IM. (1979) Alcoholism 3:46.
5. Gluckman SJ, Dvorak VC, MacGregor RR. (1977) Arch Intern Med 137:1539.
6. Lundy J, Raaf JH, Deakins S, Wanebo HJ, Jacobs DA, Lee T, Jacobowitz D, Spear C, Oettgen HF. (1975) Surg Gyn Obs 141:212.

Alcohol, Immunomodulation, and AIDS, pages 273–282
© 1990 Alan R. Liss, Inc.

SUPPRESSION OF LYMPHOCYTE ACTIVITY AFTER ACUTE MORPHINE ADMINISTRATION APPEARS TO BE GLUCOCORTICOID INDEPENDENT

Barbara M. Bayer, Monica Hernandez and Lauren Irvin

Department of Pharmacology, Georgetown School of Medicine, Washington D.C., 20007

INTRODUCTION

Chronic morphine administration has been shown to be accompanied by a generalized immunosuppression in both animals and in human addicts (Hussey and Katz, 1950; Cherubin and Brown, 1968; Louria et al., 1957; Brown, et al., 1974). The exact mechanism by which morphine may inhibit immune system activity is unknown. Recent evidence has suggested the effects of morphine may be mediated by activation of central opiate receptors (Shavit et al., 1986a; Weber and Pert, 1987).

There are several ways in which morphine may influence immune cell activities through the stimulation of central opiate receptors. For example, centrally administered morphine has been shown to increase the activity of sympathetic neurons resulting in an elevation of plasma catecholamine levels (van Loon, et al., 1981; Appel, et al., 1986). Catecholamines have been demonstrated to suppress a number of lymphocyte activities in vitro (Bourne et al., 1974; Joasoo and McKenzie, 1976). Furthermore, stimulation of sympathetic neurons innervating the spleen has been associated with a decreased immune cell function (Besedovsky et al., 1979).

Another well described consequence of central opiate receptor stimulation is the activation of the hypothalamic-pituitary-adrenal axis. The concomitant elevation of circulating neuroendocrine substances such as ACTH, TSH, β-endorphin and corticosterone also has the potential of influencing lymphocyte activity. An increase in corticosterone levels has been observed after either intracerebral (Haracz, et al., 1981) or systemic (Gibson, et al., 1979) morphine administration. Glucocorticoids have been shown to inhibit NK cell cytolytic activity (Hochman and Cudkowicz, 1979; Cox, et al., 1982) and other lymphocyte activities in vitro (Gillis, et al., 1979).

To begin to examine the mechanisms by which morphine may influence the immune system we have compared the effects of systemically administered morphine on splenic NK cell activity to those on blood and splenic mitogen-stimulated lymphocyte proliferation. Further characterization of the opioid dependency of the immunosuppressive effects of morphine was determined in naltrexone pretreated animals. Plasma corticosterone was monitored in all treatment groups to assess any possible correlation between elevated glucocorticoid levels and inhibition of immune cell activities.

METHODS AND RESULTS

Sprague Dawley rats (250-350g) were injected subcutaneously with saline or morphine at the indicated doses and sacrificed 2 hours later. Proliferation stimulated by the T cell mitogen, Concanavalin A (Con A), of both blood and splenic lymphocytes was determined. As shown in Figure 1, a dose dependent inhibition of blood lymphocyte activity was observed with morphine administration. In contrast, the splenic lymphocyte response to mitogen was not significantly depressed at any of the doses used.

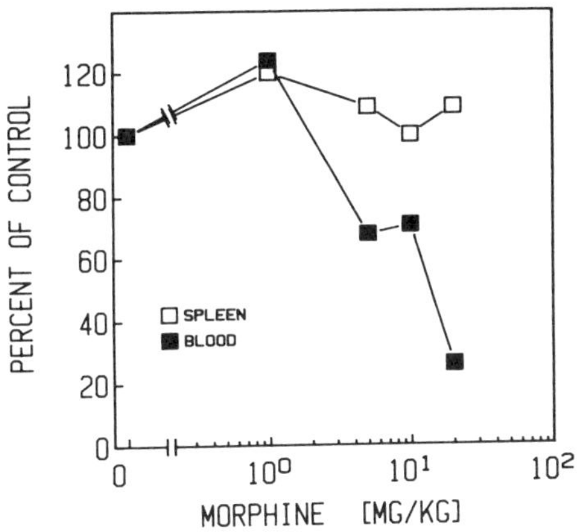

Figure 1. Effects of morphine on blood and splenic lymphocyte proliferation. Animals were injected with either saline or morphine at the indicated doses and sacrificed 2 hours later. Proliferative responses of lymphocytes were determined after 72 hours of incubation with Con A. During the final 24 hours, cultures were incubated with ^{3}H-thymidine (1μCi) and then harvested. Results are expressed as the mean ± SEM of percent of control (saline injected) for at least 3 animals per dose.

To examine whether the effect of morphine on blood lymphocyte proliferation was mediated by opiate receptors, animals were injected with the opiate antagonist, naltrexone (10 mg/kg). One hour later, half of the naltrexone treated animals received morphine (25 mg/kg) and the other half were injected with saline. Naltrexone alone had no significant effect on Con A (0.125 μg/culture) stimulated blood lymphocyte proliferation (Table 1). Morphine, on the other hand, was found to depress the blood lymphocyte response by 70 percent in saline injected controls and by only 40 percent in animals pretreated with naltrexone (Table 1). The depressed activity in animals treated with morphine alone or in combination with naltrexone was found to be significant, suggesting that pretreatment with naltrexone partially antagonized the suppression induced by morphine.

OPIOID DEPENDENT INHIBITION OF BLOOD LYMPHOCYTE PROLIFERATION INDUCED BY MORPHINE	
TREATMENT	^{3}H-THYMIDINE (CPM/CULTURE)
SALINE	32,493 ± 2,957
NALTREXONE (10 MG/KG)	28,570 ± 5,857
MORPHINE (25 MG/KG)	9,446 ± 1,137*
NALTREXONE + MORPHINE	18,568 ± 2,098*#

Table 1. Animals were treated as described in text. Results are expressed as the mean ± SEM for at least 5 animals per group. *Significantly different compared to saline treated controls ($p \leq 0.05$). #Significantly different compared to morphine treated group ($p \leq 0.05$).

We also addressed whether morphine administration would have an effect on the spontaneous lysis of a tumor cell line by NK cells. A standard cytolytic assay was used in which increasing concentrations of splenic lymphocytes were incubated with a constant number of prelabelled Cr^{51} YAC target cells. Although morphine was found to have no effect on splenic lymphocyte proliferation, splenic NK cytolytic activity was significantly inhibited at effector/target cell ratios of 25:1, 50:1 and 100:1 (Table 2). This effect was completely antagonized by pretreatment for 1 hour with naltrexone (10 mg/kg) (Table 2). Naltrexone treatment alone was found to have little effect on NK cell activity.

OPIOID DEPENDENT INHIBITION OF NK CYTOLYTIC ACTIVITY INDUCED BY MORPHINE

TREATMENT	% CYTOTOXICITY			
	EFFECTOR/TARGET RATIO			
	100:1	50:1	25:1	12.5:1
SALINE	31 ± 1.5	33 ± 0.5	25 ± 0.8	15 ± 1.2
NALTREXONE (10 MG/KG)	40 ± 2.0	36 ± 1.8	25 ± 0.7	15 ± 0.6
MORPHINE (25 MG/KG)	23 ± 3.1 *	24 ± 4.0*	18 ± 2.6 *	12 ± 2.5
NALTREXONE + MORPHINE	32 ± 1.8	35 ± 2.5	26 ± 3.3	14 ± 1.9

Table 2. Splenic cytolytic activity was determined at 4 different effector/target cell ratios as described in Methods. Results are expressed as the mean ± SEM for at least 4 animals per group. *Significantly different compared to saline treated controls ($p \leq 0.05$).

To determine if morphine and/or naltrexone treatment was accompanied by an increase in circulating plasma levels of corticosterone, animals were treated under the conditions described and plasma corticosterone was measured. As shown in Table 3, treatment with naltrexone and morphine individually, as well as their combination, resulted in significant increases in plasma corticosterone levels.

ELEVATION IN CORTICOSTERONE LEVELS WITH MORPHINE AND NALTREXONE TREATMENT

TREATMENT	CORTICOSTERONE (NG/ML)
SALINE	191 ± 74
NALTREXONE (10 MG/KG)	870 ± 91*
MORPHINE (25 MG/KG)	484 ± 88 *
NALTREXONE + MORPHINE	720 ± 140 *

Table 3. Increases in corticosterone with morphine and naltrexone. Plasma corticosterone levels were determined by radioimmunoassay. Results are expressed as the mean ± SEM for 4 to 5 animals per group. *Significantly different compared to saline treated controls ($p \leq 0.05$).

DISCUSSION

We report that both blood lymphocyte proliferation and splenic NK cytolytic activity are suppressed by acute morphine administration and that pretreatment with the opiate receptor antagonist, naltrexone, partially or completely antagonized these effects, respectively. These data suggest that the acute effects of morphine on immune cell function are mediated, at least in part, by the activation of opiate receptors. Others have demonstrated that the effects of morphine on NK cytolytic activity most likely are centrally mediated (Shavit et al., 1984; 1986a; 1986b). In these studies intracerebrally administered morphine decreased NK cell activity whereas methyl-morphine, a peripherally acting morphine analogue, had no effect when administered systemically. Supporting these observations, NK cytolytic activity was also found to be significantly suppressed following microinjection of morphine into the periaqueductal gray (PAG) but not the anterior hypothalamus, arcuate nucleus, medial amygdala, medial thalamus or dorsal hippocampus (Weber and Pert, 1987).

Although it appears that morphine can exert an effect on the immune system through stimulation of central opiate receptors, the mechanism by which this effect is transmitted to the peripheral lymphocytes remains unknown. Our data, however, suggest that the effects of morphine on lymphocyte proliferation and NK cytolytic activity are mediated by factors other than an elevation of glucocorticoids. For example, naltrexone treatment was found to be accompanied by the greatest increase in circulating corticosterone levels with no accompanying effects on either blood lymphocyte proliferation or splenic NK cytolytic activity. Thus an increase in circulating steroids, alone, was not sufficient to depress these immune cell activities within 2 hours.

It is unlikely that morphine is mediating its effects through direct interaction at opiate receptors on the lymphocyte membrane for several reasons. First, morphine has been shown to have little effect or slight stimulation on lymphocyte proliferation (Wybran, 1985a; 1985b) and NK cytolytic activity (Kay, et al., 1984; Wybran, 1985c) when added directly to cell cultures <u>in vitro</u>. We have found that <u>in vitro</u> morphine will inhibit lymphocyte proliferation and NK activity only at exceedingly high concentrations ($\geq$ 0.25 mM) (data not shown). Secondly, these <u>in vitro</u> effects were found not to be naltrexone sensitive, suggesting a direct, nonopioid effect at only high concentrations of morphine. This is in opposition to the opioid dependent suppression observed with morphine when administered <u>in vivo</u>.

We conclude that the immunosuppressive effects of morphine are most likely due to central activation of opiate receptors. Although this effect is accompanied by activation of the pituitary-adrenal axis resulting in increases in plasma corticosterone, it is apparent that additional factors are required to elicit the suppressive effects observed in morphine treated animals. These studies also illustrate that physiological increases of corticosterone are not necessarily accompanied by immunosuppressive effects. The suppressive effects of morphine on lymphocyte activity may be mediated by the release of other anterior pituitary hormones and/or through the stimulation of sympathetic neurons resulting in an elevation of plasma cathecholamines.

REFERENCES

Appel N.M., Kiritsy-Roy J.A. and van Loon G.R. (1986) Mu receptors at discrete hypothalamic and brainstem sites mediate opioid peptide-induced increases in central sympathetic outflow. *Brain Res.* **378:** 8-20.

Besedovsky H.O., del Rey A., Sorkin E., Da Prada M. and Keller H.H. (1979) Immunoregulation mediated by the sympathetic nervous system. *Cell. Immunol.* **48:** 346-355.

Bourne H.R., Lichtenstein L.M., Melmon K.L., Henney C.S., Weinstein Y. and Shearer G.M. (1974) Modulation of inflammation and immunity by cyclic AMP. *Science* **184:** 19-28.

Brown S.M., Stimmel B., Taub R.N., Kochwa S., and Rosenfield R.E. (1974) Immunologic dysfunction in heroin addicts. *Arch. Intern. Med.* **134:** 1001-1005.

Cherubin, C.E. and Brown, J. (1968) Systemic infections in heroin addicts. *Lancet* **1:** 298-299.

Cox W.I., Holbrook N.J., Grasso R.J., Specter S. and Friedman H. (1982) Suppression of the natural killer cell activity of murine spleen cell cultures by dexamethasone (41489). *Proc. Soc. Exp. Biol. Med.* **171:** 146-150.

Gibson A., Ginsberg M., Hall M., and Hart S.L. (1979) The effects of opiate receptor agonists and antagonists on the stress-induced secretion of corticosterone in mice. *Br. J.Pharmacol.* **65:** 139-146.

Gillis S., Crabtree G.R. and Smith K.A. (1979) Glucocorticoid-induced inhibition of T cell growth factor production. I. The effect on mitogen lymphocyte proliferation. *J. Immunol* **123:** 1624-1631.

Haracz J.L., Bloom A.S., Wang R.I.H. and Tseng L.F. (1981) Effect of intraventricular β-endorphin and morphine on hypothalamic-pituitary-adrenal activity and the release of pituitary β-endorphin. *Neuroendocrinology* **33:** 170-175.

Hochman P.S. and Cudkowicz G. (1979) Suppression of natural cytotoxicity by spleen cells of hydrocortisone-treated mice. *J. Immunol.* **123:** 986-976.

Hussey H.H. and Katz S. (1950) Infections resulting from narcotic addiction: report of 102 cases, *Am. J. Med.* **9:** 186-193.

Joasoo A. and McKenzie J.M. (1976) Stress and the immune response in rats. *Int. Arch. Allergy Appl. Immunol.* **50:** 659-663.

Kay N., Allen J. and Morley J.E. (1984) Endorphins stimulate normal human peripheral blood lymphocyte natural killer activity. *Life Sci.* **35:** 53-59.

Louria D.B., Hensle T. and Rose J. (1957) The major medical complication of heroin addiction, *Ann. Intern. Med.* **67:** 1-22.

Shavit Y., Lewis J.W., Terman G.W., Gale R.P., and Liebeskind J.C. (1984) Opioid peptides mediate the suppressive effect of stress on natural killer cell cytotoxicity. *Sci.* **223:** 188-190.

Shavit Y., DePaulis A., Martin F.C., Terman G.W., Pechnick R.N., Zane C.J., Gale R.P., and Liebeskind J.C. (1986a) Involvement of brain opiate receptors in the immune-suppressive effect of morphine, *PNAS* **83:** 7114- 7117.

Shavit Y., Terman G.W., Lewis J.W., Zane C.J., Gale R.P. and Liebeskind J.C. (1986) Effects of footshock stress and morphine on natural killer lymphocytes in rats: studies of tolerance and cross tolerance. *Brain Res.* **372:** 382-385.

Van Loon G.R., Appel N.M. and Ho D. (1981) β-endorphin-induced stimulation of central sympathetic outflow: β-endorphin increases plasma concentrations of epinephrine, norepinephrine and dopamine in rats. *Endocrinology* **109:** 46-53.

Weber R.J. and Pert A. (1987) Opiate action in the periaqueductal gray matter causes suppression of immune function *J. Cell Biochem.* **suppl., 12D:** 317.

Wybran J. (1985a) Enkephalins and endorphins: activation molecules for the immune system and natural killer activity. *Neuropeptides* **5:** 371-379.

Wybran J. (1985b) Enkephalins and endorphins as modifiers of the immune system: present and future. *Fed. Proc.* **44:** 92-94.

Wybran J. (1985c) Enkephalins, endorphins, substance P and the immune system. In: *Neural Modulation of Immunity* (R. Guillemin et al., Eds.), pp.157-161. Raven Press, New York.

Alcohol, Immunomodulation, and AIDS, pages 283–304
© 1990 Alan R. Liss, Inc.

EFFECT OF CHRONIC ETHANOL CONSUMPTION AND RETROVIRAL INFECTION ON CARCINOGENESIS AND ITS POSSIBLE INHIBITION BY AN IMMUNOSTIMULANT, CANTHAXANTHIN: DEFINITION OF A MURINE MODEL

Siraj I. Mufti[1] and Ronald R. Watson[2]

Departments of [1]Pharmacology and Toxicology and [2]Family and Community Medicine, University of Arizona Health Sciences Center, Tucson, Arizona 85724

INTRODUCTION

Excessive alcohol consumption is a major health problem for many societies throughout the world. There are 18 million alcohol-dependent Americans and another 40 million heavy drinkers. The cost to individuals and society, in terms of medical care and other financial and social costs, are tremendous. Between 20 to 40% of hospital beds in the U.S.A. are filled by patients whose illnesses are alcohol-related. According to an estimate of the National Institute of Alcohol Abuse and Alcoholism yearly economic costs for alcohol-related problems amount to $117 billion (Gordis et al., 1989).

Alcohol is a major risk factor for several types of cancers in humans. Sites most associated with cancers in excessive chronic drinkers are mouth, pharynx, larynx, esophagus and liver (Hakulinen et al., 1974; Monson and Lyons, 1975; Jensen, 1979; Tuyns, 1979; Rothman et al., 1980; Doll and Peto, 1981). Other sites associated with alcohol-related cancers are the pancreas (Burch and Ansari, 1968), breast (Rosenberg et al., 1982), stomach (MacDonald, 1972) and colon (Enstrom, 1977). The main lines of evidence for epidemiological studies have been a) individual patient histories of excessive alcohol consumption linked with higher rates of cancers; b) occupations with high alcohol exposure, e.g., among brewers who consume large quantities of free beer, have higher death rates from cancers; c) regions with higher per capita alcohol consumption have higher death rates.

In contrast, population groups with lower consumption, e.g., Mormons (Lyon et al., 1977) and Seventh Day Adventists (Lemon et al., 1964), have lower cancer rates. The association with cancer of the esophagus is particularly strong (Rothman et al., 1980), and 75% of esophageal cancers in the U.S.A. could be attributed to alcohol consumption. The subject of alcohol-related cancers has been extensively reviewed by others (for example, Rothman et al., 1980; Doll and Peto, 1980; NCR, 1982; Lieber et al., 1986) and recently by us (Mufti et al., 1989). Despite a preponderance of epidemiologic evidence, experimental evidence for the effect of alcohol on cancer incidence is not clear and often contradictory results have been obtained by different investigators (for a discussion, see Mufti et al., 1989).

The incidence of acquired immune deficiency syndrome (AIDS), the result of infection with a retrovirus HIV (human immunodeficiency virus), in 1984 among single men in Manhattan and San Francisco, and hemophiliacs in the United States was greater than 250/100,000 (Selwyn, 1986; Fauci, 1988). That is comparable to the yearly incidence of all cancers, i.e., approximately 330/100,000 for the general U.S. population. The economic impact of AIDS on the patient and society is very high. The average cost of caring for these patients in the USA with a comprehensive plan that emphasizes outpatient care is about $85,000 per AIDS patient (Bloom and Carliner, 1989). The cost of caring for the much more numerous HIV infected asymptomatic and ARC (AIDS-related complex) patients is not known but is of significant magnitude.

While HIV is generally regarded as the infectious agent that causes AIDS, other cofactors, including age-modulated immune functions, immunosuppression induced by alcohol, drugs and/or malnutrition (Watson, 1989) may influence the rate of development or full expression of the disease (Watson, 1989). Alcohol abuse features prominently in homosexual experience and current research has shown that alcohol in conjunction with sexual activity is conducive to AIDS (for a further discussion see papers by Cooper et al.; Doll; Hingson et al.; Leigh; Molgaard; Neff and Burge; Stall and Trocki; and Leigh in these proceedings). Individuals suffering from AIDS because of their immune deficiency are vulnerable to opportunistic cancers including Kaposi's sarcoma and squamous cell carcinomas. An increased prevalence of oral squamous cell carcinoma has been observed in homosexual males with AIDS or ARC when compared to the general population (Silverman et al., 1986). Furthermore, a lack of immune surveillance is probably responsible for aggressive behavior of Kaposi's sarcoma in many AIDS patients (Sanchez et al., 1988). However, an increase in all types of cancers has not been observed in AIDS patients, since most subjects are relatively young and in 1986 only about 10% of AIDS patients were over 50 years of age, a time by which greater opportunities for initiation and promotion have occurred.

A number of investigators including ourselves have shown that ethanol causes immunosuppression (for example, Watson 1984, 1988; Mufti et al., 1988, 1989 and Mufti, these proceedings). Our hypothesis is that increased cancer risk observed with chronic alcohol consumption is due to ethanol causing a suppression of cellular immunity. We further postulate that the cancer risk may be enhanced by HIV infection since it causes immune deficiency or dysfunction. Further that the immunosuppression and the cancer incidence caused by ethanol or retroviral infection could be overcome by supplementation with a food nutrient such as canthaxanthin that acts as immunostimulant. Preliminary data on the role of dietary materials, retinyl palmitate (vitamin A), beta-carotene and canthaxanthin, to stimulate numbers of cells involved in cellular immunity are presented here. This paper will discuss preliminary evidence for this hypothesis based on a review of the results of our previous studies. It will also define the animal model that we are utilizing for our studies.

MATERIALS AND METHODS

Experimental Animals and Their Diet. Young 4-6 week old female C57BL/6 mice are used for these studies. The animals are housed in a separate room allotted to us and maintained and cared for in the facility provided by the Division of Animal Resources, University of Arizona.

Mice are fed a nutritionally balanced, isocaloric liquid diet prepared in our laboratory according to the suggestions of American Institute of Nutrition (1977) and Lieber and DeCarli (1982) and modified according to the recommendations of the National Research Council (1978) to suit requirements of the mouse. Furthermore, the ethanol content of the diet is reduced so that it constitutes 4.0-4.5% of the total diet in gram weight (in contrast to 6-7% for the rat) and its content of destrin-maltose increased to suit long-term studies (Rao et al., 1987). In a previous pilot study with a binge type regimen, 5% ethanol was associated with some toxicity (Watson et al., 1988). A reduced level of ethanol is also suggested since ethanol at higher levels causes toxicity in mice when fed continuously. Ethanol in these studies is administered as a tumor promoter, i.e., one week after treatment with NMB_zA is completed.

The amount of ethanol and control diet consumed by the animals is recorded each time the diet is fed. Daily intake of the control diet is restricted so as to correspond to the ethanol diet consumed, that is, mice are pair-fed in effect. The blood concentration of ethanol is measured every two months by random sampling so as to verify its overall levels. The animals are examined daily and any sick, moribund, or dead animal isolated immediately. Weights are recorded every 2 weeks.

Supplementation with Canthaxanthin or Beta-Carotene. Beta-carotene or Canthaxanthin are provided on gelatin beadlets to aid absorption. Canthaxanthin and beta-carotene beadlets have been supplied to us as a kind gift by Hoffman LaRoche. Beta-carotene is a precursor of vitamin A while canthaxanthin is another carotenoid which is not converted into vitamin A. Mice receiving beta carotene or canthaxanthin as a supplement are given gelatin beadlets that contain 10% of the nutrient so that it constitutes 1% of the total diet. The diet contains 4 IU/gm of retinyl palmitate in addition to beta-carotene. Controls will receive 4 IU/gm of retinyl palmitate only with placebo beadlets. These regimens have essentially no toxicity. To verify the blood concentration of canthaxanthin or beta-carotene, samples of serum are taken every two months and analyzed for beta carotene in collaboration with Dr. Yei-Mei Peng of the Arizona Cancer Center.

Carcinogenic Treatment of Animals. Young mice are, and will be, used for these studies since DNA from growing animals that is rapidly replicating ensures that the mutagenic lesion is 'fixed'. Replicating DNA, compared to resting DNA, is more reactive with many chemical carcinogens because of its single-stranded nature (Singer and Fraenkel-Conrat, 1969). We use methylbenzyl- nitrosamine (NMB_ZA) to initiate carcinogenesis. In rats and mice, NMB_ZA has been shown to be a highly site specific carcinogen and causes a high incidence of esophageal neoplasms (Druckrey et al., 1967; Sander and Schweinsberg, 1973; Schweinsberg et al., 1977; Stinson et al., 1978).

Our objective in these studies is to determine the contribution of ethanol to the incidence of cancers. Therefore, we use a dose of the carcinogen that induces tumors in a low number of animals so that any added effects of ethanol are measurable. For this reason, we use a nitrosamine dose that induces tumors in about 25-35% of animals. Sander and Schweinsberg (1973) observed that NMB_ZA is a potent carcinogen in mice and a dose of 0.1 mg/kg/day induced esophageal tumors in 40-60% mice when given for 10-40 days. Based on these observations, we use a total of 1.4 mg/kg given over a period of 7 days (i.e., 0.2 mg/kg/day) for tumor induction.

In rats, NMB_ZA causes a high incidence of esophageal tumors regardless of the route of administration (Druckrey et al., 1967; Schweinsberg et al., 1977; Stinson et al., 1978). In mice, however, systemic administration of NMB_ZA induces forestomach and lung tumors while administration in drinking water induces tumors both in the esophagus and forestomach (Sander and Schweinsberg, 1973). Since, we are primarily interested in esophageal tumors, we administer NMB_ZA in drinking water as described above. However, the incidence of nodules/tumors in both esophagus and forestomach is determined.

Animal Model of Retrovirus Infection. We use C57BL/6 female mice for these studies because these animals can be infected with LP-BM5 murine leukemia retrovirus. Thus we can study the effect of viral infections with or without association of other experimental variables. The murine retroviral model is already in place with us at the University of Arizona (Watson et al., 1988; Watson, 1989).

The LP-BM5 murine retroviral infection is used as a

model for human AIDS. The model was developed over the last several years by Mosier, Yetter and Morse (1985, 1987). The suitability of this model has been discussed in several reviews including ours (Salzman, 1986; Watson, 1989). As against the murine model, nonhuman primates develop few of the HIV related abnormalities seen in man (Salzman, 1986). Furthermore, the availability of murine retroviral model provides a rapid and economical system for a study of immune stimulation and to investigate cofactors that are involved in the pathogenesis of AIDS and related diseases. NIH has designated LP-BM5 a nonhuman pathogen and it is not transmitted naturally to uninfected mice cohoused in the same room (Salzman, 1986; Mosier et al., 1987; Watson et al., 1988). These studies are done in collaboration with Dr. Robert A. Yetter, Chief Research Virologist of the Baltimore Veterans Administration Medical Center who has been associated with us in the past. A 0.1 mg inoculum of the virus is injected, i.p., per mouse. The disease runs its course in five to six months with death due to either pulmonary lymphodenopathy or sometimes opportunistic infections as cancers. Therefore, viral infections are done about 5 months before animals are terminated.

The virus is a mixture of ecotropic, xenotropic and mink cell focus (MCF) murine type C retrovirus. The characteristics of the infection are that the animals develop hypergammaglobulinemia (IgM, IgG and IgE), lymphadenopathy, T-cell and B-cell immunodeficiency, and later neurological signs including paralysis as well as opportunistic infections (hepatitis and *Pneumocystis carinii*, etc.). The viral infection involves macrophages, B-cells and to a lesser extent T-cells. The infection also causes B-cell lymphomas and we will study the added effect of ethanol on their development.

The similarities between this murine model for AIDS and early stages of AIDS are striking in many respects (Watson, 1989). There is an early phase of B-cell hyperactivity and polyclonal activation in both. The order of loss of T-cell function is similar with helper T-cell function loss occurring well before cytotoxic/suppressor T-cell function. In the mouse while there is not a clear loss in numbers of T-helper cells, there is a rapid loss of T-helper activity. There are few early changes in other hematopoietic elements in the mouse model. Unlike other animal models for AIDS, LP-BM5 MuLV infection does not result in a general depression of bone marrow function. The mouse model diverges from AIDS in humans in the extent of B-cell lymphoproliferation and in the absence of a long latent phase of infection. For immunologic studies, the murine model has many advantages including a more accurate reflection of the early stages of AIDS, availability of genetically-identical inbred animals, defined immunologic parameters, and the ability to reproduce disease in large numbers of mice within a relatively short time.

Processing of animals for Nodules/Tumors. We have previously evaluated esophageal lesions (Mufti et al., 1989) according to the recommendations of Napalkov and Pozhariski (1969), Van Rensburg (1981), and Van Rensburg et al. (1985). Since with time nodules progress into tumors and are numerically equivalent, Van Rensburg et al. (1985) concluded that early appearing nodules were preneoplastic lesions. The model has been successfully utilized by a number of investigators including Newberne and his colleagues (for example, Gabrial et al., 1982). The lesions are visible macroscopically on the esophageal epithelium. Esophageal nodules usually seen after 10-20 weeks of treatment with the carcinogen, appear as whitish plaques. All such areas $>$ 0.5 mm in size on visual examination are counted. They are then confirmed by histological examination. Initial abnormality shows a thickening of the epithelium, especially of the prickly cell layer with concomitant hyperplasia of the basal cell layer and hyperkeratosis is evident in almost all areas. Presence or absence of dysplasia in these lesions is evaluated which is normally apparent at later times after treatment as carcinogenesis progresses. Tumors exhibit various extents of gross morphological and histological abnormalities apparent as disorderly growth with a three-dimensional structure. They are characterized by extensive proliferation of the basal cells into the lumen of the esophagus. Frank malignancies are diagnosed by demonstrating histologic invasion into the surrounding tissue i.e. the lamina propia. Tissues from oropharynx and forestomach are also taken for histological examination when gross observations indicate the presence of lesions.

According to the modified procedure followed in our

laboratory, esophageal tissues are fixed in phosphate buffered 4% formaldehyde-1% gluterldehyde (McDowell and Trump, 1976). The tissue specimens are collected from all presumptive lesions and embedded in paraffin or glycol methacrylate. Sections are stained with basic fuschin, methylene blue, hematoxylin and PAS (periodic acid Schiff) for histopathological examination (McManus, 1948). The same procedure is followed for evaluating lesions in the forestomach.

Numerical and Functional Assays of the Immune System in the Mouse: These studies measure T-lymphocytes and their subpopulations, macrophages and NK cells. We measure T-cell and macrophage functional abilities as we have previously done (Moriguchi et al., 1985; Gensler et al., 1987; Watson et al., 1987; Mufti et al. 1988): (a) direct contact killing of tumor cells by macrophages, (b) phagocytosis of unopsonized and opsonized sheep red blood cells labeled with chromium 51, (c) using flow cytometry to identify T-cell subsets, macrophages, activated macrophages and lymphocytes, (d) production of immunoregulators, IL-1, and (e) mitogenesis of T-cells.

Identification of T-Cell Subsets and Evidence of Activation. Isolated splenic lymphocytes at 5×10^6 cells/ml in 0.2 ml RPMI 1640 containing 2% Neonatal Calf Serum (NCS) will be stained with 5 ul of the appropriate primary monoclonal antibody (MoAb) as done previously by us in retrovirally-infected mice (Watson et al., 1988). These will include anti-mouse L3T4 for T-helper cells, Lyt-23 as a measure of T-suppressor cells, and Thy-1 as a measure of total T-cells. We will use antisera for IL-2 receptor, and transferrin or albumin as markers of lymphocyte activation. Antisera to Mac-1 will measure monocytes and to Mac-2 for evidence of their activation or stimulation.

A conjugate control will contain 5 ul of the antibody suspension buffer. The tubes will be agitated, sealed with parafilm and incubated on ice for 30 minutes. The cell-MoAb suspension will be carefully layered over 0.5 ml of NCS tubes and centrifuged at 200 x g for 5 minutes at 4°C. The NCS will be decanted and 0.2 ml of diluted fluorescein conjugated goat anti-rat immunoglobulin will be added. This solution will be agitated and incubated on ice for 30 minutes. After incubation, the cell-antibody solution is again overlayed onto 0.2 ml of NCS and centrifuged as before. The fluorescein labeled conjugate will be carefully removed with a Pasteur pipette and any remaining conjugate decanted. Cells are then counted on an EPICs flow cytometer.

RESULTS

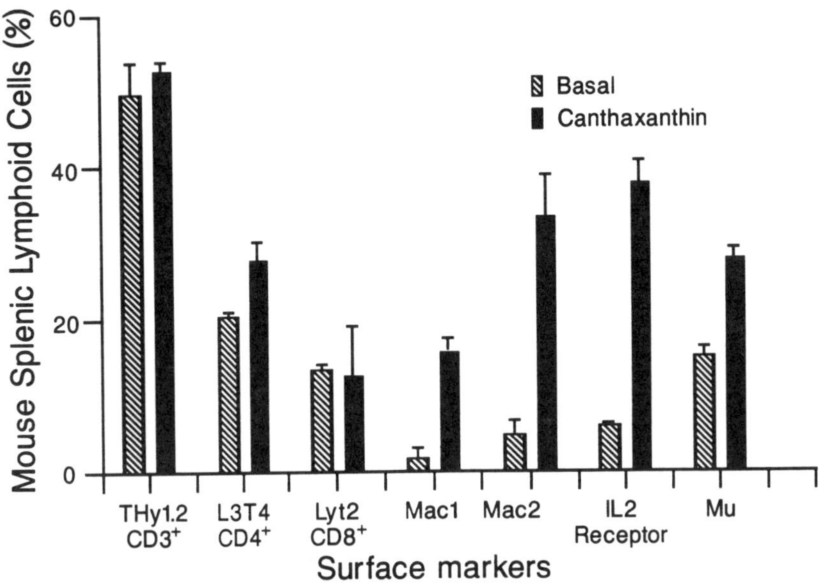

Figure 1. Effects of canthaxanthin on C57BL/6 mouse spleen lymphoid cell types. Placebo or canthaxanthin beadlets incorporated into the AIN76A synthetic mouse diet (at 10% w/w to give a final concentration of 1% canthaxanthin) were fed for 12 weeks ($n = 5$, $p < 0.05$).

We have carried out a number of experiments on the effects of retinoids and carotenoids on the immune system of uninfected mice. The results of our preliminary studies on canthaxanthin are presented in Fig. 1 and the corresponding results for vitamin A are presented in Fig. 2. These results show that canthaxanthin, and to a lesser extent vitamin A as retinyl palmitate in the diet stimulated the number of some spleen cells. Both retinyl palmitate and canthaxanthin significantly stimulated macrophages, activated lymphocytes ($IL2^+$) and increased T helper cells in mice. There was no significant change in the number of cells with surface markers for total T cells ($CD3^+$) and T-suppressor cells ($CD8^+$). However, as shown in Fig. 1 and 2 the effects were not universal on all lymphoid subsets. Results of our studies on other carotenoids and retinoids are discussed in the next section.

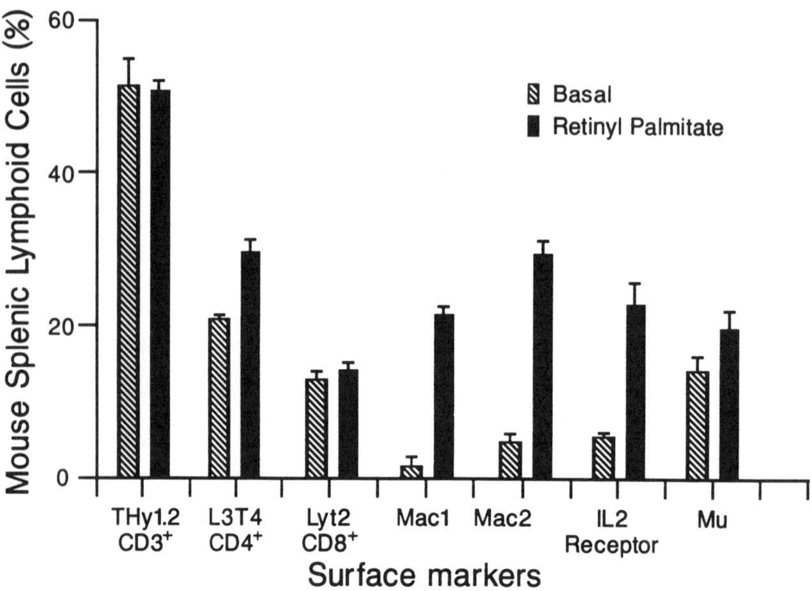

Figure 2. Effects of dietary vitamin A, as retinyl palmitate (RP), on mouse spleen cell types. RP at 120 IU/gm and 4 IU/gm was added for 12 weeks in AIN76A diet fed to C57BL/6 female mice. The diets contained gelatin beadlets at 10% w/w with the RP in the beadlets ($n = 5$, $p < 0.05$).

DISCUSSION

Since both ethanol consumption and retrovirus infection lead to immune dysfunction, it would be beneficial to employ agents that have immunorestorative properties. Once we have characterized combined interactions of ethanol and retroviral infection, supplementation with a retinoid or carotenoid will be investigated because of (a) their general immunostimulatory actions which we have helped define (Moriguchi et al., 1985; Gensler et al., 1987; Watson et al., 1987; Moriguchi et al., 1988), (b) their likelihood of use by HIV infected people including ARC and AIDS patients (Johnson and Williams, 1986), and (c) our observation that retinol could cause immunostimulation in ethanol stressed rats (Watson et al., 1986), and (d) our finding that they effectively stimulate suppressed immune functions resulting in increased survival of young, LP-BM5 MuLV infected mice (Watson et al., 1988).

Results of our preliminary studies on immunostimulation by canthaxanthin and retinyl palmitate presented in Figure 1 and 2 showed an increase in the numbers of activated lymphocytes and macrophages which could have key roles in immunosurveillance of newly initiated tumors. Our other studies have shown that other carotenoids and retinoids also stimulate characteristic cellular immune functions in normal, young animals (Watson, 1984; Watson and Mohs, 1984; Watson and Moriguchi, 1985; Watson, 1986; Watson and Rybski, 1988; Moriguchi et al., 1988). Our preliminary studies with oral leukoplakia patients who are heavy tobacco and alcohol users suggest that their immune functions can be stimulated dramatically by beta carotene supplementation (Prabhala and Watson, 1989). Particularly encouraging are the results of another study where we treated aged, normal and healthy volunteers (Watson et al., 1989) and 11 HIV infected patients (Watson et al., 1989) for 4 months with 30 mg/day of beta-carotene. Beta-carotene supplementation produced increased T-helper cells and strongly stimulated NK cells and activated (interleukin-2 receptor^{+}) lymphocytes. We also found that retinoids and carotenoids stimulate macrophage cytotoxic action in vitro (Moriguchi et al., 1985, 1988). High intakes of retinyl palmitate (vitamin A) were found to stimulate human and mouse macrophages in vivo (Moriguchi et al., 1985; Watson, 1986; Moriguchi et al., 1988). We observed that increased dietary intakes of retinyl palmitate stimulated production of interleukin-1 by peritoneal macrophages as well as in vitro phagocytosis of opsonized and unopsonized sheep red blood cells (Moriguchi et al., 1985). Our data also show increased production of a new tumor cytotoxic factor in vitro and in vivo by beta-carotene treatment of macrophages (April et al., 1989). In papilloma bearing mice, macrophage functions were enhanced with intakes of retinyl palmitate, selenium plus retinyl palmitate, and to a much lesser degree with 13-cis retinoic acid (Gensler et al., 1987; Watson et al., 1987). Reduction in papilloma growth was dose-dependent on supplemental dietary retinyl palmitate and in general corresponded with enhanced phagocytosis (Gensler et al., 1987; Watson et al., 1987).

Recently, we completed studies on animal models of alcohol-related cancers that could explain the contradictory data obtained by other investigators as well as provide basis for an understanding of epidemiologic observations. These studies were based on the following postulates. Since ethanol by itself is not carcinogenic, ethanol enhancing effects must be explained in terms of its modifying the effects of other carcinogens that frequent human environment, e.g., nitrosamines in tobacco. Thus, ethanol may either modify the initiation stage of carcinogenesis, or alternatively, act as a tumor promoter and thus enhance the effect of initiating carcinogens. Our results show that when ethanol was administered before and during initiation by methylbenzyl-nitrosamine, a potent esophagus specific carcinogen, it inhibited tumor incidence. Ethanol enhanced tumor incidence only when it was administered as a tumor promoter after initiation by the carcinogen was completed (for a discussion of these studies see Mufti et al., 1989, also Mufti, these proceedings). Another significant observation was that ethanol appears to act during progression stage by increasing tumors that developed from initiated lesions. This order of events is in consonance with the suggestion that ethanol-induced immunosuppression may have a role in enhancing cancer incidence. These studies were performed using rat as a model animal. We will now like to extend these results to another species, i.e., the mouse as the experimental model. The use of mouse also allows us to understand the role of immunosuppression due to retroviral infection on this process. We will thus be able to determine the effect of ethanol-related immunosuppression both on chemically and retrovirally induced tumors.

Also, we recently reported a study of ethanol and cellular immune functions and summarized our findings on ethanol use in vitro and in vivo on T-cells, macrophages and NK cells (Mufti et al., 1988; also see Mufti, these proceedings). In vitro, an ethanol metabolite, acetaldehyde, in extremely low concentrations was found to suppress some functions and numbers of human T-lymphocytes from peripheral blood. By comparison ethanol itself, other alcohols and another ethanol metabolite, acetate, had much less effect on T-cells numbers and functions. In agreement with other investigators (Bernstein et al., 1974; Lundy et al., 1975; Pelletier et al., 1984; Perrin et al., 1984; Jerrells et al., 1986), we found that in vivo chronic ethanol consumption caused a loss of T-lymphocytes. A significant decrease in size and weight of lymphoid organs was also observed. We also found that in vitro very low amounts of ethanol stimulated natural killer cell function but with increasing levels this small stimulation was overcome and some suppression occurred at physiological levels. This confirms some in vivo studies of NK cells done by others (Saxena et al., 1981) which found increased NK activities at low levels of dietary ethanol. Furthermore, we observed that rats fed 1% or 7% of diet as ethanol showed a functional suppression of their macrophages to phagocytize sheep red blood cells after twelve weeks of ethanol consumption (Mufti et al., 1988, Mufti, 1989). In studies with mice, we have observed changes in immunoarchitecture with reductions in T cell localities after 1 week of consumption of 7% ethanol. There was significant suppression in cellular immune functions as well as changes in numbers and positioning of T helper cells in the spleen. A suppression of macrophage cell function was observed by in vivo microscopy (unpublished data), and of in vitro phagocytosis, after 8 days of ethanol exposure in mice.

We have also measured the effects of alcohol abuse on cellular immune functions in adult men (Watson et al., 1985). In these studies, previous abusers, current abusers, and patients with alcoholic cirrhosis or pancreatitis were age-matched to controls. It was observed that T-lymphocyte mitogenesis stimulated by phytohemagglutinin and concanavalin A was generally reduced in peripheral blood lymphocytes of current and previous alcohol consumers. While the cells with T-suppressor surface antigens in controls amounted to 27%, those in the blood of alcoholic cirrhosis or pancreatitis subjects were 16%, a significant suppression. On the other hand, in people currently consuming alcohol, plasma corticosteroid levels were significantly increased to levels which could cause immunosuppression.

We have already initiated studies on the effect of LP-BM5 virus infection on immune functions in C57BL/6 mice (Watson, et al., 1988). Studies carried out by Dr. R. Yetter show that LP-BM5 retroviral infection caused increase in serum IgM and a marked increase in spleen weight and the use of potential anti-HIV drugs including AZT significantly slowed the increase indicating drug efficacy (communication of unpublished data by R. Yetter). Other mice that were given binge or chronic ethanol, had significantly reduced survival and the percentage of cells with activation markers was also reduced (Watson et al., 1988).

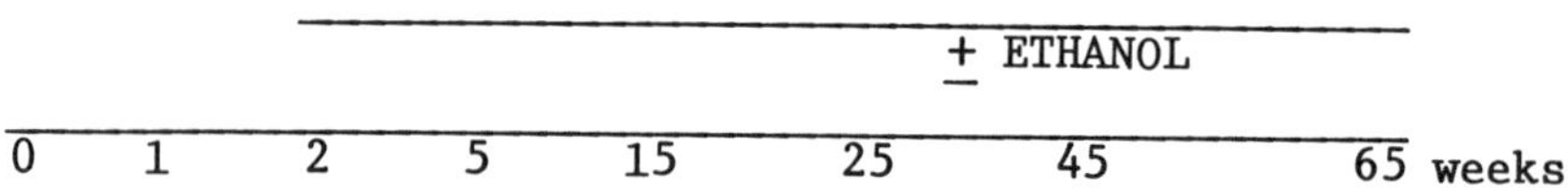

Figure 3. Animal Model for studies of alcohol, AIDS and cancer incidence. For studies of chemically induced carcinogenesis, young 5 week old C57BL/6 female mice will be treated with NMB_zA at time 0 until week 1 (0.2 mg/kg/day for 7 days). Ethanol administration will start at week 2. For the study of effect of canthaxanthin, diet will be supplemented with the nutrient at week 1. For studies of retroviral infection, mice will be infected with LP-BM5, i.p., at a dose of 0.1 mg/mouse at week 45. Experiments will be terminated at 5, 15, 25, 45, 55 and 65 weeks.

Determinations:

1. Incidence of preneoplastic/neoplastic lesions and tumors.
2. Immunological assays. Samples from peripheral blood,

peritoneal and lung lavage, spleen, liver and possibly target tissue(s) analyzed for numbers and/or functions of T-lymphocytes and their subpopulations, monocytes/macrophages and natural killer cells.
3. Incidence of preneoplastic/neoplastic lesions and tumors correlated with the immune response.

Based on the above observations, we propose the following animal model for studies of alcohol, AIDS and cancer incidence. For these studies mice, strain C57BL/6, will be used because as discussed earlier these mice can be infected with LP-BM5 which is a model virus for AIDS. The mice will be fed 4-4.5% ethanol as part of a nutritionally balanced isocaloric liquid diet as discussed in "Materials and Methods". The effect of chronic ethanol consumption and retroviral infection will be determined on the incidence of preneoplastic/ neoplastic lesions and tumors with and without prior chemical induction. For chemical induction, a site specific carcinogen such as methylbenzylnitrosamine (NMB_zA) that induces tumors in the esophagus (refer to discussion in "Materials and Methods") will be used. Ethanol will be administered as a tumor promoter and started a week after treatment with the carcinogen is completed. For studies of the effect of retrovirus LP-BM5, infections will be carried out 20-25 weeks before experiments are terminated because of probable death of infected animals. Immune surveillance is important for body defenses and a slackening or impairment of immunity would provide conditions that are conducive to pathogenesis/carcinogenesis (for a review, see Burnett, 1971; Mufti et al., 1989, Mufti, these proceedings). The effect of canthaxanthin supplementation on restoration of immune resistance and on inhibition of chemically or retrovirally induced preneoplastic/ neoplastic lesions and tumors will be determined. To determine effect of canthaxanthin, mice diet will be supplemented with the nutrient starting one week before ethanol administration is started. This is to build up body supplies of canthaxanthin; ethanol intake is known to deplete reserves of vitamin A and retinoids (Smith et al., 1975; Leo and Lieber, 1982). Use of canthaxanthin as immunostimulant will be particularly useful because whereas most retinoids including vitamin A are associated with toxicity (Olson, 1984), carotenoids, beta-carotene and canthaxanthin have very low or almost no toxicity.

The goal of immunostimulation is to overcome the immunosuppression induced by alcohol and/or retroviral infection causing AIDS and of their contribution to cancer incidence.

Acknowledgments. Research described in this paper was supported by a specialized Alcohol Research Center grant (AA08037), NIH grant DA04827, and a National Institute of Environmental Health Sciences grant (No. E503438).

REFERENCES

American Institute of Nutrition (1977). Report of the American Institute of Nutrition Ad Hoc Committee on standards for nutritional studies. J Nutr 107:1340-1348.

April ER, Rybski JA, Scuderi P, Watson RR (1989). Beta-carotene stimulates human monocyte secretion of a novel tumorcidal cytokine. J Leuk Biol 45:255-261.

Bernstein IM, Webster KH, Williams RC, Strickland RG (1974). Reduction in circulating T-lymphocytes in alcoholic liver disease. Lancet ii:488-490.

Bloom DE, Carliner G (1988). The economic impact of AIDS in the United States. Science 239:604-610.

Burch GE, Ansari A (1968). Chronic alcoholism and carcinoma of pancreas: a correlative hypothesis. Arch Intern Med 122:273-275.

Burnett FM (1971). Immunological surveillance in neoplasia. Transplant Rev 7:3-25.

Doll R, Peto (1981). The causes of cancer: quantitative estimates of avoidable risks of cancer in the United States today. J Natl Cancer Inst 66:1191-1308.

Druckrey H, Preussmann R, Ivankovic S, Schmahl D (1967). Organstrope carcinogene Wirkungen bei 65 verschiedenen N-nitroso-Verbindungen an BD-Ratten. Z. Krebsforsch 69:103-201.

Enstrom JE (1977). Colorectal cancer and beer drinking. Br J Cancer 35:674-683.

Fauci AS (1988). The human immunodeficiency virus: infectivity and mechanisms of pathogenesis. Science 239:617-622.

Gabrial GN, Schrager TF, Newberne PM (1982). Zinc deficiency, alcohol and a retinoid: association with esophageal cancers in rat. J Natl Cancer Inst 68:785-789.

Gensler HL, Watson RR, Moriguchi S, Bowden GT (1987). Effects of dietary retinyl palmitate or 13-cis-retinoic acid on the promotion of tumors in mouse skin. Cancer Res 47:967-970.

Gordis E, Lewis M, Warren L (1989). Alcoholism. "Medical and Health Annual," Encyclopedia Britannica, pp 266-270.

Hakulinen T, Lehtimaki L, Lehtonen M, Teppo L (1974). Cancer morbidity among two male cohorts with increased alcohol consumption in Finland. J Natl Cancer Inst 52:1711-1714.

Jensen OM (1979). Cancer morbidity and causes of death among Danish brewery workers. Int J Cancer 23:454-563.

Jerrells TR, Marietta CA, Eckardt MJ, Majchrowicz E, Weight FF (1986). Effects of ethanol administration on parameter of immunocompetency in rats. J Leuk Biol 39:499-520.

Johnson RD, Williams R (1986). Immune responses in alcoholic liver disease. Alcohol Clin Exp Res 10:471-486.

Lemon FR, Walden RT, Woods RW (1964). Cancer of the lung and mouth in Seventh-Day Adventists. Preliminary report on a population study. Cancer 17:486-497.

Leo MA, Lieber CS (1982). Hepatic vitamin A depletion in alcoholic liver injury. N Eng J Med 307:597-601.

Lieber CS, DeCarli LM (1982). The feeding of alcohol in liquid diets: two decades of applications and 1982 update. Alcohol Clin Exp Res 6:523-531.

Lieber CS, Garro AJ, Leo MA, Mak KM, Werner T (1986). Alcohol and Cancer. Hepatology 6:1005-1019.

Lundy J, Raff JH, Deakins S, Wanebo HJ, Jacobs DA, Lee T, Jacobowitz V, Spear C, Dettgen HF (1975). The acute and chronic effects of alcohol on the human immune system. Surg Gynecol Obstet 141:212-218.

Lyon JL, Gardner JW, Klauber MR, Smart CR (1977). Low cancer incidence and mortality in Utah. Cancer 39:2608-2018.

MacDonald WC (1972). Clinical and pathological features of adenocarcinoma of the gastric cardia. Cancer 29:724-732.

McDowell EM, Trump BF (1976). Histologic fixatives suitable for diagnostic light and electron microscopy. Arch Pathol Lab Med 100:405-414.

McManus JFA (1948). Histological and Histochemical uses of periodic acid. Stain Tech 23:99-108.

Monson RR, Lyons JL (1975). Preoportional mortality among alcoholics. Cancer 36:1077-1079.

Moriguchi S, Werner L, Watson RR (1985). High dictary vitamin A (retinyl palmitate) and cellular immune functions in mice. Immunology 56:169-177.

Moriguchi S, Kohge M, Kishino Y, Watson RR (1988). In vitro effect of retinol and 13-cis retinoic acid on cytotoxicity of human monocytes. Nutr Res 8:255-264.

Mosier DE, Yetter RA, Morse HC (1985). Retroviral induction of acute lymphoproliferative disease and profound immunosuppression in adult C57BL/6 mice. J Exp Med 161:766-784.

Mosier DE, Yetter RA, Morse HC (1987). Functional T lymphocytes are required for a murine retrovirus-induced immunodeficiency disease (MAIDS). J Exp Med 165:1737-1742.

Mufti SI, Prabhala R, Moriguchi S, Sipes IG, Watson RR (1988). Functional and numerical alterations induced by ethanol in the cellular immune system. Immunopharmacol 15:85-94.

Mufti SI (1988). Ethanol metabolites as indicators of alcohol abuse. In Watson RR (ed): "Diagnosis of Alcohol Abuse," Boca Raton FL: CRC Press, in press.

Mufti SI, Darban HR, Watson RR (1989). Alcohol, cancer, and immunomodulation. CRC Crit Rev Hematol Oncol, in press.

Mufti SI, Garewal HS, Watson RR (1989). Role of environment, drug of abuse, and nutritional factors in the etiology and prevention of cancers of the oral cavity and esophagus. In Watson RR (ed): "Focus on Biochemistry and Physiology of Drugs of Abuse," Boca Raton FL: CRC Press, in press.

Mufti SI, Becker G, Sipes IG (1989). Effect of chronic dietary ethanol consumption on the initiation and promotion of chemically-induced esophageal carcinogenesis in experimental rats. Carcinogenesis 10:303-309.

Mufti SI (1989). An evaluation of laboratory tests of alcoholisms and alcohol abuse and suggestions for improvement. In Watson RR (ed): "Focus on Biochemistry and Physiology of Drug Abuse," Boca Raton FL: CRC Press, in press.

Mufti SI (1989). An animal model of immune response associated with alcohol-related cancers, these proceedings.

Napalkov NK, Pozhariski KM (1969). Morphogenesis of experimental tumors of the esophagus. J Natl Cancer Inst 42:927-940.
National Research Council (1978). Nutrient Requirements of Domestic Animals, No. 10. Nutrient Requirements of Laboratory Animals, 3rd revised edition.
National Research Council (1982). Diet, Nutrition and Cancer. The Committee on Diet, Nutrition and Cancer, Assembly of Life Sciences, National Academy Press, Washington, DC.
Olson JA (1984). Vitamin A. In Machin LS (ed): "Handbook of Vitamins: Nutritional, Biochemical, and clinical Aspects," New York: Marcel Dekker Inc., p 1.
Pelletier G, Segond P, Attali P, Briantais MJ, Ettiene JP (1984). T-lymphocyte subpopulations in alcoholic liver disease. Gastroenterol Clin Biol 8:911-914.
Perrin D, Bignon JD, Braugard E, Cheneau ML (1984). T-lymphocyte populations in peripheral blood of patients with alcoholic cirrhosis. Gastroenterol Clin Biol 8:907-910.
Prabhala R and Watson RR (1989). Immunomodulation by beta-carotene: Role of cytokine. Submitted for publication.
Rao GA, Riley DE, Larkin EC (1987). Dietary carbohydrate stimulates alcohol diet ingestion, promotes growth and prevents fatty liver in rats. Nutr Res 7:81-87.
Rosenberg L, Shapiro S, Slone D, Kaufman DW, Helmrich SP, Miettinen DS, Stolley PD, Levy M, Rosenshein NB, Schottenfeld D, Engle RL (1982). Breast cancer and alcoholic-beverage consumption. Lancet 1:267-271.
Rothman K, Garfinkel L, Keller AZ, Muir CS, Schottenfeld D (1980). The proportion of cancer attributable to alcohol consumption. Prev Med 9:174-179.
Salzman LA (ed) (1986). "Animal Models of Retrovirus Infection and Their Relationship to AIDS." New York: Academic Press.
Sanchez MA, Ames ED, Erhardt K, Auer GU (1988). Analysis of DNA distribution in Kaposi's sarcoma in patients with and without the acquired immune deficiency syndrome. Anal Quant Cytol Histol 10:16-20.
Sander J, Schweinsberg F (1973). Tumorinduktion bei Mausen durch N-Methylbenzyl-nitrosamin in niedriger Dosierung. Z. Krebsforsch 79:157-161.

Saxena QB, Saxena RK, Adler WH (1981). Regulation of natural killer activity in vivo. IV. High natural killer activity in alcohol drinking mice. Ind J Exp Biol 19:1001-1006.

Schweinsberg F, Schott-Kollat P, Burkle G (1977). Veranderung der Toxizitat und Carcinogenitat von N-Methyl-N-nitrosobenzylamine durch Methylsubstitution am Phenylrest bei Ratten. Z. Krebsforsch 88:231-236.

Selwyn PA (1986). AIDS: What is now known. I. History and Immunovirology. Hospital Prac 21:67-76, 81-82.

Silverman S, Migliorati CA, Lozada-Nur F, Greenspan D, Conaut MA (1986). Oral findings in people with or at high risk for AIDS: a study of 375 homosexual males. J Am Dent Assoc 112:187-192.

Singer D, Fraenkel-Conrat HM (1969). The role of conformation in chemical mutagenesis. In Davidson JN, Cohn WE (eds): "Progress in Nucleic Acid Research and Molecular Biology," New York: Academic Press, Vol 9, pp 1-29.

Smith JC, Brown ED, White Sc, Finkelson JD (1975). Plasma vitamin A and zinc concentration in patients with alcoholic cirrhosis. Lancet 1:1251-1252.

Stinson SF, Squire RA, Sporn MB (1978). Pathology of esophageal neoplasms and associated proliferative lesions induced in rats by N-methyl-N-benzylnitrosamine. J Natl Cancer Inst 6:1471-1475.

Tomita Y, Himenok, Nomoto K, Endo H, Hirohata T: (1982). Combined treatments with vitamin A and 5-fluorouracil and the growth of allotransplantable and sygenic tumors in mice. J Natl Cancer Inst 68:823-827.

Tuyns AJ (1979). Epidemiology of alcohol and cancer. Cancer Res 39:2840-2843.

Van Rensburg SJ (1981). Advances in experimental cancer of the oesophagus. S Afr Cancer Bull 25:66-76.

Van Rensburg SJ, Hall JM, Bruyn DuB (1985). Effect of various dietary staples on esophageal carcinogenesis induced in rats by subcutaneously administered N-nitrosomethylbenzylamine. J Natl Cancer Inst 75:561-566.

Watson RR (1984). Alcohol and immune functions. In Watson RR (ed): "Nutrition, Disease Resistance, and Immune Function," New York: M. Dekker, pp 313-329.

Watson RR, Mohs ME (1984). New approaches to determine requirements for nutrients like zinc and vitamin A with critical roles in lymphocyte functions. Nutr Res 4:951-955.
Watson RR, Jackson JC, Hartmann B, Sampliner R, Mobley D, Eskelson C. (1985). Cellular immune functions, endorphins, and alcohol consumption in males. Alcohol Clin Exp Res 9:248-254.
Watson RR, Moriguchi S (1985). Cancer prevention by retinoids: Role of immunological modification. Nutr Res 5:663-675.
Watson RR (1986). Immunological enhancement by fat-soluble vitamins, minerals and trace metals: a factor in cancer prevention. Cancer Diet Prev 9:67-77.
Watson RR, Mohs M, Sampliner D, Eskelson C, Hartmann B (1986). Identification of alcohol abuse and alcoholism with biological parameters. Alcohol Clin Exp Res 10:364-385.
Watson RR, Rybski JA (1988). Immunological response modification by vitamin A and other retinoids. In Chandra RK (ed): "Nutrition and Immunology," Publishers, pp 87-99.
Watson RR (1988). Diagnosis of alcohol abuse by modulation of immune response. In Watson RR (ed): "Diagnosis of Alcohol Abuse." Boca Raton FL: CRC Press, in press.
Watson RR, Prabhala RH, Abril E, Smith TL (1988). Changes in lymphocyte subsets and macrophage functions from high, short-term dietary ethanol in C57BL/6 mice. Life Sci 43:865-870.
Watson RR, Prabhala RH, Darban HR, Yahya MD, Smith TL (1988). Changes in lymphocyte and macrophage subsets due to morphine and ethanol treatment during a retrovirus infection causing murine AIDS. Life Sci 43:v-xi.
Watson RR, Yahya MD, Darban HR, Prabhala RH (1988). Enhanced survival by vitamin A supplementation during a retrovirus infection. Life Sci 43:i-iv.
Watson RR (1989). A murine retrovirus model for studies of the role of cofactors, ethanol and vitamin A in AIDS development. NIDA publication of Conference held 31 Oct. - 2 Nov 1988, in press.
Watson RR (1989). Murine models for Acquired Immune Deficiency Syndrome. Life Sci 44:i-iii.
Watson RR (ed) (1989). "Cofactors in HIV-1 Infection and AIDS." Boca Raton FL: CRC Press, in press.

Watson RR, Garewal H, Ampel N, Prabhala R, Allen V, Dols C and Hicks MJ (1989). Abstract, Vth International AIDS Conference. Immunostimulatory effects of beta-carotene on T-cell activation markers and NK cells in HIV infected patients. Submitted for publication.

Watson RR, Prabhala R, Sayers S, Alberts DS, Plezia P (1989). Dose response of beta-carotene on lymphocyte subpopulations in aging humans. Submitted for publication.

Zetterman RK, Sorrell MF (1981). Immunologic aspects of alcoholic liver disease. Gastroenterology 81:616-624.

Alcohol, Immunomodulation, and AIDS, pages 305–312
© 1990 Alan R. Liss, Inc.

RECEPTOR MODULATION AS A PRIMARY TARGET OF THE IMMUNOLOGICAL EFFECTS OF ALCOHOL AND OTHER DRUGS OF ABUSE

Robert M. Donahoe

Departments of Psychiatry and Pathology, Laboratory of Psychoimmunology, Emory University, Georgia Mental Health Institute, 1256 Briarcliff Road, Atlanta, Georgia 30306

There is a growing body of evidence which supports the notion that abuse of addicting substances like alcohol and opiates may be a contributing factor in development of immune deficiency (Jerrells et al., 1988; Donahoe, 1988). Since individuals at high risk for AIDS often are abusers of addictive substances, their risk of immunological deficit may be directly influenced by their drug abuse. Such a situation would obviously contribute to the morbidity of drug abuse and threaten the public health since a main means for contraction of AIDS by heterosexuals is through contact with infected drug abusers.

Our laboratory has devoted much of its effort to descriptions of the immunological effects of opiates and street heroin addiction. We have also delineated immunological effects of alcohol abuse and the interactive effects of heroin, cocaine and alcohol on immune parameters in heroin addicts. A common theme has emerged from these studies, that the immunological deficits associated with the use of addicting substances are related to their ability to modulate the expression of receptors on the surface of T-cell lymphocytes. The data which support this contention and the implications of these data are the subject of this brief review.

In 1972, Falek et al., reported that heroin addicts had elevated levels of chromosomal aberrations. The immunological relevance of this finding stems from the fact that cytogenetic analyses are conducted with T-lymphocytes that are stimulated to divide in vitro by lectin mitogens.

These data were contemporaneous with several other studies that showed immunological deficits in heroin addicts (Brown et al., 1974; Louria 1974), including the inability of addict T-cells to appropriately respond to mitogenic stimulation in vitro (Brown et al., 1974) Consequently, Falek and associates (McDonough et al., 1980) surveyed heroin addicts for immunological deficits, finding that their T-cells were frequently severely deficient in the ability to form rosettes with sheep erythrocytes (E). Notably, the depressed E-rosette formation was reversible by treatment with the opiate antagonist naloxone in vitro and others (Wybran et al., 1979) had shown that morphine induced naloxone-reversible depression of E-rosette formation in vitro. Collectively, these findings led to several important conclusions: 1) that addicts probably have the common experience of suffering immune depression; 2) that T-cells appear to have physiologically relevant opiate receptors; 3) that T-cell opiate receptor activity may downregulate E-receptor expression.

At the time opiate effects on E-rosette formation were first described, there was considerable debate as to the immunological relevance of the E-rosetting phenomenon. Though it was clear that the E-rosette formation was based on an unusual type of receptor-ligand interaction through cell-to-cell contact of E with T-cells and that depressed E-rosetting represented a clinical means of identifying depressed immunocompetency (Kerman and Geis, 1976; Kerman et al., 1980), it was equally evident that E-rosetting was not a universal predictor of immune status and that there was poor understanding about the role of E-receptors in immune phenomena. This situation led us to study in detail the kinetics of E-rosette formation in the presence of opiates, and, later, other drugs of abuse, to define the nature of drug effects on E-rosette formation.

By manipulating the conditions of the assay to measure E-rosette formation to allow for kinetic analyses, we were able to determine the nature of the E-rosetting process and the ability of morphine to inhibit the process. In essence, we found (Donahoe et al., 1985a), as did Bernard et al. (1982), that T-cells possess a pool of cryptic E-receptors within their cell membrane that are expressed after crosslinking and capping of the E-receptor by E. By interfering with expression of these dormant E-receptors, morphine apparently limits their availability for E-rosette formation and, thus, depresses E-rosette formation.

When the kinetic E-rosette-formation assay was used to examine formation of E-rosettes with T-cells from pregnant women who were abusing alcohol, it was found that their rate of E-rosette formation was elevated relative to control subjects who were not consuming alcohol and that this effect could also be duplicated by exposing lymphocytes to alcohol (0.1%) in vitro (Madden et al., 1984). We hypothesized that this E-rosette-enhancing effect of alcohol was due to its ability to increase the fluidity of the T-cell membrane making dormant E-receptors more viable for E-rosette formation.

Taken together the effects of morphine and alcohol on E-rosette formation had one seemingly important commonality. That is, both substances exerted their effects through modulation of expression of the E-receptor on the T-cell surface. This led to the generalized concept that receptor modulation is the common effector mechanism by which addictive substances exert changes in neuroendocrinological and immunological behaviors. This unifying concept led to further examination of the membrane modulating properties of substances of abuse.

We first examined the interactive effects of alcohol and cocaine on the ability of opiates to depress E-rosette formation in heroin addicts and found that cocaine use by heroin addicts totally reversed depression of E-rosette formation (Donahoe, et al., 1986). As in past studies (McDonough et al., 1980), we also found that alcohol use by heroin addicts did not alter their normally depressed state of E-rosetting. However, if addicts were abusing all three drugs (heroin, alcohol and cocaine), they generally had an intermediate level of depression of E-rosette formation as compared with addicts who used heroin alone or heroin plus alcohol (depressed E-rosetting) and those who used heroin and cocaine (normal to enhanced E-rosetting). Thus, alcohol modulated the effects of cocaine on E-rosette formation in heroin addicts.

Such observations are very pertinent, since street addiction commonly involves polydrug abuse. It is remarkable that the interactive effects of addicting substances on E-receptor expression and E-rosette formation are very similar to their behavioral properties in that, for instance, heroin is perceived as a emotional depressant just as it depresses E-rosette formation, while cocaine is an emotional stimulant which enhances E-rosette formation and counters E-rosette depression by opiates. Such observations lend credence to the hypothesis that receptor modulation is equally responsible for the behavioral changes associated with drug use as it is for the immunological changes.

The advent of the use of monoclonal antibodies and cytofluorometry as a means of typing leukocytes through detection of their surface antigenic markers gave us the opportunity to extend our studies beyond analyses of E-rosette formation to examine the effects of abused substances on E-receptor expression at the molecular level (the CD2 molecule) as well as other T-cell surface markers that are relevant to immunoresponsiveness. In the latter respect, we were initially interested in the antigenic markers that characterize T-helper-inducer (Th) and T-suppressor-cytotoxic (Ts) cells, the CD4 and CD8 molecules respectively.

We found (Donahoe et al., 1987; Donahoe and Falek, 1988) that heroin addiction depresses the ratio between Th and Ts cells which is an indication of immunodepression. Along with the work of Des Jarlais, et al. (1985), we showed that this effect was not related to infection with AIDS viruses and that heroin addicts who did not experience depression of Th/Ts as a group had elevated levels of circulating Th (CD4+) cells that correlated with their duration of heroin use. Moreover, we found (Donahoe et al., 1985a) that alcohol use by heroin addicts and control subjects tended to enhance expression of CD4, but not CD8 markers. Inasmuch as the CD4 is the only known viroreceptor for HIV1 (Dalgleish et al., 1986; Klatzman et al., 1986), this information is of particular relevance to understanding how drugs of abuse may modulate host resistance to HIV1 and AIDS.

Because of the complexity of the addiction milieu, it is very difficult to ascertain the role of drugs independent of other factors that might modulate immunoresponsiveness such as nutritional and stress factors, polydrug abuse, and the repeated exposure of addicts to antigenic and infectious insults. For this reason, we attempted to correlate the in vivo data regarding modulation of the molecular expression of CD2, CD4 and CD8 markers with in vitro evidence of opiate modulatory effects. By adapting the kinetic analyses of morphine effects in the E-rosetting assay to molecular analyses via use of epitope-specific monoclonal antibodies and cytofluorometry, we showed (Donahoe et al., 1987;

Donahoe and Falek, 1988) that morphine could modulate CD2, CD4 and CD8 expression in vitro, a finding corroborated indirectly by Puppo et al. (1985) who showed that endorphin also modulates CD4 expression in vitro.

Thus, there is ample evidence that opiates, alcohol and cocaine can modulate expression of T-cell antigenic markers that are involved in regulation of immunoresponsiveness. Since Wybran et al. (1979) showed that enkephalins enhance E-rosette formation in vitro, and Puppo et al. (1985) that endorphins downregulate CD4 expression, it is probable that both endogenous and exogenous behaviorally active substances influence immune function through regulation of receptor expression on the surface of T-cells. This is important because it reflects on the issue of whether the immunological effects of substances of abuse are mediated directly or indirectly.

To address this issue of direct versus indirect effects, it must be appreciated that the immunological system is not independent of other organ systems influenced by substances of abuse. From a holistic standpoint, consideration needs to be given to the fact that substances of abuse must interact with the immune system in vivo through their comprehensive influence over the psychoneuro-immunological intersystemic network as shown in Figure 1. This point has been documented by the work of Shavit et al. (1984, 1986), who have shown that opioids exert their control over NK cell activity through a stress-mediated, centrally-controlled axis.

In conclusion, a major effect of exposure of a host to abused substances is to alter expression of the antigenic markers on the surface of T-cells that are so pertinent to immunoregulation and immunoresponsiveness. This effect is likely to be mediated by abused substances both through direct interaction with T-cells (and other cells of the immune system) and through their systemic effects on the psychoneuroimmunological network. Thus, a major battleground for future studies on the immunological effects of drugs of abuse is going to involve efforts to achieve better understanding of the effects of abused substances on the cell membrane of immune cells themselves. The challenge is to determine how the immune system balances (or, as the case may be, falls out of balance in the presence of substances of abuse) multiple neuro-immunoendocrinological signals at the cellular level.

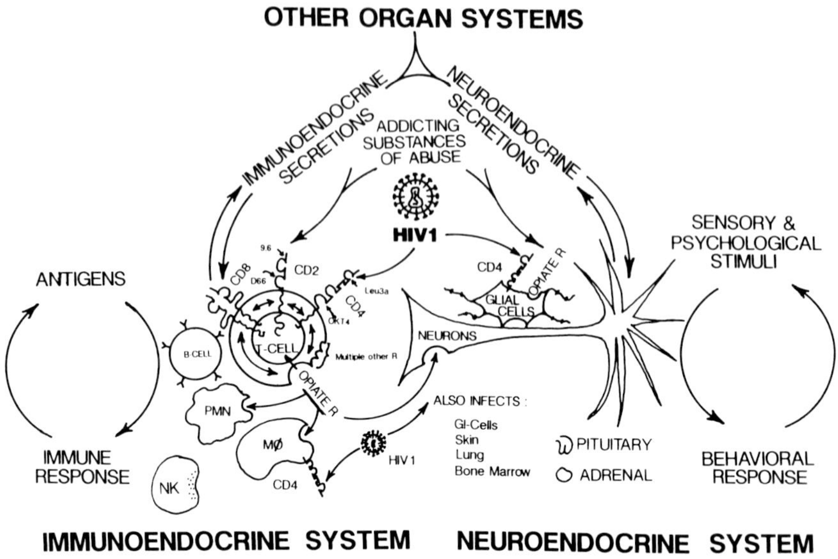

Figure 1. Interactive effects of substances of abuse within the psychoneuroimmunological network and potential points of influence over HIV1 infection. The ultimate immunological influence of abused substances on T-cell function within the network is through modulation of receptor expression at the cell (T cell) surface.

REFERENCES

Bernard A, Gelin C, Raynal B, Pham D, Gosse, C, Boumsell L (1982). Phenomenon of human T cells rosetting with sheep erythrocytes analyzed with monoclonal antibodies. "Modulation" of a partially hidden epitope determining the conditions of interaction between T cells and erythrocytes. J Exp Med 155:1317-1333.

Brown SW, Stimmel B, Taub RN, Kochwa S, Rosenfield RE (1974). Immunological dysfunction in heroin addicts. Arch Intern Med 134:1001-1006.

Dalgleish AG, Beverley PCL, Clapham PR, Crawford DH, Greaves MF, Weiss RA (1984). The CD4 (T4) antigen is an essential component of the receptor for AIDS retrovirus. Nature 312:763-767.

Des Jarlais DC, Friedman SR, Hopkins W (1985). Risk reduction for the acquired immunodeficiency disease syndrome among intravenous drug users. Ann Intern Med 103:755-759.

Donahoe RM (1988). Opiates as immunocompromising drugs: the evidence and possible mechanisms. NIDA Res Monogr 90:105-114.

Donahoe RM, Bueso-Ramos C, Donahoe F, Madden JJ, Falek A, Nicholson JKA, Bokos P (1987). Mechanistic implications of the findings that opiates and other drugs of abuse moderate T-cell surface receptors and antigenic markers. Ann NY Acad Sci 496:711-721.

Donahoe RM, Falek A (1988). Neuroimmunomodulation by opiates and other drugs of abuse: relationship to HIV infection and AIDS. Adv Biochem Psychopharmacol 44:145-158.

Donahoe RM,.Madden JJ, Holingsworth F, Shafer DA, Falek A (1985a). Morphine depression of T cell E-rosetting: Definition of the process. Fed Proc 44:95-99.

Donahoe RM, Madden JJ, Hollingsworth F, Shafer DA, Falek A, Nicholson JKA, Bokos P (1985b). Immunomodulation by behaviorally active drugs provides a paradigm for connecting AIDS-like processes and psychoneuroimmunology. In: Neuroimmunomodulation: Proceedings of the First International Workshop on Neuroimmunomodulation, edited by NH Spector, pp. 201-204. International Working Group on Neuroimmunomodulation, Bethesda, MD.

Donahoe RM, Nicholson JKA, Madden JJ, Donahoe F, Shafer DA, Gordon D, Bokos P, Falek A (1986). Coordinate and independent effects of heroin, cocaine and alcohol abuse on T-cell E-rosette and antigenic marker expression. Clin Immunol Immunopathol 41:254-264.

Falek A, Jordan RB, King BJ, Arnold PJ, Skelton WB (1972). Human chromosomes and opiates. Arch Gen Psychiat 27:511-515.

Jerrells TR, Marietta CA, Bone G, Weight FF, Eckardt MJ (1988). Ethanol associated immunosuppression. Adv Biochem Psychopharmacol 44:173-185.

Kerman RH, Floyd M, Van Buren CT, Kahan BD (1980). Improved allograft survival of strong immune responder-high risk recipients with adjuvant antithymocyte globulin therapy. Transplantation 30:450-454.

Kerman RH, Geis WP (1976). Total and active T cell dynamics in renal allograph recipients. Surgery 79:398-407.

Klatzman D, Champagne E, Chamarets S, Greust J, Guetard D, Hercend T, Gluckmon JC, Montagnier L (1986). T-lymphocyte T4 molecule behaves as the receptor for human retrovirus LAV. Nature 312:767-768.

Louria DB (1974). Infectious complications of nonalcoholic drug abuse. Annu Rev Med 25:219-231.
Madden JJ, Donahoe RM, Smith IE, Martinson DE, Moss-Wells S, Klein L, Falek A (1984). Increased rate of E-rosette formation by T-lymphocytes of pregnant women who drink alcohol. Clin Immunol Immunopathol 36:67-79.
McDonough RJ, Madden JJ, Falek A, Shafer DA, Pline M, Gordon D, Bokos P, Kuehnle JC, Mendelson J (1980). Alteration of T and null lymphocyte frequencies in the peripheral blood of human opiate addicts: in vivo evidence of opiate receptor sites on T lymphocytes. J. Immunol 125:2539-2543.
Puppo F, Corsini G, Mangini P, Bottaro L, Barreca T (1985). Influence of B-endophin on phytohemagglutanin induced lymphocyte proliferation and on expression of mononuclear cell surface antigens in vitro. Immunopharmacology 10:119-125.
Shavit Y, DePaulis A, Martin FA, Terman GW, Pechnick RN, Zanc CJ, Gale RP, Liebeskind JC (1986). Involvement of brain opiate receptors in the immune suppressive effect of morphine. Proc Natl Acad Sci 83:7114-7117.
Shavit Y, Lewis JW, Terman GW, Gale RP, Liebeskind JG (1984). Opioid peptides mediate the suppressive effect of stress on natural killer cell cytotoxicity. Science 223:188-190.
Wybran J, Appleboom T, Famaey JP, Govaerts A (1979). Suggestive evidence for receptors for morphine and methionine-enkephalin on normal human blood T lymphocytes. J. Immunol 123:1068-1070.

Alcohol, Immunomodulation, and AIDS, pages 313–320
© 1990 Alan R. Liss, Inc.

ETHANOL INDUCED ALTERATION OF IMMUNE FUNCTION MAY INVOLVE HORMONES OF THE HYPOTHALAMIC-PITUITARY-ADRENAL AXIS

Eva Redei, William R. Clark and
Robert F. McGivern
Department of Psychiatry (E.R.), University of Pennsylvania, Philadelphia and Departments of Biology (W.R.C.) and Medicine (R.F.M), UCLA, Los Angeles

Prolonged and excessive consumption of ethanol lowers many aspects of host defenses, resulting in an increased susceptibility to infection (Wands, 1979). Prolonged administration of ethanol to experimental animals as well as alcohol abuse in humans results in a number of immunological abnormalities including a decrease in spleen and thymus weights and cell numbers (Jerrels et al., 1986) and a reduction in the number of circulating leukocytes (Watson et al., 1985). Chronic exposure to ethanol has also been found to result in impaired humoral antibody response (Jerrels et al., 1986; Smith et al., 1980) and in impaired cell-mediated immune responses (Mutchnick and Horchang, 1988; Roselle and Mendenhall, 1984). However, no studies to date have assessed the underlying mechanisms by which chronic alcohol exposure compromises immune function.

Drugs and environmental challenges that induce stress are known to suppress immune function. Current evidence indicates that bidirectional communication via a common set of hormones and associated receptors exists between neuroendocrine systems and the immune system (see Berczi, 1986 for review). A number of endocrine hormones, including hormones of the hypothalamic-pituitary-adrenal (HPA) axis, such as glucocorticoids and endogenous opiates, modulate immune function either by acting directly on lymphocytes or through mediators such as lymphokines. Thus glucocorticoids, which are elevated in response to both acute and chronic exposure to alcohol (Ellis, 1966; Mendelson et al., 1971; Stokes, 1973), produce a variety of effects on the immune system. These effects are similar to those caused by alcohol consumption and include involution of the thymus (Dougherty, 1952), redistribution of T-cells (Fauci, 1975) and monocytes (Thompson and Vanfurth, 1970) and the diminution of the proliferative response (Fauci, 1976; Lee, 1977).

Since alcohol alters production of hormones which affect immune function, we hypothesize that the immune suppression reported in chronic alcoholics is mediated in part by such hormonal alterations. The present study provides some circumstantial evidence for this hypothesis.

In experimental animals, several methods of administration have been used to study the effects of ethanol on the immune system: ethanol-containing liquid diet, ethanol drinking solution, incubation or inhalation of ethanol. Some effects of ethanol on the immune system have been found to vary with the route of alcohol administration (see Marietta et al., 1988 for review). In our studies, we have chosen to administer ethanol as part of a liquid diet, as a model for human alcohol consumption. We have measured mitogen-induced lymphocyte blastogenesis as a measure of immune function, and the plasma and tissue content of corticotropin releasing factor (CRF), corticotropin (ACTH) and corticosterone hormones. Pituitary ACTH and hypothalamic CRF contents are sensitive indicators of the prolonged elevations in blood glucocorticoid levels that are known to occur during alcohol consumption and known to alter immune competence.

Adult male rats were placed on a liquid alcohol diet <u>ad libitum</u> containing 35% ethanol-derived calories or on an isocaloric liquid diet without ethanol. Ethanol consumption averaged 10.4 ± 1.59 g/kg BW.day, which has been shown to produce blood alcohol levels of 79 mg/100 ml 6 hr after lights on and 127 mg/100 ml 3 hr after lights off (Redei et al., 1988).

At the end of the 14 day diet there were no differences in body weight, spleen or adrenal weight between the groups. However, thymus weight of ethanol-fed rats were significantly lower compared to pair-fed controls (1.01 ± 0.07(E) vs. 1.365 ± 0.09(PF) mg/g body weight; $p<0.01$).

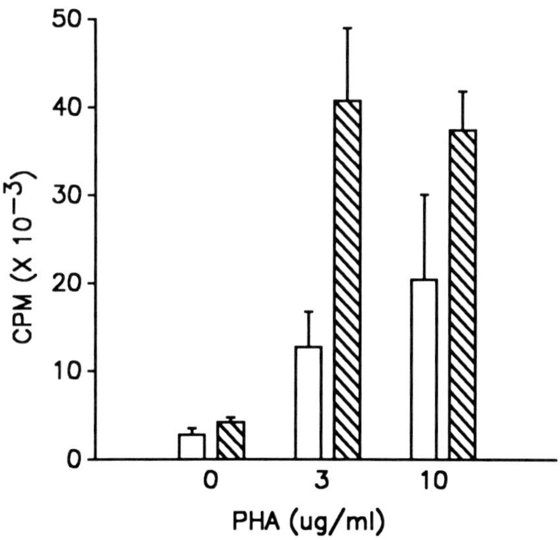

FIGURE 1: **Splenic lymphocyte response to PHA (3 or 10 ug/ml) in two-week ethanol exposed (hatched bars) and pair-fed (open bars) adult male rats. Data shown are mean ± SEM of six animals per group.**

Results depicted in Figure 1 show a significant increase in lymphocyte proliferation induced by phytohemagglutinin (PHA) in the alcohol-treated group compared to pair-fed controls. These results, obtained after 2 weeks of exposure, are similar to those observed in human chronic alcohol abusers without liver disease (Bonanno et al., 1983), in which an enhanced pokeweed mitogen and concanavalin A-induced lymphocyte proliferation was observed. A stimulation of delayed cutaneous hypersensitivity response was also observed with low dose, short duration alcohol treatment in rats (Dehne et al., 1989).

Table 1 shows endocrine parameters of chronic alcohol exposed and pair-fed males, some of which were used in the lymphocyte proliferation experiment. There were no differences from controls in the plasma ACTH and corticosterone levels in the ethanol-treated rats (57.7 ± 5.8 (PF) vs. 52.3 ± 6.5 (E) pg/ml ACTH; 198.1 ± 25.7 (PF) vs.154.1 ± 36.9 (E) ng/ml corticosterone). By contrast, the ethanol group had lower ACTH content in the pituitary and hypothalamus and a lower CRF content in the hypothalamus than the pair-fed rats (Table 1). In the light of no change in plasma ACTH levels after alcohol exposure, the decreased ACTH and CRF content in the pituitary and hypothalamus is probably not a reflection of increased hormone release, but rather of decreased hormone synthesis.

TABLE 1: Hypothalamic CRF and ACTH, and Pituitary ACTH Content of Ethanol Exposed (E) and Pair-Fed (PF) Adult Males

Group	ACTH[a]	ACTH[b]	CRF[b]
PF (6)	662.1±45.6	2.06±0.38	8.70±0.27
E (6)	406.1±70.3*	0.97±0.13**	6.77±0.59*

***p<.05; **p≤.01 from PF controls.**
[a] ng/pituitary; [b] ng/hypothalamus

Evidence suggests that such results reflect the past history of the endocrine homeostasis of the animal. Thymic involution and decreased ACTH and CRF biosynthesis (Dallman et al., 1985) are known to result from past elevations in blood glucocorticoid concentrations. After a one-day of immobilization stress thymic involution reaches its maximum at 3-4 days post-stress (Teshima et al., 1987), and thymic weight returns to pre-stress values only by day 7. Similarly, hypothalamic content of CRF remains elevated a week after cessation of continuous i.c.v. administration of corticosterone antiserum, reflecting the past history of decreased negative corticosterone feedback inhibition on CRF synthesis (VanZuylen et al., 1986). In our experiments the plasma levels of ACTH and corticosterone were not different in the ethanol-treated rats at the end of the 2 week diet. Such data are consistent with the idea that the thymic involution and hypothalamic content of CRF does not reflect the present, but rather the past, glucocorticoid environment of the animal.

Therefore, it seems that chronic alcohol treatment of a short, two week, duration induces stimulation in splenic lymphocyte mitogenesis even though glucocorticoids may have been temporarily elevated at some point during alcohol exposure.

Longer, five weeks, exposure to ethanol resulted in significantly elevated levels of plasma ACTH and corticosterone (92.7 $\pm$ 8.6 (E) vs. 44.9 $\pm$ 1.3 (PF) pg/ml ACTH, $p<0.001$; 198.6 $\pm$ 25.1 (E) vs. 67.8 $\pm$ 13.9 (PF) ng/ml corticosterone, $p<0.001$). Thymus was involuted and adrenals were significantly hypertrophied in the ethanol-treated animals (Thymus weight: 1.10 $\pm$ 0.05 (E) vs. 1.83 $\pm$ 0.11 (PF) mg/g BW, $p<0.001$; Adrenal weight: 17.15 $\pm$ 0.67 (E) vs. 12.42 $\pm$ 0.59 (PF) mg/100g BW, $p<0.001$) suggesting permanent stimulation of the adrenal cortex. Long term exposure to ethanol has also been shown to result in diminution of the proliferative response (Jerrels et al, 1986) indicating that the permanent elevations in glucocorticoid levels may be responsible for the suppressed T-cell function.

An underlying mechanism by which ethanol can either enhance or suppress T cell function can be hypothesized. Leukotrienes, the endogenously produced arachidonic acid (AA) metabolites, seem to be critical to T cell proliferation (Goodwin et al, 1986). Short term exposure to ethanol in vivo or in vitro may increase the production of leukotrienes, while long term exposure in vivo or in vitro without exogenous AA may deplete the releasable pool of AA, the precursor of leukotrienes (Wescott and Murphy, 1983). Since long-term exposure to ethanol results in permanently elevated glucocorticoid levels, and glucocorticoids are known to inhibit the release of AA from membrane phospholipids (Gryglewski et al, 1975; Flower et al, 1978), the direction of ethanol-induced changes in lymphocyte proliferation, suppression or enhancement, would depend on the amount of available AA to form leukotrienes. Studies are currently underway in our laboratory to investigate the mechanism of interactions between ethanol-induced perturbations in the HPA activity and immune function.

REFERENCES

Berczi I (1986). "Pituitary Functions and Immunity." CRC Press, Boca Raton.

Bonanno G, Bocchini G, Canevari A, Pieri F, Ferrini S, Melioli G (1983). Immunological imbalance in uncomplicated chronic alcoholism. Drug Alcohol Depend 12:189-196.

Dallman MF, Makara GB, Roberts JE,Levin N, Blum M (1985). Corticotrope response to removal of releasing factors and corticosteroids in vivo. Endocrinology 117:2190-2197.

Dehne NE, Mendenhall CL, Roselle GA, Grossman GJ (1989). Cell-mediated immune responses associated with short term alcohol intake: Time course and dose dependency. Alcohol Clin Exp Res 13:201-205.

Dougherty TF (1952). Effects of hormones on lymphatic tissue. Physiol Rev 32:379-401.
Ellis FW (1966). Effect of ethanol on plasma corticosterone levels. J Pharmacol Exp Therap 153:121-127.
Fauci AS (1976). Mechanism of corticosteroid action of lymphocyte subpopulations. II. Differential effects of in vivo hydrocortisone, prednisone and dexamethasone on the in vitro expression of lymphocyte function. Clin Exp Immunol 24:54-62.
Fauci AS (1975). Mechanism of corticosteroid action on lymphocyte subpopulation. I. Redistribution of circulating T and B lymphocytes to the bone marrow. Immunology 28:669-676.
Flower RJ, Blackwell GJ (1978). Anti-inflammatory steroids induce biosynthesis of a phospholipase A2 inhibitor which prevents prostaglandin generation. Nature 278:456-458.
Goodwin JS, Atluru D, Sierakowski S, Lianos EA (1986). Mechanism of action of glucocorticoids. J Clin Invest 77:1244-1250.
Gryglewski RJ, Panczenko B, Korbut R, Grodzinska L, Ocetkiewica A (1975). Corticosteroids inhibit prostaglandin release from perfused mesenteric blood vessels in rabbits. Prostaglandins 10:343-354.
Jerrels TR, Marietta CA, Eckardt MJ, Majchrowicz E, Weight FF (1986). Effects of ethanol administration on parameters of immunocompetency in rats. J Leuk Biol 39:499-510.
Lee KC (1977). Cortisone as a probe for cell interactions in the generation of cytotoxic T cells.I. Effects on helper cells, cytotoxic T lymphocytes, precursors and accessory cells. J Immunol 119:1836-1848.
Marietta CA, Jerrels TR, Meagher RC, Karonian JW, Weight FF, Eckardt MJ (1988). Effects of long-term ethanol inhalation on the immune and hematopoietic systems of the rat. Alcohol Clin Exp Res 12:211-214.

Mendelson JH, Ogata M, Mello NK (1971). Adrenal function and alcoholism. Psychosom Med 33:145-157.
Mutchnick MG, Horchang HL (1988). Impaired lymphocyte proliferative response to mitogen in alcoholic patients. Absence of a relation to liver disease activity. Alcohol Clin Exp Res 12:155-158.
Redei E, Branch BJ, Gholami S, Lin EYR, Taylor AN (1988). Effects of ethanol on CRF release in vitro. Endocrinology 123:2736-2743.
Roselle GA, Mendenhall CL (1984). Ethanol-induced alterations in lymphocyte function in the guinea pig. Alcohol Clin Exp Res 8:62-67.
Smith WI, Van Thiel DH, Whiteside T, Janoson B, Magovern J, Puet T, Rabin BS (1980). Altered immunity in male patients with alcoholic liver disease: Evidence for defective immune regulation. Alcohol Clin Exp Res 4:199-206.
Stokes PE (1973). Adrenocortical activation in alcoholics during chronic drinking. Ann NY Acad Sci 215:77-83.
Teshima H, Sogawa H, Kihara H (1987). Changes in populations of T-cell subsets due to stress. In Jankovich BD, Markovich BM, Spector NH (eds): "Neuroimmune Interactions," Ann NY Acad Sci, pp 496-459.
Thompson J, Vanfurth R (1970). The effect of glucocorticoids on the kinetics of mononuclear phagocytes. J Exp Med 131:429-432.
VanZuylen JE, Taylor AN, Gholami S, Redei E (1986). ACTH response to stress after continuous intraventricular administration of corticosterone antiserum. Soc Neurosci Abstr 12:782.
Wands JR (1979). Ethanol and the immune response. In Noble EP (ed): "Biochemistry and Pharmacology of Ethanol," Plenum Press, New York, pp 641-658.
Watson RR, Jackson JC, Hartmann B, Sampliner R, Mobley D, Eskelson C (1985). Cellular immune functions, endorphins and alcohol consumption in males. Alcoholism Clin Exp Res 9:248-254.
Wescott JY, Murphy RC (1983). The interaction of ethanol and exogenous arachidonic acid in the formation of leukotrienes and prostaglandin D2 in mastocytoma cells. Prostaglandins 26:223-239.

Alcohol, Immunomodulation, and AIDS, pages 321–332
© 1990 Alan R. Liss, Inc.

CELL-MEDIATED IMMUNITY IN ALCOHOLIC LIVER DISEASE

Antonio Chedid, Charles L. Mendenhall, and the Veterans Administration Cooperative Study #275 Department of Pathology, (A.C.) and Medicine, (C.L.M.), University of Health Sciences/The Chicago Medical School, North Chicago, IL, Veterans Administration Hospital, and University of Cincinnati, College of Medicine, Cincinnati, OH

INTRODUCTION

In this country the number of chronic alcoholics is estimated to be between 9-10 million and in large metropolitan areas cirrhosis of the liver is the fourth most common cause of death between the ages of 35 and 54 (5). Alcoholic hepatitis is believed to be a reversible stage of alcoholic liver injury frequently preceding development of cirrhosis. In the most recent study of alcoholic hepatitis (6), of the initial 995 alcoholics who were screened, with disease severe enough to require hospitlization, almost 34% of those studied by biopsy had alcoholic hepatitis. The total prevalence was expected to be higher since mild or asymptomatic patients were not evaluated by biopsy.

ETHANOL CONSUMPTION AND THE IMMUNE SYSTEM

Many reports have appeared describing immune alterations in the chronic alcoholic. The alterations affect several cell types including B and T cells (7). Of considerable more interest in the pathogenesis of the disease have been the reported alterations in cell-mediated immunity (1, 2,8). These include: decreased number (9,10) of peripheral rosette-forming lymphocytes (CD-3$^+$, CD-11$^+$) and decreased peripheral blood helper lymphocytes (T4, CD-4$^+$). In addition there is an increased activity of cytotoxic T lymphocytes (CD-8$^+$, T_8, CTL) and possibly natural killer (NK) cells (CD-16$^+$) or lymphocyte activated (LAK) killer cells when tested in vitro with autologus hepatocytes, Chang cells (11) and allogeneic hepatocytes (12). Concanavalin A (Con-A)-

induced suppressor cell activity in patients with ALD is markedly impaired (12) but the monocyte-macrophage system is intact. In ALD the following changes have been reported: a decrease in CD-4 positive lymphocytes with alteration of the CD-4/CD-8 ratio (13) as well as activation of the Fc-receptor bearing lymphocytes (14) with the capacity to kill antibody-coated target cells. Finally cell-mediated immunologic response to alcoholic hyalin (2) has been postulated to occur in ALD although its significance in the pathogenesis remains unknown.

Immunological alterations have been proposed as responsible factors in the initiation and progression of ALD even after discontinuation of ethanol ingestion. The evidence now indicates that the immune system is altered in alcoholic hepatitis: circulating antibodies directed against alcoholic hyalin have been found in all cases of severe ALD and in up to 42% of patients with mild or moderate disease (15). Although circulating immune complexes have been suggested to play a role (16-18) the consensus now favors the participation of cell-mediated immunity (1,2) in the pathogenesis of alcoholic liver injury: lymphocyte sequestration has been shown to occur in the liver (19) associated with a decrease in number of circulating T lymphocytes (9,10). Furthermore, studies in ALD using the immunoperoxidase technique (20,21) have shown increase in T4 cells ($CD\text{-}4^+$) and perhaps NK cells in the portal tracts and T8 cells ($CD\text{-}8^+$, CTL) in the parenchyma along the sinusoidal walls in direct contact with hepatocytes. The hepatocytes have been shown by immunofluorescense to be coated with IgA (16-18) and in all patients with acute alcoholic hepatitis, by immunoperoxidase, the HLA-class I antigens (22) have been shown to be present focally or diffusely on the cell membrane of the hepatocytes. The presence of CTLs on IgA-coated surfaces of hepatocytes expressing MHC-I molecules certainly suggests that CTL-mediated killing of hepatocytes is the main event in alcoholic hepatitis. Following the initial episode of polymorphonuclear inflammation in ALD, a lymphocytic population predominates to the extent that a disease morphologically indistinguishable from chronic active (autoimmune) hepatitis has been described (23) in the alcoholic. The lymphocytic population and its hormone modulators in the liver tissue still need to be properly characterized and correlated with clinical manifestations and progression of ALD. This is the objective of this study.

The unique responsiveness of T cells to alcoholic hyalin (1,2) and the cytolytic activity of certain subsets of lymphocytes to liver cells in culture (2,8) has led to the suggestion that a hypersensitivity reaction (24) or a graft versus host phenomenon (10) may be operating in the pathogenesis of ALD.

A. Antigen recognition and cytolysis

The antigen presenting cell (macrophage, plasma cell, dendritic cell, Kupffer cell, and Langerhans' cells) processes the antigen (25), a fragment of which is transported to the cell surface where in combination with an HLA class II molecule (26) is recognized by the T_4 helper lymphocyte. This recognition is mediated by the T cell surface receptor (27) that binds to two ligands: the peptide derived from the processed antigen and a glycoprotein (the MHC-class II molecule) present on the cell surface of the antigen presenting cell (APC). The subset of T cells that turns on the immune response, helper T cells, and the T cells responsible for specific destruction of target cells, cytotoxic T lymphocytes, express a T cell receptor. The latter is a molecular complex that consists of an α and β subunits that mediate antigen recognition. They are associated with three CD3 subunits that mediate signal transduction when the T cells are activated by receptor binding. However, this molecular complex recognizes antigen only when it is associated on the surface of the target cell with a molecule encoded by the MHC. The antigen binds first with the MHC molecule (28) and later the T cell receptor binds the antigen (29). The latter has been subdivided into two components: the aminoacid residue that interacts with the T cell receptor (epitope) and the aminoacid residue that interacts with the MHC molecule (agretope) (30). The CTL reacts with the APC through an MHC class I molecule. This triggers T_8 cell differentiation. The APC then secrets IL-1 that stimulates T_4 cells to proliferate. This, in turn, brings about production by the T_4 cell of several other cytokines: IL-2 that stimulates T_8 as well as T_4 cell proliferation; IL-4 that stimulates growth and differentiation of B and T cells (31-35); and γ IFN that acts as a macrophage-activating factor and increases the expression of MHC-class II molecules in a variety of cell types. The growth and differentiation of CTLs is thus regulated by both IL-2 and IL-4 (36).

At the other end of the sequence, the final event of target cell killing by CTL's (or NK cells) appears to involve either the release of pore-forming molecules (37) [perforins] or the triggering of an internal mechanism on the target cell that facilitates their own death (38).

Antigen specific T lymphocyte-mediated killing is a process involving antigen recognition and adhesion of the CTL to the target cell (39, 40). Three cell surface antigens associated with the CTL-target cell interaction have been identified and termed lymphocyte function-associated (LFA) antigens (41,42). LFA-1 is an antigen widely distributed in lymphoid tissues that participates in NK cell mediated cytolysis in addition to T lymphocyte-mediated cytotoxity and proliferation. LFA-2 is expressed in CTL lines but not on B cells. Monoclonal antibodies (43) to LFA-1 and LFA-2 inhibit their function by binding to effector cell surface molecules. Lymphocyte function-associated antigen 3 (LFA-3) is a cell surface glycoprotein found on epithelial, hematopoietic and other cell types (42) that interacts with the T lymphocyte CD-2 membrane glycoprotein and this ligand-receptor pair mediates intercellular adhesion between LFA-3^+ cells and NK cells, CTL's and mature T lymphocytes. Anti-LFA-3 antibodies block adhesion by binding to the target cell. Another set of molecules that seems to play a role in LFA antigen-mediated cell-cell adhesion is known as intercellular-adhesion molecules (ICAM). They exist in several tissues. Recent studies indicate that ICAM-1 is a ligand for LFA-1 in antigen-independent B- and T-cell adhesion and in cytotoxic T cell recognition (44). Furthermore ICAM-1 seems to be homologous to the neural cell adhesion molecule [NCAM] (45), which in turn is homologous with CD-2. LFA-1 (CD11a/CD-18) is a receptor for ICAM-1 (CD54). Induction of ICAM-1 (56) on epithelial cells mediates LFA-1-dependent adhesion of lymphocytes. A second LFA-1 ligand (ICAM-2) has been identified, it appears to mediate adhesion to endothelial cells and is an integral membrane protein with two immunoglobulin-like domains while ICAM-1 has five. The role of ICAM-2 is yet to be investigated.

B. Necrosis of hepatocytes

Cytotoxic cell killing involves adhesion of CTL's to a target cell followed by delivery of a lethal hit and cytolysis. Monoclonal antibodies to LFA-1, LFA-2, LFA-3, and HLA-

DR inhibit target cell killing in cell-mediated response to viruses, tumor cells and allografts (43). As stated earlier, CTL's and T_4 (helper) cells recognize antigens bound to MHC-I or MHC-II molecules attached to short peptides (46). The peptides can inhibit lysis by binding to the T cell or facilitate lysis by binding to HLA-class I molecules on the target cell.

The distribution of the major histocompatibility complex (MHC) antigens on different cellular components of the liver has been studied recently with varying results (47,48). In normal liver HLA-II antigens were detected in Kupffer cells but not in hepatocytes while HLA-class I antigens were found in bile duct epithelim and sinusoid-lining cells. This contrasts with the results obtained in acute alcoholic hepatitis in which HLA-I antigens were detected on the membrane of the hepatocytes in all patients (22). It has been demonstrated that ethanol acts as an enhancer of MHC antigen expression (49) in several cell lines thus leading to the speculation that alcohol induces (48) an increase in MHC-I antigen expression in hepatocytes, a feature that may have implications in the development and progression of alcoholic hepatitis. Evidence obtained in other human liver diseases such as chronic type B hepatitis (50) and primary biliary cirrhosis (51) indicates that under pathologic conditions, HLA, class I or II molecules, are expressed on the membrane of hepatocytes. Thus the expression of HLA class I and II, IL-1, IL-2, IL-4, IL-6, and γ IFN in the alcoholic liver would argue in favor of cell-mediated participation in the pathogenesis of ALD. The findings reported here represent our initial preliminary observation in order to confirm this possibility.

METHODS AND RESULTS

Liver Biopsies: Pre-randomization liver biopsies with adequate tissue and appropriate fixation (frozen sections) were available on 63 patients. Each patient is evaluated with clinical and laboratory parameters. In our laboratory one HE stain is done on each liver biopsy used for frozen section together with the immunoperoxidase procedures for the cell markers. This HE is used to assign each patient to the appropriate group (i.e. group I, alcoholic hepatitis only and group II, alcoholic hepatitis plus cirrhosis). If the tissue is insufficient for proper evaluation, the regular HE stain done on the paraffin-embedded block of the same biopsy is used. This has been the case very infrequently.

Each biopsy consists of two portions. One portion is processed by conventional stains for routine diagnosis. The second portion is used for the study of lymphocyte subsets. Hospitalized patients diagnosed as having moderate to severe alcoholic hepatitis comprise the patient population. Initial and follow-up biopsies are obtained percutaneously in order to complement the clinical, nutritional and biochemical evaluation of these patients. Lymphocyte surface antigens are determined in the liver with the use of commercially available monoclonal antibodies using an immunoperoxidase method (53,54) applicable to the liver and slightly modified by us. The method used is the avidin-biotin peroxidase complex (ABC method). When applied to the liver its main difficulty arises from the fact that a substantial degree of nonspecific staining is present. The latter is due mainly to the presence of a high concentration in the liver of biotin, a B vitamin, otherwise widely distributed in other mammalian tissues. Avidin-biotin systems have become quite popular for a variety of purposes including the detection of T and B cell antigens in natural or pathologic lymphocytes. The ABC method has been applied to liver biopsies (54) to characterize lymphoid malignancies based on previous observations (55) that in the liver, incubation of frozen sections prior to an avidin-horseradish peroxidase stage with either avidin alone or avidin followed by biotin eliminates any excess of endogenous biotin. Human liver incubated sequentially with avidin, biotin, monoclonal primary and secondary antibody and avidin-peroxidase complex, suppresses endogenous biotin. The hepatic background is thus eliminated when free avidin and biotin are used as blocking agents of endogenous biotin. The method employs (54,55) excess free avidin (dilution 1:10) to block endogenous biotin and excess free biotin (undiluted) the block any excess of bound avidin. We found that at the blocking stage the best results were obtained when the sections were exposed for 30 minutes to avidin and following PBS washings, exposure for another 30 minutes to biotin. Preliminary results are now available in 63 biopsies for the following surface markers: Pan T (anti-CD-3, anti-Leu 1, anti-Leu 4), Pan B (anti-B1 and anti-B4), natural killer (NK) cells (anti-Leu 11b, NKH-1); helper cells (anti-CD-4, anti Leu 3a + 3b); cytotoxic lymphocytes (anti-CD-8). MHC, class I, (anti-HLA-ABC) and class II (anti-HLA-

DR, anti-DP and anti-DQ) have now been tested in most biopsies.

Quantitation of lymphocytes in liver biopsies: For each liver biopsy the slides made include a control HE and a negative control. Each slide is examined with a light microscope equipped with an ocular grid of 1 cm dimension divided in square compartments (5x5) and used at a magnification of x400. Cells positioned within the grid area are counted. At least five different microscopic fields are examined for each antigen marker. Biopsy size permitting the grid is positioned in portal areas as well as other portions of the lobule in order to enumerate cells either scattered throughout the lobule or in dense infiltrates. Total numbers of each cell type are logged per biopsy in a "records book" where patient's name, specimen number, medical center of origin and diagnosis are recorded. The data are analyzed and presented as a mean number of lymphocytes per five high power fields per biopsy and CD-4/CD-8 ratios are calculated. Negative and positive controls are done simultaneously on tonsils and lymph node sections. The preliminary results show that B cells are present in conspicuously low numbers, Leu 11b stains macrophages with phagocytized material, NKH-1 outlines bile ducts and ductules but NK cells are not present. T_4 and T_8 are easily demonstrable. (Table 1.)

The MHC-I is strongly positive on the cell membrane of the hepatocytes. HLA-DR, -DP and -DQ stain prominently the sinusoid-lining cells as well as collagens type I (mature) and III (reticulin). At the stage of alcoholic hepatitis, after the initial polymorphonuclear infiltration has subsided, the infiltrate consists almost exclusively of cytotoxic T lymphocytes (CD-8) in the portal areas, in the periportal zone of piecemeal necrosis and in the aggregates observed within the lobule. This seems to be true, although not to the same extent, of the CD-4 cells as well. The number of CD-4 positive cells is higher than CD-8 and approaches significance. When alcoholic micronodular cirrhosis is already established, the CD-4/CD-8 ratio is higher and equally significant in cirrhosis ($p < 0.05$) when compared with alcoholic hepatitis. This data are shown in the table.

TABLE 1

		T4	T8	T4/T8
ALCOHOLIC HEPATITIS	(19)	38.4 ± 5.3	40.4 ± 3.9	1.07 ± 0.13
CIRRHOSIS	(44)	47.8 ± 4.3	38.3 ± 3.3	1.40 ± 0.10
T-Test:	t	-1.37	0.40	-1.97
	p	ns	ns	0.05

Values given are Mean ± SEM of (n) cases and the p value is from a 1-tailed Student's t test.

FIGURE 1. Photomicrograph of a representative cluster of CTL's (magnification x400). Note the absence of non-specific background. ABC method.

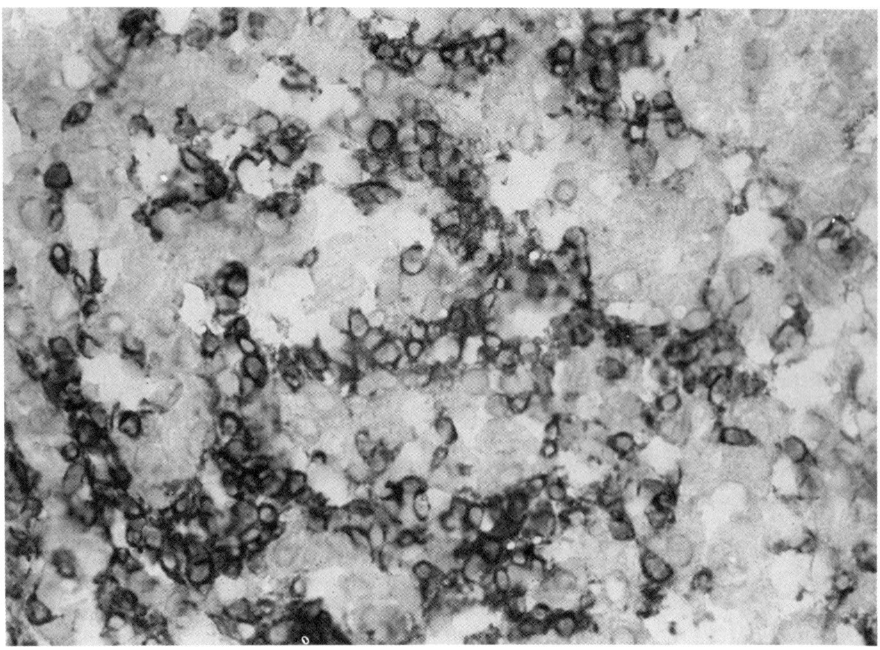

DISCUSSION AND CONCLUSIONS

Our data suggest that in ALD the humoral arm of immunity does not probably play any significant role in the pathogenesis of hepatocyte injury since B cells are, as a rule, almost never present or in very small numbers. NK cells are not observed either.

The role played by lymphocytes in the mechanism of hepatocyte necrosis is unknown. In several cell systems (39, 40) the interaction of the cytotoxic T lymphocyte (CTL, T_8) and the target cell involves antigen recognition, cell adhesion, release of cytolytic molecules and necrosis. The results of our preliminary data suggest that in alcoholic hepatitis the CTL is most likely responsible for the lethal hit that ends in necrosis of the hepatocyte but the numbers are still too small to establish this with statistical certainty. The absence of NK cells from our liver specimens, in contrast to our controls (tonsils and lymph nodes), indicates that perhaps these do not play a major role in hepatocyte necrosis in ALD. This is in agreement with experiments showing that antibodies that inhibit perforin-mediated lysis do not inhibit T-cell mediated (in contrast to NK-cell mediated) lysis (52).

It is unclear from the literature which subsets of lymphocytes (53) are present in the liver of the alcoholic. In our biopsies we have been unable to demonstrate the presence of NK cells using the two best (commercially available) monoclonal antibodies that work in other organs or systems such as peripheral blood, tonsils, lymph nodes or spleen. NKH-1 stains the bile duct epithelium but Leu 11b stains pigment-containing macrophages. It does seem that this is an indication that NK cells are not present in the liver of the alcoholic (53). B cells appear occasionally to be present in very small numbers with the pan B monoclonal antibodies commercially available. However a quite extensive evaluation in a larger number of specimens is necessary in order to ascertain the extent of their frequency. This is necessary in order to establish the relationship of these cells to the various clinical and pathologic process, i.e., necrosis, inflammation and fibrosis. The staining of bile duct epithelial cells with NKH-1 invalidates any claims, made on flow cytometry studies using liver treated with collagenase, that NK cells do play a role in the liver damage of ALD since immunohistochemistry shows those cells to be not NK but bile duct cells. The HLA-ABC antigen expression is enhanced on the hepatocyte cell membrane in the chronic alcoholic and in addition, MHC class II molecules are also expressed on sinusoid-lining cells and collagens. Thus we propose the following series of events to explain these observations: the APC, bearing class II antigens (HLA-DR, DP, DQ) or class I (HLA-ABC) are recognized by CD-4+ and CD-8+ cells respectively. The helper T cell (CD-4+) interacts with the class II antigen leading to the release of IL-1 by the APC. IL-1 promotes proliferation of CD-4+ cells and the release of IL-2 from these cells. IL-2 promotes further proliferation of CD-4+ cells and helps CD-8+ cells to undergo differentiation. In addition, CD-4+ cells secrete IL-4 and IL-6 that induce B-cell differentiation as well as γIFN. Furthermore, lymphotoxin, a soluble factor secreted by activated T cells enhances in vitro B cell proliferation. γIFN exerts a feedback effect on the APC and IL-4 induces further differentiation of CD-8+ cells. At the target site, cells are destroyed by CTL's with the participation of at least an intercellular adhesion molecule (ICAM-1) and lymphocyte-function-associated antigens LFA-1 and LFA-3. This is a sequence of events likely to occur in ALD with the nature of the initiating antigen being still unknown.

REFERENCES

1. Mihas AA, Bull DM, Davidson CS (1975). The Lancet i: 951-953.
2. Zetterman RK, Luisiada-Oper A, Leevy CM (1976). Gastroenterology 70:382-384.
3. Mendenhall CL (1987). Alcoholic hepatitis. In Schiff L, Schiff ER (eds): "Diseases of Liver" 6th edition: pp 669-687.
4. Popper H (1977). Am J Pathol 87:228-264.
5. Cancer Statistics Ca (1988). A Cancer J for Clinicians 38:5-22.
6. Mendenhall CL (1981). Clinics in Gastroenterology Chapter 10; 10:417-441.
7. Feitz T (1968). Gut 9:193-198.
8. Sorrell MF, Leevy CM (1972). Gastroenterology 63:1020-1025.
9. Berstein IM, Webster KH, Williams Jr RC, Strickland RG (1974). The Lancet ii:488-490.

10. Zetterman RK, Leevy CM (1975). Bull NY Acad Med 51:533-544.
11. Kakumu S, Leevy CM (1977). Gastroenterology 72:594-597.
12. Kawanishi H, Tavassolie H, McDermott RP, Sheagren JN (1981). Gastroenterology 80:510-517.
13. Alexander GJM, Nouri-Aria KT, Eddleston ALWF, Williams R (1981). The Lancet i:1191-1293.
14. Sanchez-Tapias J, Thomas HC, Sherlock S (1977). Gut 18: 472-475.
15. Chen T, Kanagasundaram N, NcNakumus S (1975). Gastroenterology 61:A-13/813 (abstract).
16. Kater L, Jobsis AC, Baart EHF-K, Vogten AJM, Grijm R (1975). Am J Clin Pathol 71:51-57.
17. Goldin RD, Cattle S, Boylston AW (1986). J Clin Pathol 39:1181-1185.
18. Swerdlow M, Chowdhury L, Horn T (1982). Am J Clin Pathol 77:259-266.
19. French SW, Burbige EJ, Tarder G, Bourke E, Harken CG, Denton T (1979). Arch Pathol Lab Med 103:146-152.
20. Si L, Whiteside TL, Schade RR, Van Thiel D (1983). Alcoholism: Clin Exp Res 7:431-435.
21. Si L, Whiteside TL, Van Thiel DH, Rabin BS (1984). BS Lab Invest 50:341-347.
22. Barbatis C, Woods J, Morton JA, Fleming KA, McMichael A, McGee J'O (1981). Gut 22:985-991.
23. Goldberg SG, Mendenhall CL, Connell AM, Chedid A (1977). Gastroenterology 72:598-604.
24. Leevy CM, Chen T, Zetterman R (1975). Ann NY Acad Sci 252:106-115.
25. Unanue ER, Allen PM (1987). Science 236:551-557.
26. Germain RN (1986). Nature 322:687-689.
27. Reinherz EL (1987). Nature 325:660-663.
28. Babbitt BP, Allen PM, Matsueda G, Haber E, Unanue ER (1985). Nature 317:359-361.
29. Rao A, Fass SJ, Cantor H (1984). Cell 36:889-895.
30. Schwartz RH (1985). Rev Immunol 3:239-263.
31. Barry MR, Woloski NJ, Guller GM (1985). Proc Natl Acad Sci USA 82:1443-1447.
32. Garman RD, Jacobs KA, Clark SC, Raulet DH (1987). Proc Natl Acad Sci USA 84:7269-7633.
33. Gauldic J, Richards C, Harnish D, Lansdorp P, Baumann H (1987). Proc Natl Acad Sci USA 84:7251-7255.
34. Lotz M, Jiyik F, Kabouridis P, Tsoukas C, Hirano T, Kishimoto T, Carson DA (1988). J Exp Med 167:1253-1258.
35. Yamashi K, Taga T, Hinata Y, Yawata H, Kawanishi Y, Seed B, Taniguchi T, Hirano T, Kishimot T (1988). Science 241:

825-828.
36. Widmer MB, Grabstein KH (1987). Nature 326:795-798.
37. Young J D-E, Leong LG, Liu CC, Damiano A, Cohn ZA (1986). Proc Natl Acad Sci USA 83:5668-5672.
38. Ucker DS (1987). Nature 327:62-64.
39. Sanchez-Madred F, Krensky AM, Ware CF, Robbins E, Strominger JL, Burakoff SJ, Springer TA (1982). Proc Natl Acad Sci USA 79:7489-7493.
40. Krensky AM, Robbins E, Springer TA, Burakoff SJ (1984). J Immunology 132:2180-2182.
41. Seed B (1987). Nature 329:840-842.
42. Dustin ML, Selvaraj P, Mattaliano RJ, Springer TA (1987). Nature 329:846-848.
43. Krensky AM, Sanchez-Madrid F, Robbins E, Nagy JA, Springer TA, Burakoff SJ (1983). J Immunology 131:611-616.
44. Makgoba MW, Sanders ME, Ginther Luce GE, Dustin ML, Springer TA, Clark EA, Mannoni P, Shaw S (1988). Nature 331:86-88.
45. Simmons D, Makgoba MW, Seed B (1988). Nature 331:624-627.
46. Clayberger C, Parham P, Rothband J, Ludwig DS, Schoolnik GK, Krensky AM (1987). Nature 330:763-765.
47. Lautenschlager I, Taskinen E, Inkinen K, Leho V-P, Virtanen I, Hayry P (1984). Cell Immunol 85:191-200.
48. Fukusato T, Gerber MA, Thung SN, Ferrone S, Schaffner F (1986). Am J Pathol 123:264-270.
49. Parent LJ, Ehrlich R, Matis L, Singer DS (1987). FASEB J 1:469-473.
50. Chu C-M, Shyu W-C, Kuo R-W, Liaw Y-F (1987). Hepatology 7:1311-1316.
51. Gores GT, Moore SB, Fisher LD, Powell FC, Dickson ER (1987). Hepatology 7:889-892.
52. Goldstein P (1987). Nature 327:12.
53. Paronetto F, Colucci G, Columbo M (1986). "Progress in Liver Disease", Chapter 11, Vol VIII:191-208.
54. Verdi CJ, Grogan TM, Protell R, Richter L, Rangel C (1986). Hepatology 6:6-13.
55. Wood GS, Warnke R (1981). J Histoch & Cytoch 29:1196-1204.
56. Staunton DE, Dustin ML, Springer TA (1989). Nature 339:61-64.

Alcohol, Immunomodulation, and AIDS, pages 333–340
© 1990 Alan R. Liss, Inc.

IMMUNE RESPONSE TO ACETALDEHYDE ADDUCTS

Lynell W. Klassen, D.S. Xu, Dean J. Tuma

Department of Internal Medicine, University of Nebraska Medical Center, and Omaha VA Medical Center, Omaha, Nebraska 68105

INTRODUCTION

It has long been postulated that alcohol induced organ damage may be initiated or maintained by abnormal immune responses. Several groups have shown that metabolically derived acetaldehyde can complex with macromolecules forming stable adducts (Medina et al, 1985). Others have demonstrated that acetaldehyde/protein adducts can act as immunogens in heterologous systems (Israel et al, 1986). Recent work has described the presence of antibodies with anti-acetaldehyde adduct specificity in the sera of alcoholics (Anthony et al, 1983; Niemela et al, 1987). Metabolically derived acetaldehyde adduct formation has been shown to directly interfere with hepatocyte protein metabolism, protein secretion, plasma membrane assembly, receptor mediated endocytosis, and cytoskeletal protein structure. Thus it is clear that metabolically derived acetaldehyde/protein adducts can alter cellular function and act as immunogens.

The current investigations are based on the hypothesis that humoral and/or cellular immune responses are directed against acetaldehyde/protein adducts on cell surface determinants and can result in tissue damage and dysfunction. The initial research approach has been to develop a panel of polyclonal and monoclonal antibodies that recognize specific chemically defined acetaldehyde adduct-related epitopes formed under varying conditions.

METHODS

Anti-aldehyde adduct antibody production and assay. Bovine brain tubulin and bovine serum albumin (BSA) was incubated with 5 mM aldehyde in PBS under reducing conditions utilizing 10 mM of cyanoborohydride for two days or under non-reducing conditions by incubation in PBS at pH 7.4 for five days. C57Bl/6 mice were immunized and boosted with 75 ug. of appropriate immunogen in Freund's adjuvant at three-week intervals. Sera was separated, heat-inactivated and serially diluted for testing in a specific ELISA antibody assays. Optimum serum dilution was usually at 1:500. The ELISA assay was performed by immobilizing aldehyde-protein adducts on Immulon II microtiter plates at 1 ug. protein per well. Non-specific binding sites were blocked with 1% gelatin solution and after appropriate washing the diluted sample serum added. Plates were incubated overnight at room temperature, and the binding of IgG antibody detected using a secondary peroxidase-conjugated sheep anti-mouse IgG antibody. The amount of secondary antibody present was detected by the addition of ABTS and reading the optical transmission in a spectrophotometer. Relative O.D. was determined by dividing the specific O.D. value by a given reference protein.

Quantification of aldehyde adducts on BSA protein. The relative number of adducts formed for each aldehyde agent studied was determined by incorporation of ^3H from $NaCNBH_3$. Final incubation conditions included 5 mM acetaldehyde with 30 mM ^3H-$NaCNBH_3$. The adducts present were expressed as pM ^3H incorporated per mg. of protein.

Inhibition assay for epitope specificity of anti-acetaldehyde adduct antibodies. Classic antigen/antibody inhibitor assays were used to determine the specificity of anti-acetaldehyde antibodies found in the serum of immunized animals. Diluted sera (1:500) was incubated with varying aldehyde/BSA adducts for 15 minutes at 37° followed by 45 minutes at 4°. This mixture was then assayed for residual non-bound antibodies by the standard ELISA system used above.

RESULTS

Specificity of aldehyde adduct antibodies. Antibodies developed against reduced acetaldehyde/tubulin adducts were tested against a variety of different aldehyde adducts complexed with bovine serum albumin (BSA). The results are:

TABLE I: Specificity of Acetaldehyde/Tubulin Produced Antibodies

Aldehyde/Protein Conjugation	Relative O.D.
BSA-acetaldehyde	1.000
BSA-propionaldehyde	0.802
BSA-butyraldehyde	0.531
BSA-crotonaldehyde	0.162
BSA-benzaldehyde	0.131
BSA-2-ethyl-2-hexenaldehyde	0.112

These results confirm that the specificity of acetaldehyde adduct antibodies is carrier protein independent. In addition, the antibodies induced by one specific chemical aldehyde may or may not cross-react with other aldehyde protein adducts. The intermediate crossreactivity seen when acetaldehyde-induced antibodies were assayed on butyraldehyde adducts raises the possibility of differences in epitope (adduct) density, alterations in antibody affinity to a variety of aldehyde adducts, or the presence of different but multiple epitopes on various aldehyde adduct conjugates.

Relative frequency of aldehyde/BSA adducts formed under reducing conditions. In order to answer the question of differences in epitope density, the amounts of adduct formed on three crossreacting antigens were quantitated:

TABLE II: Relative Frequency of Aldehyde/BSA Adducts Formed Under Reducing Conditions

Conjugation	pM ^{3}H Incorporation/mg. Protein
BSA-acetaldehyde	9.2 ± 1.9*
BSA-propionaldehyde	8.1 ± 2.1
BSA-butyraldehyde	11.3 ± 11.4

*Mean plus standard deviation

Thus the difference in binding of an antibody derived to acetaldehyde adducts to other aldehyde/protein conjugates cannot be due to a quantitative decrease in the available epitopes.

Epitope specificity determined by antigen/antibody inhibition studies. Competetive antigen inhibition studies were used to look for the presence of multiple shared epitopes on the chemically different aldehyde adducts formed to tubulin conjugates and assayed on aldehyde/BSA conjugates. Anti-reduced acetaldehyde/tubulin sera was diluated at 1:500 prior to incubation with different soluble adduct protein antigens at a variety of protein concentrations. The results are as follows:

TABLE III: Crossreactivity of Antibodies Made to Reduced Acetaldehyde/Tubulin

Inhibiting Soluble Antigen	Percent Control O.D. Assayed on Reduced Acetaldehyde/BSA Antigen
BSA	
10 mg/ml	1.000
25 mg/ml	0.953
50 mg/ml	1.103
250 mg/ml	0.987
Butyraldehyde/BSA	
10 mg/ml	0.830
25 mg/ml	0.759
50 mg/ml	0.747
250 mg/ml	0.648
Propionaldehyde/BSA	
10 mg/ml	0.761
25 mg/ml	0.628
50 mg/ml	0.283
250 mg/ml	
Acetaldehyde/BSA	
10 mg/ml	0.685
25 mg/ml	0.355
50 mg/ml	0.166
250 mg/ml	0.142

Antibodies made to acetaldehyde/tubulin adducts are completely absorbed by both acetaldehyde/BSA and propionaldehyde/BSA antigen. Soluble butyraldehyde/BSA antigens absorb some, but not all, of the antibodies suggesting a variety of epitopes present on the acetaldehyde adduct.

Epitope specificity for reduced versus non-reduced acetaldehyde/protein adducts. There appears to be antigenic differences in adducts made under varying biochemical conditions. The specificity of antibodies raised against acetaldehyde adducts made under chemically reduced versus chemically non-reduced conditions was determined as shown:

TABLE IV. Epitope Specificity for Reduced Versus Non-Reduced Acetaldehyde/Protein Adducts

	ELISA Antigen		
Antisera Against	**Tubulin**	**Non-Reduced Acetaldehyde/ Tubulin**	**Reduced Acetaldehyde/ Tubulin**
Tubulin	90*	50	100
Non-Reduced Acetaldehyde/ Tubulin	120	1500	250
Reduced Acetaldehyde/ Tubulin	100	450	900

*Reciprocal serum titer at O.D. greater than 3 S.D. from control mouse serum.

It appears that there may well be different antigenic epitopes expressed by reduced and non-reduced acetaldehyde adducts that can be detected by specific antibodies.

DISCUSSION

These studies have confirmed that antibodies to aldehyde/protein adducts can be readily developed using an adjuvant system in a murine experimental model. It appears that antibodies to aldehyde/protein adducts demonstrate a variety of unique epitopes that are unrelated to the carrier protein itself. This confirms the pioneering studies of others (Steinbrecher et al, 1984). In addition, antibodies produced against specific aldehyde/protein adducts may or may not crossreact with chemically disimilar aldehyde adducts. Of interest is that the specific antigen-antibody inhibition studies suggest the presence of more than one epitope on antibodies made to reduced acetaldehyde protein conjugate adducts. This may explain some differences in detection of anti-acetaldehyde adduct antibodies in the literature.

The variety of unique shared and non-shared specificities seen in aldehyde/protein adducts may be analogous to the epitopes seen on other macromolecules such as MHC antigens. Epitopes seen by the polyclonal anti-aldehyde adduct anti-sera appear to recognize "public" epitopes shared on a variety of chemically different aldehyde adduct as well as "private" epitopes seen only on specific aldehyde protein adducts.

It also appears that epitope specificity exists for reduced versus non-reduced acetaldehyde/protein adducts. Thus the biological significance of any detected anti-acetaldehyde adduct antibodies in patients must be interpreted in the settings of the differences seen by adducts formed under chemically reduced versus non-reduced conditions. The availability of epitope specific antibody probes will be helpful in demonstrating which adducts are formed in situ.

Ongoing efforts are directed at developing a panel of monoclonal antibodies that recognize the aldehyde/protein adducts demonstrated in the polyclonal antisera. It is hoped that this panel of monoclonal antibodies can differentiate antigens by biochemical class, as well as by reduced versus non-reduced conjugate formation. Such monoclonal antibodies can be used as probes to define the role of cell surface acetaldehyde adduct antigens in alcohol-related tissue damage.

REFERENCES

Anthony RS, Farquharson M, MacSween R (1983). Liver membrane antibodies in alcoholic liver disease. II. Antibodies to ethanol-altered hepatocytes. J Clin Path 36: 1302.

Israel Y, Hurwitz E, Niemela O, et al (1986). Monoclonal and polyclonal antibodies against acetaldehyde-containing epitopes in acetaldehyde-protein adducts. Proc Natl Acad Sci 83: 7923.

Medina VA, Donohue TM, Sorrell MF, Tuma DJ (1985). Covalent binding of acetaldehyde to hepatic proteins during ethanol oxidation. J Lab Clin Med 105: 5.

Niemela O, Klajner F, Orrego H, Vidins E, Blendis L, Israel Y (1987). Antibodies against acetaldehyde-modified protein epitopes in human alcoholics. Hepatology 7: 1210.
Steinbrecher UP, Fisher M, Witztum JF, et al (1984). Immunogenicity of homologous low density lipoprotein after methylation, ethylation, acetylation, or carbamylation: Generation of antibodies specific for derivatized lysine. J Lipid Res 25: 1109.

Alcohol, Immunomodulation, and AIDS, pages 341–350
© 1990 Alan R. Liss, Inc.

IN VIVO MICROSCOPY OF THE LIVER FOLLOWING ACUTE ADMINISTRATION OF ETHANOL

R.S. McCuskey, P.A. McCuskey, H. Eguchi, E.G. Crichton, R. Urbaschek, and B. Urbaschek

Dept. of Anatomy, College of Medicine, Univ. of Arizona, B.W. Zweifach Microcirculatory Laboratories, VA Medical Center, Tucson, Arizona 85724, and Dept. of Immunology and Serology, Institute for Hygiene and Medical Microbiology, University of Heidelberg, 6800 Mannheim, West Germany

INTRODUCTION

Following the ingestion of alcohol, significant alterations occur in host defense mechanisms including depressed reticuloendothelial (RES) function as well as altered immune, lymphocyte, granulocyte and platelet functions. These increase the host's susceptibility to infection (Adams and Jordan, 1984; Louria, 1963; Nolan, 1965).

Kupffer cells are one of the cellular compoments of the sinusoids in the liver and are a major part of the RES. Several studies have demonstrated that Kupffer cell function is affected by alcohol in both experimental animals and man. Clearance of microaggregated albumin and endotoxin is depressed in rats following both acute and chronic administration of alcohol (Ali and Nolan, 1967; Nolan et al., 1980; Nolan and Camara, 1982). Acute human alcoholics with no evidence of liver disease also have a depressed RES which returns to normal several days following alcohol withdrawal (Liu, 1979). Furthermore, patients also have been reported to have a depressed RES as evidenced by reduced clearance of microaggregated albumin (Cooksley et al., 1973); and, another group lacked a concentration gradient of immune complexes between portal and hepatic veins (Kaufman et al., 1982). Finally, elevated levels of systemic, circulating endotoxin have been reported in humans intoxicated with alcohol (Bode et al., 1987) and during alcoholic liver disease (Bode et al., 1987; Liehr, 1983; Nolan and Camara, 1982) suggesting spill-over of gut-derived endotoxin no longer being cleared by alcohol-depressed hepatic Kupffer cells. As a result, Kupffer cell dysfunction and endotoxin have been implicated in the etiology of alcoholic liver disease (Liehr, 1983; Nolan and Camara, 1982; Nolan et al., 1980). This concept is further supported by recent animal studies which demontrated that, in the presence of alcohol, normally innocuous doses of endotoxin become toxic and result in severe liver damage (Bhagwandeen et al., 1987). Hypoxia, such as reported for centrilobular hepatocytes in rats acutely dosed with ethanol (Sato et al., 1987), also potentiates the hepatotoxicity of endotoxin (Shibayama, 1987).

Endotoxins, lipopolysaccharides of the cell walls of gram-negative bacteria, have manifold toxic and, in low concentrations, beneficial effects (reviewed in Nowotny, 1983; Schlessinger, 1980; Szentivanyi, 1986; Urbaschek, 1987). Kupffer cells are the principal site for the removal of circulating endotoxins from the blood (Mairer and Ulevitch, 1981; Mathison and Ulevitch, 1979; McCuskey et al., 1987; Munford, 1978; Ruiter et al., 1981). Following the endocytosis of endotoxin, a variety of toxic and beneficial mediators are released from Kupffer cells, as well as other macrophages. Among the mediators produced are tumor necrosis factor (TNF), interleukin-1 (IL-1), eicosanoids, and reactive free radicals. These are thought to participate in the host response to endotoxin (reviewed in McCuskey et al., 1987). Although high concentrations of endotoxins, such as are found during gram-negative sepsis, usually precipitate a toxic response, low levels of gut-derived endotoxin such as normally found in the portal blood, may contribute to non-specific resistance by modulating Kupffer cell activity (reviewed in McCuskey et al., 1987). Unfortunately, little is known about the role of these substances in mediating blood vessel and cellular injury in the liver during health as well as in the presence of alcohol and/or infection.

As indicated above, a variety of evidence implicates Kupffer cells and endotoxin in the etiology of alcoholic liver disease (Liehr, 1983; Nolan and Camara, 1982; Nolan et al., 1980) as well as hepatic microvascular and parenchymal dysfunction during sepsis and shock (McCuskey et al., 1987; Munford, 1978; Nolan and Camara, 1982; Nolan et al., 1980). Surprisingly, only a limited number of in vivo microscopic studies have been reported on the basic hepatic microcirculatory response to alcohol (Sato et al., 1987a,b). Due to this lack of knowledge concerning the microvascular pathyphysiology induced in the liver by acute and chronic alcohol alone of in the presence of endotoxin and/or infection, we initiated studies to elucidate the hepatic microvascular responses, including Kupffer cell function, during these conditions. This paper reports our initial results obtained by high resolution in vivo microscopy of the dynamic responses of hepatic microvasculature to acute intragastric ethanol administration in mice.

MATERIALS AND METHODS

Male NMRI, C_3H/HeJ and C57Bl/6 mice weighing 20-30 gm were used as experimental animals. All animals were provided food and water ad libitum. The mice were administered ethanol intragastrically at doses of 1-5 gm/kg bw. Animals similarly dosed with equivalent volumes of either sterile water or isocaloric sucrose in sterile water served as controls. Each experimental group contained at least six animals.

The animals were anesthetized with 20% urethane (0.3 ml ip) and the hepatic microvascular responses studied at intervals up to three hours using high resolution in vivo microscopic methods (reviewed in McCuskey, 1986b). Kupffer cell function was assessed by observing the phagocytosis of 1.0 μm fluorescent latex particles by individual cells (McCuskey et al., 1983; McCuskey, 1986a,b). The latex was diluted 1:10 with sterile saline and administered intravenously in the tail. Each mouse received 0.1 ml (10^5 particles). To assess the number of phagocytic Kupffer cells, the number of cells that had phagocytosed latex was counted in 10 consecutive microscopic fields in each liver 15 min after each mouse had received the latex solution. In addition, the relative adequacy of blood perfusion through the sinusoids was evaluated by counting the number of sinusoids containing blood flow in the same 10 microscopic fields. Since reduced perfusion of individual sinusoids can reduce the delivery of the latex particles to Kupffer cells in these vessels, the ratio of Kupffer cells that phagocytosed latex to sinusoids containing blood flow also was used as a measure of Kupffer cell activity (McCuskey, 1986a,b; McCuskey et al., 1983). The data were evaluated statistically by analysis of variance, with

P<0.05 considered significant.

In addition, the blood levels of ethanol and transaminases (SGOT, SPGT) were measured as a function of time following single intragastric dosing of C57Bl/6 male mice with 1-5 gm/kg bw ethanol. Animals similarly dosed with isocaloric sucrose in water served as controls. Comparisons also were made between changes in ethanol levels in portal vs systemic blood. The assays were done spectrophotmetrically using appropriate diagnostic kits obtained from Sigma Chemical Co., St. Louis, MO.

RESULTS

Initial experiments using endotoxin-sensitive NMRI mice dosed intragastrically with 1 or 5 gm/kg ethanol demonstrated an increase in the numbers of phagocytic Kupffer cells/microscopic field one hour after ethanol ingestion (Table 1). However, 5 gm/kg intragastric ethanol resulted in a slight reduction in phagocytic Kupffer cells (Table 1). In contrast, 5 gm/kg ethanol elicited an increase in the number of phagocytic Kupffer cells in endotoxin non-responding C_3H/HeJ mice (Table 1).

TABLE 1. Effect of Ethanol on Kupffer Cells in NMRI and C_3H/HeJ Mice After 1 Hr.

Number of Phagocytic Kupffer Cells/Microscopic Field*

Dose	NMRI Mice	C_3H/HeJ Mice
Sterile Water	11.33 ± 1.35	8.6 ± 1.06
1 gm/kg Ethanol	14.77 ± 0.71**	------
5 gm/kg Ethanol	9.23 ± 0.19**	11.23 ± 0.59**

* Mean ± S.E.
** P<0.05 compared to control

Encouraged by the above experiments, more extensive experiments were conducted to better define the hepatic microvascular responses to different doses of ethanol and relate these to blood ethanol levels in C57Bl/6 mice.

Doses of 1 gm/kg bw ethanol in C57Bl/6 mice produced systemic blood ethanol levels of 0.1% 30 min after dosing. Portal levels were not significantly higher than levels in systemic blood; by 3 hrs no detectible blood ethanol was found. In contrast, 4 gm/kg bw ethanol resulted in blood levels of 0.35% by 30 min, these levels were still evident at 3 hrs but had dropped to 0.1% by 6 hrs. Only modest changes in transaminases were detected even at the highest doses (5 gm/kg bw) of acute ethanol administration with these values remaining in the normal range.

Based on these results, the hepatic microvascular responses to a single acute, low (1 gm/kg bw) and high dose (4 gm/kg bw) of intragastric ethanol was studied in more detail by high resolution in vivo microscopy at 30 min and 3 hrs after dosing. Similar examinations were made of control animals dosed with isocaloric sucrose in water. The high dose of ethanol (4 gm/kg) elicited hepatocellular damage as evidenced by the formation of vacuoles and/or swollen organelles, endothelial cellular swelling, and transient plugging of sinusoidal blood flow by leukocytes. Following challenge with a standardized i.v. dose of 1.0 μm latex particles, there appeared to be less uptake by Kupffer cells although the number of phagocytic cells was not significantly different from controls (Table 2). The low dose of ethanol elicited considerably less change in the microcirculation as well as enhanced phagocytosis of latex particles by Kupffer cells. The number of phagocytic Kupffer cells also increased (Table 2), particularly by 3 hrs when the blood ethanol level had returned to undetectable levels.

TABLE 2. Effect of Ethanol on Kupffer Cells in C57Bl/6 Mice After 30 Min and 3 Hr.

Ratio of Numbers of Phagocytic Kupffer Cells to Sinusoids with Blood Flow per Microscopic Field*

Dose	30 Minutes	3 Hours
1 gm/kg Ethanol	1.00 ± 0.06	1.38 ± 0.13**
Isocal. Sucrose	0.89 ± 0.07	0.97 ± 0.09
4 gm/kg Ethanol	0.91 ± 0.06	1.21 ± 0.09
Isocal. Sucrose	0.88 ± 0.11	1.00 ± 0.17

* Mean ± S.E.M.
** P<0.05 compared to isocaloric sucrose control at same time interval.

DISCUSSION

Ethanol ingestion produces increased hepatic oxygen consumption, fatty liver, hepatomegaly, hepatocellular damage and, with prolonged consumption, hepatitis, fibrogenesis and cirrhosis may result. Alterations in hepatic blood flow accompany these responses. Acutely administered ethanol increases hepatic blood flow (Castenfors et al., 1960; Shaw et al., 1977). The acute vasodilatory effect of ethanol is not thought to be a result of vascular actions of metabolites of ethanol, acetalaldehyde or acetate (Altura and Altura, 1982; Altura and Gebrewold, 1981; Carmichael et al., 1986, 1987), but is suggested to be due to adenosine (Carmichael et al., 1987). The potential role of vasoactive mediators released from Kupffer cells, however, has not been evaluated.

At the microcirculatory level, limited knowledge exists about alcohol-induced alterations in the hepatic microvasculature, how such alterations are exacerbated in the presence of endotoxemia and/or infection, and the role played by Kupffer cells in these processes. The few published in vivo microscopic studies report that acute, oral administration of ethanol to rats increases both portal and hepatic arterial blood flow resulting in an average net increase in the velocity of erythrocyte flow through the sinusoids (Sato et al., 1982a,b). The increased flow in the sinusoids, however, was heterogeneous, with some sinusoids exhibiting dramatic increases in cellular velocity while others had little or no increase and some a decrease. As a result, some centrivenular areas became hypoxic while others exhibited an increase in oxygenation (Sato et al., 1987a,b). There are no reports of in vivo microscopic examination of livers in animal chronically ingesting ethanol.

The current studies demonstrate that an acute single dose of ethanol differentially affects the hepatic microvascular system, including Kupffer cell phagocytic function, in a dose dependent manner. Many of the events, e.g., endothelial cellular swelling, leukocyte adhesion and plugging of sinusoids, mimic responses elicited by injection of endotoxin and tumor necrosis factor alpha (TNFα), as well as sepsis (McCuskey, 1986a; McCuskey et al., 1984a,b, 1987, 1988, 1989). This suggests that endotoxin and/or mediators released from Kupffer cells may be responsible for the intravascular events elicited by ethanol. That ethanol affects Kupffer cell function is evident from enhanced phagocytic activity elicited by low doses of ethanol and the lack of affect or suppression of phagocytosis with high doses. Since the latter responses were not seen in endotoxin non-responsive mice where enhanced phagocytosis was observed instead, the effects of ethanol on phagocytic activity appear to depend on the state of Kupffer cell activation which is low in C_3H/HeJ mice (McCuskey et al., 1982, 1984b). Differential, dose dependent effects on Kupffer cell phagocytic function also are elicited by both endotoxin and TNFα (McCuskey, 1986; McCuskey et al., 1984a,b, 1987, 1988, 1989).

ACKNOWLEDGEMENTS

These studies were supported by NIAAA Alcohol Center Grant 1P50AA08037 and the A.v. Humboldt Stiftung (U.S. Senior Scientist Award to RSM).

REFERENCES

Adams HG, Jordan C (1984) Infections in the alcoholic. Med Clin of NA 68:179-200.

Ali MV, Nolan JP (1967) Alcohol induced depression of reticuloendothelial function in the rat. J Lab Clin Med 70:295-301.

Altura BM, Altura BT (1982) Microvascular and vascular smooth muscle actions of ethanol, acetaldehyde, and acetate. Fed Proc 41:2447-2451.

Altura BM, Gebrewold A (1981) Failure of acetaldehyde or acetate to mimic the splanchnic arteriolar or venular dilator actions of ethanol: direct in situ studies on the microcirculation. Br J Pharmacol 73:580-582.

Bhagwandeen BS, Apte M, Manwarring L, Dickeson J (1987) Endotoxin induced hepatic necrosis in rats on an alcohol diet. J Pathol 152:47-53.

Bode C, Kugler V, Bode JC (1987) Endotoxemia in patients with alcoholic and non-alcoholic cirrhosis and in subjects with no evidence of chronic liver disease following acute alcohol excess. J Hepatol 4:8-14.

Carmichael FJ, Saldivia V, Israel Y, Orrega H (1986) Does acetaldehyde (ACT) mediate the ethanol (E) induced increase in liver blood flow? Hepatol 6:1125.

Carmichael FJ, Saldivia V, Israel Y, Orrega H (1987) Effect of acetate on splanchnic hemodynamics. Hepatol 7:1061.

Castenfors H, Hultman E, Josephson B (1960) Effect of intravenous infusions of ethyl alcohol on estimated hepatic blood flow in man. J Clin Invest. 39:776-781.

Cooksley WGE, Powell LW, Halliday JW (1973) Reticuloendothelial phagocytic function in human liver disease and its relationship to haemolysis. Brit J Haematol 25:147-152.
Kaufman RL, Hoefs JC, Quismorio FP Jr (1982) Immune complexes in the portal and systemic circulation of patients with alcoholic liver disease. Clin Immunol Immunopath 22:44-54.
Liehr H (1983) Endotoxins and alcoholic hepatitis. In Cosmos G, Thaler H (eds): "Clinical Hepatology", Berlin: Springer Verlag, pp 336-339.
Liu YK (1979) Phagocytic capacity of reticuloendothelial system in alcoholics. J Reticuloendothel Soc 25:605-613.
Louria DB (1963) Susceptibility to infection during experimental alcohol intoxication. Trans Assoc Amer Physicians 76:102-112.
Mairer RV, Ulevitch R (1981) The response of isolated rabbit hepatic macrophages (H-MO) to lipopolysaccharide (LPS). Circ Shock 8:165-181.
Mathison JC, Ulevitch R (1979) The clearance, tissue distribution and cellular localization of intravenously injected lipopolysaccharide in rabbits. J Immunol 123:2133-2143.
McCuskey RS (1986a) Hepatic microvascular dysfunction during sepsis and endotoxemia. In Tsuchiya M (ed): Cytoprotection and Cytobiology, Vol 3", Amsterdam: Excerpta Medica, pp. 3-17.
McCuskey RS (1986b) Microscopic Methods for Studying the Microvasculature of Internal Organs. In Baker CH, Nastuk WF (eds), "Physical Techniques in Biology and Medicine Microvascular Technology", New York: Academic Press, pp. 247-264.
McCuskey RS, McCuskey PA, Urbaschek R, Urbaschek B (1984a) Hepatic microvascular alterations during sepsis. Circ Shock 13:88-89.
McCuskey RS, McCuskey PA, Urbaschek R, Urbaschek B (1987) Kupffer cell function in host defense. Rev Infect Dis 9(suppl 5):S616-619.
McCuskey RS, Urbaschek R, McCuskey PA, Sacco N, Stauber W, Pinkstaff CA, Urbaschek B (1982) Studies of Kupffer cells in mice sensitized or tolerant to endotoxin. In Knook DL, Wisse E (eds), "Sinusoidal Liver Cells", Amsterdam: Elsevier/North Holland, pp. 387-392.
McCuskey RS, Urbaschek R, McCuskey PA, Sacco N, Stauber WT, Pinkstaff CA, Urbaschek B (1984b) Deficient hepatic phagocytosis and lysosomal enzymes in the low endotoxin-responder, C3H/HeJ mouse. J Leukocyte Biol 36:591-600.

McCuskey RS, Urbaschek R, McCuskey PA, Urbaschek B (1983) In vivo microscopic observations of the responses of Kupffer cells and the hepatic microcirculation to Mycobacterium bovis BCG alone and in combination with endotoxin. Infect Immun 42:362-367.

McCuskey RS, Urbaschek R, McCuskey PA, Urbaschek B (1988) Microvascular responses to tumor necrosis factor. FASEB J 2, A1873

McCuskey RS, Urbaschek R, McCuskey PA, Urbaschek B (1989) Hepatic microvascular responses to tumor necrosis factor. In Decker K, Knook DL, Wisse E (eds), "Cells of the Hepatic Sinusoids, II", Leiden: Kupffer Cell Foundation, In press.

Munford RS (1978) Endotoxins and the liver. Gastroenterology 75:532-535.

Nolan JP (1965) Alcohol as a factor in the illness of University service patients. Amer J Med Sc pp 249:135-142.

Nolan JP, Camara DS (1982) Endotoxin, sinusoidal cells, and liver injury. Prog Liver Diseases 7:361-376.

Nolan JP, Leiborwitz A, Vladutiu AL (1980) Influence of alcohol on Kupffer cell function and possible significance in liver injury. In Liehr H, Grun M, (eds), "The Reticuloendothelial System and the Pathogenesis of Liver Disease", Amsterdam: Elsevier/North Holland Press, pp 125-136.

Nowotny A (ed) (1983) "Beneficial Effects of Endotoxins", New York: Plenum Press.

Ruiter DJ, van den Maulen J, Brouwer A, Hummel MJR, Mauer BJ, von den Ploeg JCM, Wisse E (1981) Uptake by liver cells of endotoxin following its intravenous injection. Lab Invest 45:38-45.

Sato N, Eguchi H, Takei Y, Hijioka T, Tsuji S, Matsumura T, Hayashi N, Kawano S, Kamada T (1987a) Microcirculatory aspects for the mechanism of alcoholic liver disease-sinusoidal blood flow and oxygenation at periportal regions of hepatic lobules in rats. In Tsuchiya M, Asano M, Mishama Y, Oda M (eds) "Microcirculation -- An Update, Vol. 2", Amsterdam: Excerpta Med, pp 345-348.

Sato N, Matsumura T, Kawano S, Kamada T (1987b) Hepatic microcirculation and hepatic cellular-metabolism. In Tsuchiya M, Asano M, Mishama Y, Oda M (eds) "Microcirculation--An Update, Vol. 2", Amsterdam: Excerpta Med, pp 345-348.

Schlessinger D (ed) (1980) "Endogenous mediators in host responses to bacterial endotoxin, Microbiology-1980", Washington: American Society for Microbiology.

Shaw S, Heller EA, Friedman HS (1977) Increased hepatic oxygenation following ethanol administration in the baboon. Proc Soc Exp Biol Med 156:509-513.
Shibayama Y (1987) Enhanced hepatotoxicity of endotoxin by hypoxia. Pathol Res Pract 182:390-395.
Szentivanyi E, Nowotny A, Friedman H (eds) (1986) "Immunobiology and Immunopharmacology of Bacterial Endotoxins", New York: Plenum Press.
Urbaschek B ed. (1987) Perspectives on Bacterial Pathogenesis and Host Defense. Rev Infect Dis 9 (Suppl 5); S431-659.

Alcohol, Immunomodulation, and AIDS, pages 351–358
© 1990 Alan R. Liss, Inc.

EFFECTS OF ALCOHOL INGESTION ON IN VITRO SUSCEPTIBILITY OF PERIPHERAL BLOOD MONONUCLEAR CELLS TO INFECTION WITH HIV-1 AND ON CD4 AND CD8 LYMPHOCYTES

Omar Bagasra*, Patricia Whittle*, Andre Kajdacsy-Balla+, and Harold W. Lischner°

*Dept. Micro, Univ. of Med. and Dent. of N.J., Camden, NJ 08103, +Dept. Path., Univ. of Oklahoma, OK 73190 and °Dept. of Ped. & Micro & Immun., Temple Univ. School of Med., Philadelphia, PA 19140

INTRODUCTION

An increase in chronic heavy alcohol (EtOH) use and EtOH use during sexual activity has been associated with AIDS in epidemiological studies of gay men (Siegel, 1986; Stall et al, 1986), but not of intravenous substance abusers (Lake-Bakaar et al, 1988). One explanation for this association could be that gay men who engage in behavior placing them at a risk for AIDS also drink heavily (Israelstam et al, 1986). Since chronic EtOH consumption has been shown to profoundly affect various functions of the immune system (Bagasra, Kajdascy et al, 1988; Jerrells et al, 1988; Bagasra et al, 1988), another hypothesis is that EtOH reduces resistance to human immunodeficiency virus (HIV) infection. Such an effect might be masked in the case of substance abusers because of parallel effects of various drugs on the immune system (Donahoe et al, 1986; Watson et al, 1983). If heavy EtOH use is a factor in resistance to HIV, this might be secondary to the malnutrition, liver disease or other factors. On the other hand if EtOH has a direct effect on resistance to HIV infection, this would be expected to manifest during or after any use; even occasional users might be expected to be at increased risk if their consumption occurred during or shortly before or after an activity associated with exposure to HIV.

It is presumed that infection with HIV occurs by attachment of virus budding from the surface of transferred infected cells or free virus to the CD4 molecules on the surfaces of CD4+ lymphocytes, mononuclear phagocytes or other cells (Fauci, 1988; Tschachler et al, 1987; Bagasra, Freund et al, 1988). Latent infection of the cell results from production of a DNA copy of the retrovirus utilizing viral reverse transcriptase and host cell transfer RNA as a primer (Nabel, 1988). Little is known about factors which may influence the likelihood of primary infection, but a variety of co-factors as well as immunologic responses are thought to influence the activation of latent infection - that is, replicative production of complete RNA virus (Mock et al, 1987; Koyanagi et al, 1958, Nabel, 1988). EtOH may be such a co-factor and/or may influence progression of HIV infection by modulating immunologic functions involved in control of such infection (Mock et al, 1987).

Monocytes and CD4+ T lymphocytes are the primary, if not exclusive, targets for HIV in peripheral blood (Fauci, 1988) and the helper/inducer (CD4+) and suppressor (CD8+) subgroups of T lymphocytes are the primary regulators of immunologic responses (Reinertz et al, 1980). We conducted a pilot test of the hypothesis that moderate consumption of alcoholic beverage influences susceptibility of these cells to HIV infection or modulates lymphocyte functions which might be involved in natural resistance to activation of such infection. In our preliminary studies, PBM were isolated from six normal volunteers before and after they drank 30-110 ounces of beer or an equivalent dose of ethanol in other beverages. The PBM were exposed in vitro to HIV-1 without Phytohemagglutinin. Alcohol consumption was associated with a consistent increase in HIV-1 replication in PBM as assessed by indirect syncytium formation after culture for

30 days (Fig. 1; p<.001) and by the levels of

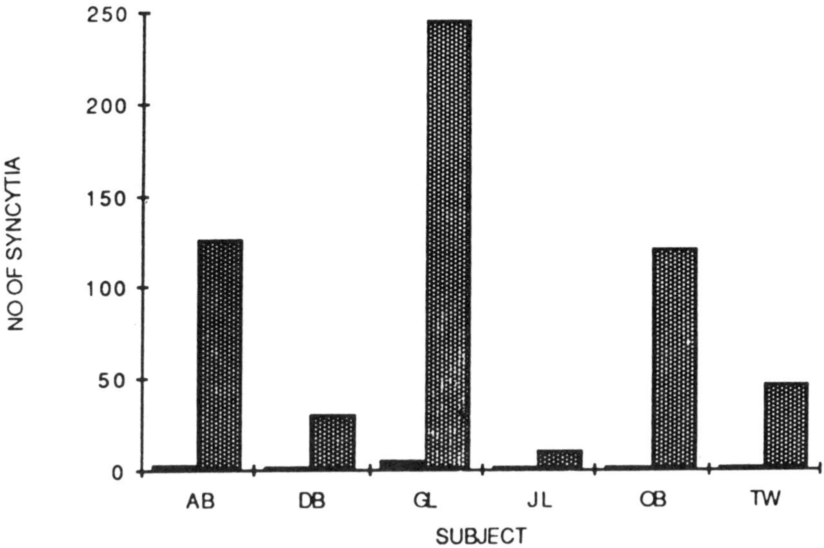

Figure 1. Overnight syncytium formation between SUP-T_1 indicator cells and PBMC pre-cultured 28 days in the presence of IL-2 and 1:3 dilution of 100X HIV concentrate from supernate of 3rd passage H_9/HTLV-IIIB cells. The means of the number of syncytia and syncytial ghose cells observed in 12 wells are shown before and 13-17 h after ingestion of alcoholic beverage. Mean numbers of syncytia and ghosts formed was 1 ± 2 cells/well before and 96 ± 87 cells/well after ETOH intake (p<0.002).

p24 antigen released into the culture supernates (not shown, p<.001). When cultured for 48 hours in the presence of optimal concentrations of Concanavalin A, PBM isolated after alcohol ingestion had decreased ability to secrete interleukin-2 (Fig. 2; $p<.001$) and soluble immune

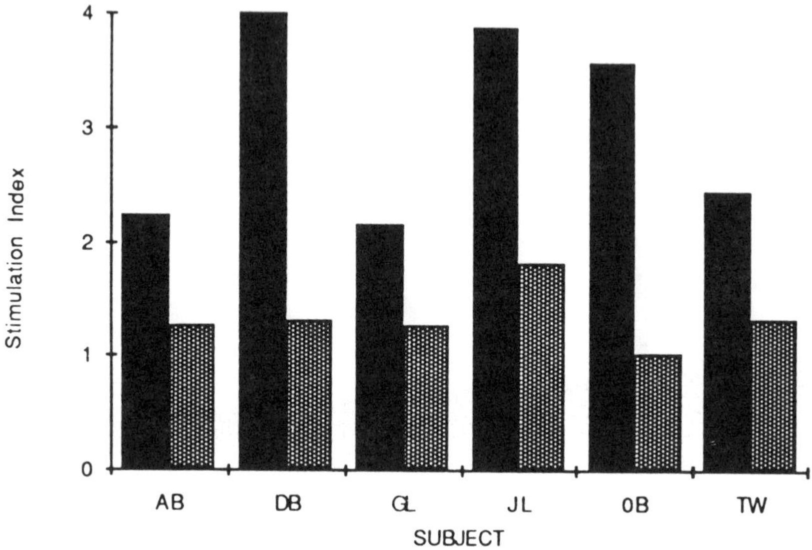

Figure 2. IL-2-like activity in 48 h supernates of Con A-stimulated PBMC. Presumptive IL-2 activity is shown as the stimulation index: [^{3}H]TdR uptake induced in autologous lymphoblasts by the supernates, at 1:4 dilution, divided by that induced by TCM without supernate or IL-2. The stimulation induced by supernates obtained from cultures of PBMC harvested prior to ingestion of alcoholic beverage, is compared to that induced by supernates from cultures of cells drawn 13-17 h after alcohol intake for each subject. The mean stimulation indices for the 6 subjects were 3.1 ± 0.9 and 1.3 ± 0.2, respectively ($p<.003$).

response supressor (Fig. 3; $p<.001$). Synthesis of the

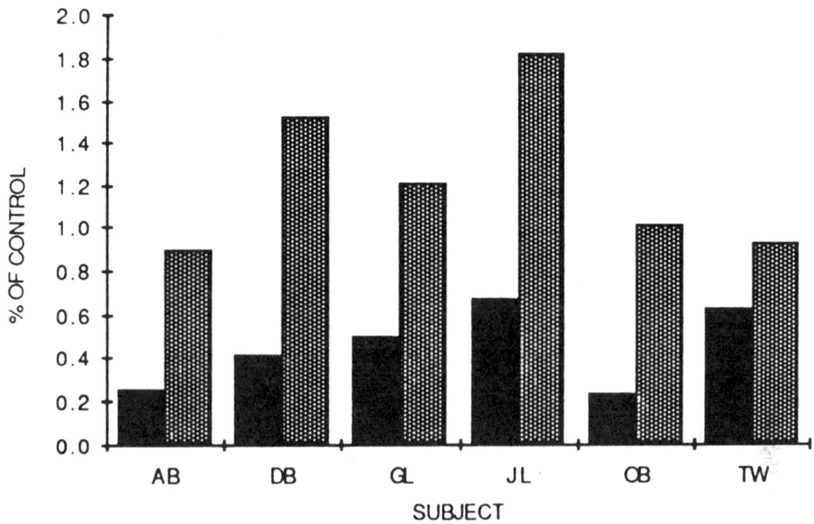

Figure 3. SIRS activity induced by 28 h culture of PBMC with Con A. SIRS activity was measured as the percent of control [^{3}H]TdR incorporation induced by a 1:4 dilution of 28 h supernate from Con A-stimulated PBMC. The indicator cells were fresh autologus PBMC cultured in TCM/2-ME containing 10 μg/ml of Con A. The control wells contained only TCM/2-ME. The test wells contained ¼ part of supernate. In each case, the SIRS activity measured in supernates from cells harvested prior to intake of alcoholic beverage are compared to that from cells harvested 13-17 h after EtOH ingestion. The mean percent of control for the 6 subjects was 45 $\pm$ 19% before and 119 $\pm$ 31% after EtOH ingestion ($p<.001$), the latter indicating no SIRS activity.

latter by CD4+ (T4) and CD8+ (T8) cells, respectively, is also depressed in chronic alcohol abuse. Studies now in progress from PBM of 60 volunteers support our earlier studies. One of the mechanisms of alcohol-associated enhancement of HIV-1 replication seems to be the loss of CD8+ lymphocyte functions due to alcohol or its metabolites (Fig. 4). Role of CD8 cells in resistance

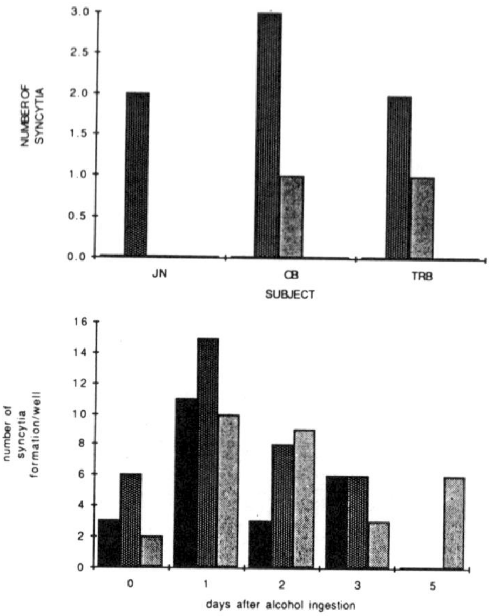

Figure 4. Susceptibility of PBMC to HIV infection followed for 5 days in three volunteers in a separate experiment and role of CD8+ cells were analyzed. Top: infection of PBMC was detected by syncytia formation as in figure 1. No syncytia were detected in any wells prior to alcohol ingestion. Bottom: CD8+ cells were depleted by two cycles of panning. Note significant increase in number of syncytia formed after CD8 depletion.

against HIV in human (Walker et al, 1986) and against SIV in monkeys (Kanngi et al, 1988) have been described.

REFERENCES

Bagasra O, Freund M, Weidmann J, Harley G (1988). Interaction of human immunodeficiency virus with human sperm in vitro. J AIDS 1:431.

Bagasra O, Howeedy A, Kajdacsy-Balla A (1988). Macrophage

function in chronic experimental alcoholism. I. Modulation of surface receptors and phagocytosis. Immunology 65:405.

Bagasra O, Kajdascy-Balla A (1988). Ethanol induced immunomodulation in chronic alcoholism. Clin Immunol Newslet 9:9.

Donahoe RM, Nicholson JKA, Maddem JJ, Donahoe F, Shafer DA, Gordon D, Bokos P, Falek A (1986). Coordinate and independent effects of heroin, cocaine and alcohol abuse on T-cell E-rosette formation and antigenic marker expression. Clin Immunol Immunopathol 41:254.

Fauci AS (1988). The human immunodeficiency virus: Infectivity and mechanisms of pathogenesis. Science 239:617.

Israelstam S, Lambert S (1986). Homosexuality and alcohol: Observations and research after the psychoanalytic era. Intern J Addict 21:509.

Jerrells TR, Marietta CA, Bone G, Weight FF, Eckhardt MJ (1988). Ethanol-associated immunosuppression. In Bridge TP, Mirsky AF, Goodwin FK (eds): "Neuro-psychiatric and Substance Abuse Aspects of AIDS," New York: Raven Press, p 173.

Kannagi M, Chalifour LV, Lord CI, Letrin NL (1988). Suppression of Simian immunodeficiency views in vitro by CD8+ lymphocytes. J Immunol 140:2237.

Koyanagi Y, O'Brien WA, Zhao JQ, Golde DW, Gasson JC, Chen ISY (1988). Cytokines alter production of HIV-1 from primary mononuclear phagocytes. Science 241:1673.

Lake-Bakaar G, Gupta N, Beidas S, Straus EW (1988). Alcohol and the acquired immunodeficiency syndrome in intravenous drug addicts, in Abstracts of 4th International Congress on AIDS, Stockholm, Sweden, p 454.

Mock DJ, Roberts NJ Jr (1987). Proposed immunopathogenic factors associated with progression from human immunodeficiency virus seropositivity to clinical disease. J Clin Microbiol 24:1817.

Nabel GJ (1988). Activation of human immunodeficiency virus. J Lab Clin Med 111:495.

Reinertz EL, Schlossman SF (1980). The function and differentiation of human T cells. Cell 19:821.

Siegel L. (1986). AIDS: Relationship to alcohol and other drugs. J Substance Abuse Treat 3:271.

Stall R, McKusick L, Wiley J, Coates TJ (1986). Alcohol

and drug use during sexual activity and compliance with safe sex guidelines for AIDS: The AIDS behavioral research project. Health Educ Quart 13:359.

Tschachler E, Groh V, Popovic M, Mann DL, Konrad K, Safai B, Eron L, diMarzoVeronese F, Wolff K, Stingl G (1987). Epidermal Langernans cells: A target for HTLV-III/LAV infection. J Invest Dermatol 88:233.

Walker CM, Moody DJ, Stiles DP, Lery JA (1986). CD8+ lymphocytes can control HIV infection in vitro by suppressing virus replication. Science 234:1563.

Watson ES, Murphy JC, Elsohly HN, Elsohly MA, Turner CE. (1983). Effects of the administration of coca alkaloids on the primary immune responses of mice: Interaction with delta-9-tetrahydrocannabinol and ethanol. Toxico Appl Pharmacol 71:1.

Alcohol, Immunomodulation, and AIDS, pages 359–371
© 1990 Alan R. Liss, Inc.

AN ANIMAL MODEL OF IMMUNE RESPONSE ASSOCIATED WITH ALCOHOL-RELATED CANCERS

Siraj I. Mufti

Departments of Pharmacology and Pharmacology and Toxicology, University of Arizona Health Sciences Center, Tucson, Arizona 85724

INTRODUCTION

Alcohol is a major risk factor for cancers in humans. Sites most associated with alcohol-related cancers are mouth, pharynx, larynx, esophagus and liver (for example, Hakulinen et al., 1974; Monson and Lyons, 1975; Jensen, 1979; Tuyns, 1979; Rothman et al., 1980; Doll and Peto, 1981). The association with esophageal cancers is particularly strong and 75% of esophageal cancers in the U.S.A. are attributable to alcohol consumption (Rothman et al., 1980). The subject of alcohol-related cancers has been extensively reviewed by others (for example, Doll and Peto, 1981; NCR, 1982; Lieber et al., 1986) and recently by us (Mufti et al., 1989a,b).

There is good deal of evidence showing that ethanol acts as an immunosuppressive factor. The subject has been discussed in several recent reviews including ours (Zetterman and Sorrell, 1981; Johnson and Williams, 1986; MacGregor, 1986; Watson, 1984,1988; Mufti et al., 1988). A suppression or impairment of immunity would be favorable for increased incidence or severity of malignancy since it would undoubtedly affect the host defense mechanisms that resist pathogenesis or carcinogenesis. For an initial report of the studies discussed here please refer to Mufti et al. (1988, 1989c). Based on the literature reviewed and observations presented, this report offers suggestions for an animal model for the study of cellular immunity in its relation to the development of preneoplastic lesions and tumors.

MATERIALS AND METHODS

Experimental Animals and Their Diet. Male Sprague-Dawley rats weighing 70-120 grams, purchased from Harlan Laboratories (IND), were used for these studies. After arrival, the rats were allowed an adjustment period of 5-7 days and then housed in suspended cages is a room with regulated temperature (23°C) and humidity (30-40%). The animals were maintained and cared for in the facility provided by the Division of Animal Resources, University of Arizona.

Rats were fed a nutritionally balanced isocaloric liquid diet prepared in our laboratory according to the recommendations of American Institute of Nutrition (1977) and Lieber and DeCarli (1982). Ethanol constituted 7% or 1% of diet in gram weight, as indicated. The animals were pair-fed, i.e. the controls were restricted in their feeding so that they received no more diet than their ethanol-fed counterparts.

Rats on carcinogenesis studies were administered ethanol, either (a) only for a period of 12 weeks before and during treatment with the carcinogen, or (b) a week after treatment with the carcinogen was completed and continued receiving ethanol until terminated. Rats in study (a) were maintained on regular laboratory chow diet after the initial 12-week administration of ethanol until their termination. Rats on immunological studies were not treated with any carcinogen but were administered ethanol after the initial adjustment period until their termination at 12 weeks or 13 months of ethanol feeding, as indicated.

Carcinogenesis Studies. Rats on a preliminary study of the effect of ethanol on preneoplastic lesions were treated with methylbenzylnitrosamine (NMB_zA), purchased from Ash Stevens (Chicago, ILL), at a dose of 2.5 mg/kg, i.p., twice a week for 3 weeks. Following this study the dose was readjusted for tumor studies and the animals were treated with NMB_zA at a dose of 2.5 mg/kg three times a week for 3 weeks. The animals were killed by cervical dislocation at 30 weeks for the study of preneoplastic lesions or at 20 months of age for tumor studies and their esophagi carefully excised. The esophagi were visually examined initially and confirmed under a dissecting microscope for the presence of nodules and tumors as described by Van Rensburg (1981) and Van Rensburg and his colleagues (1985). All lesions $>$ 0.5 mm were counted. The lesions were subsequently confirmed by a histological examination.

Immunological Studies. The body and tissue weights of rats terminated after 12 weeks of 1% or 7% ethanol feeding were recorded. Alveolar macrophages (AM) were collected from these rats by tracheopulmonary lavage. The viability of cells was determined by staining with trypan blue. The AM collected from lavaged fluid were layered on multi-well plates. The nonadherent cells, removed by washing with HBBS, were incubated in RPMI-1640 containing fetal bovine serum, then opsonized sheep red blood cells (SRBC) labeled with 200 uCi $Na_2\,^{51}CrO_4$ were added to them and incubated for 24 hr at 37°C. The culture, lysed with 1 N NaOH, was measured for radioactivity and the difference in counts of the target cells in the presence of AM determined.

Spleens of rats that received 7% ethanol for 13 months were excised, cut into half and passed through an 80-mesh stainless-steel sieve into RPMI-1640 medium. The cells obtained after filtration were centrifuged and resuspended in a lysing buffer consisting of 154 mM ammonium chloride, 10 mM potassium bicarbonate and 0.1 mM tetrasodium EDTA to separate splenocytes. The cells were washed and resuspended in the RPMI-1640 medium and then counted for total cells. Subpopulations of lymphocytes were characterized from these cells by binding to the rat antibodies, i.e. T-w3/13, H-w3/25 and S-ox8 (Sera Laboratories, Westbury, NY) as total T-lymphocytes, T-helper and T-suppressor lymphocytes respectively. The unbound cells were removed and the bound cells were incubated for 30 min with fluorescent- labeled goat anti-rat immunoglobins and the stained cells analyzed in an EPICS flow cytometer.

RESULTS

1. Effect of ethanol on carcinogenesis.

The aim of these studies was to determine the effects of ethanol on initiation or promotion of carcinogenesis.

Therefore, ethanol was either administered for a period of 12 weeks before and during treatment with methylbenzylnitrosamine (NMB_zA), the esophagus specific carcinogen, to determine the effect of ethanol on initiation of carcinogenesis; or alternatively, ethanol was administered a week after treatment with NMB_zA to determine the effect of ethanol on promotion of carcinogenesis. Preliminary experiments terminated at 30 weeks for a study of preneoplastic lesions showed that 13 out of a total of 27 or 48% of animals that received ethanol had nodules compared to 4 out of 12 or 33% of the controls. A typical preneoplastic nodule had a thickened epithelium with a hyperplastic basal cell layer (Mufti et al., 1989c). However, since a low dose of NMB_zA (2.5 mg/kg, 2 times a week for 3 weeks) was used, it resulted in nonparametric distribution and differences in the two incidences were not significant. It is, therefore, important to repeat this experiment with a higher dose of nitrosamine in order that the effect of ethanol on incidence of preneoplastic lesions could be ascertained.

Table 1. Effect of Ethanol on Promotion of NMB_zA-induced Esophageal Lesions

Treatment	# of rats	Lesions/rat (mean ± SE)	Size (mm)/ lesion (mean ± SE)	# of rats with nodules only	# of rats with nodules and tumors
Ethanol	75	8.75 ± 1.07	1.02 ± 0.09	61	14
Control	32	10.94 ± 1.49	1.32 ± 0.13	31	1

For experimental details, see text. Differences between ethanol and control treatments are significant at $P < 0.05$.

The above experiment was followed by a adjustment of NMB_zA dose (2.5 mg/kg, 3 times a week for 3 weeks) for long term studies. Experiments were then terminated at 20 months of age and the incidence of persistent nodules and tumors determined. From the results presented in Table I it appears that when ethanol was used as a promoter of carcinogenesis, it neither enhanced the mean frequency nor the mean size of esophageal lesions. Rather, such a treatment, it appears, caused an atrophy of persistent nodules. However, the number of lesions that developed into tumors were markedly increased with ethanol consumption, tumors were characterized by gross morphological abnormalities, i.e. a 3-dimensional structure associated with histological abnormalities including extensive hyperplasia and proliferation of basal cells into the lumen of the esophagus (Mufti et al., 1989c). Fourteen of 75 ethanol-receiving had tumors while only one out of 32 of control animals had a small tumor. Moreover, two of the ethanol-consuming animals had multiple (two and four) tumors. Therefore, while ethanol administered as a tumor promoter caused an atrophy of persistent nodules, it enhanced the number of tumors that developed from persistent nodules.

Table 2 Effect of Ethanol Administered Before and During Initiation of NMB_zA-induced Esophageal Lesions.

Treatment	# of rats	Lesions/rat (mean ± SE)	Size (mm)/ lesion (mean ± SE)	# of rats with nodules only	# of rats with nodules & tumors
Ethanol	13	8.04 ± 3.04	1.44 ± 0.27	10	3
Control	26	12.41 ± 2.12	0.92 ± 0.17	16	10

For experimental details, see text. Differences between ethanol and control treatments are significant at $P < 0.05$.

The results of the effect of ethanol on initiation of carcinogenesis are presented in Table 2. Here rats were administered ethanol for a period of 12 weeks only, before and during treatment with NMB_zA. The data show that this treatment significantly decreased the mean frequency of esophageal lesions. Furthermore, although the mean size of lesions was somewhat increased, the number of lesions that developed into tumors were significantly decreased. While 10 out of 26 control rats had tumors, only 3 out of 13 ethanol-fed rats had tumors. Therefore, ethanol administered before and during initiation significantly inhibited incidence of persistent nodules as well as significantly inhibited development of the nodules into tumors.

We would like to note another observation in the data given in Tables 1 and 2. It appears that with the administration of defined liquid diet, the incidence of tumors was relatively low in the rats that were fed control diet (Table 1). On the other hand, the incidence of tumors in rats that were fed regular laboratory chow (after treatment with the carcinogen) was relatively high (Table 2). Apparently, ingredients in the chow diet acted to enhance the tumor incidence.

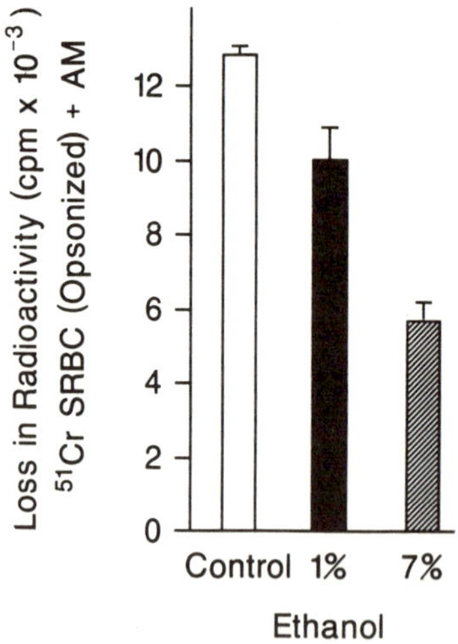

Fig. 1. Effect of ethanol on phagocytosis by alveolar macrophages (AM) isolated from Sprague-Dawley rats. The AM (concentration 2.8-3.2 x 10^6) were collected and treated with ^{51}Cr-labeled SRBC as described in text. The loss in radioactivity was calculated from the difference in c.p.m. counts in the presence of AM.

2. Effect of ethanol on cellular immunity.

Body and organ weights of rats fed 1% or 7% ethanol were determined after 12 weeks. While ethanol did not significantly affect body, liver and spleen weights (data not shown), the weight of thymus was significantly decreased. The thymus from control-fed rats weighed 0.40 ± 0.07 grams, and the thymus from 1% and 7% ethanol-fed rats weighed 0.28 ± 0.03 and 0.27 ± 0.08 grams respectively ($P < 0.05$, n = 5). Alveolar macrophages were isolated from these rats and their activity determined by their ability to release radioactivity from ^{51}Cr-labeled SRBC. The data presented in Fig. 1 show that there was a significant decrease in loss of radioactivity from the target cells when macrophages from the ethanol-fed rats were used. Furthermore, the loss in phagocytic activity was proportional to the concentration of ethanol in the diet.

Splenocytes were isolated from rats that were fed 7% ethanol for 13 months and number of cells counted. There were $115.6 \pm 34 \times 10^6$ cells in spleen of rats fed control-diet, the number of such cells decreased to $60.6 \pm 11 \times 10^6$ cells in ethanol-fed rats and the differences were significant ($p < 0.05$, n = 4). Therefore chronic ethanol consumption caused a significant decrease in number of cells in this lymphoid tissue.

DISCUSSION

Since ethanol by itself is not carcinogenic, the increase in cancer incidence observed with alcohol consumption must be explained in terms of ethanol modifying of the effect of other carcinogens that frequent human environment, e.g. nitrosamines in tobacco. Therefore, ethanol may either influence the initiation stage of carcinogenesis or alternatively ethanol may act as a tumor promoter, thus exacerbating the effect of initiating carcinogen(s). The results discussed above show that when ethanol was administered before and during initiation, it inhibited incidence of persistent nodules and development of tumors. An explanation for this observation is provided in that ethanol acts as a competitive inhibitor of the microsomal demethylase enzyme that is involved in the metabolism and activation of nitrosamines (Phillips et al., 1977). Ethanol, in our studies, was found to enhance tumor incidence remarkably but only when it was administered as a tumor promoter after initiation by the carcinogen was completed. For a detailed discussion of the effect of ethanol on initiation and promotion of carcinogenesis, please refer to Mufti et al. (1989b,c). A significant observation of these studies was that ethanol appears to act during the long progression stage by increasing tumors that developed from persistent nodules. This order of events is in accord with the suggestion that immunosuppression induced by ethanol may have a role in enhancing cancer incidence.

Details of ethanol causing immunosuppression are provided in several recent reviews (Zetterman and Sorrell, 1981; Johnson and Williams, 1986; MacGregor, 1986; Watson, 1984, 1988; Mufti et al., 1988, 1989a) which summarize how ethanol-induced immunosuppression could increase incidence of oral/esophageal and other cancers. These reviews indicate that high, prolonged ethanol consumption in man is associated with suppression of important cellular immune functions. Studies discussed above indicate that ethanol intake reduced the weight of lymphoids and numbers of lymphocytes in rodents. Our other in vitro studies on human lymphocytes discussed by Mufti et al (1988) show that a higher than 0.1% concentration of ethanol and acetaldehyde and acetate, the metabolites of ethanol, caused a decrease in the formation of lymphocyte rosettes with sheep erythrocytes. This indicates an impaired functioning of lymphocytes. Studies discussed here have shown that ethanol intake also impairs functioning of macrophages.

Understandably, a proper functioning of different immune components is critical in providing the body with a surveillance system against pathogenesis/ carcinogenesis. Ever since Burnett (1971) proposed a role for immune surveillance, a number of studies have provided such evidence. For example, there is a 100-fold increase in cancer incidence rate in patients with a primary immunodeficiency disease compared to the general population (Gatti and Good, 1971; Kersey et al., 1973). Similarly, patients who are iatrogenically immunosuppressed, for example, to inhibit graft rejection in transplantation, have markedly increased risk of developing malignancy (Penn and Starzl, 1972). Although, there is general agreement that immune system is involved in the development of malignancy, it is not clear whether neoplasia is due to a lack of immune recognition mechanism or is due to a failure in immune response (Klein, 1976).

Since cancer, in general, is an age-associated phenomenon, it has been hypothesized that cancers are due in part to an impaired immune response or an immune dysfunction (Mufti et al., 1989a).

In addition, existing evidence supports the concept that functioning of lymphoid cells is involved in offering resistance to cancer. Experimental and clinical studies have shown that NK cells may play an important role in resistance to development of tumors in vivo since they possess the capacity to spontaneously lyse neoplastic cells. Defective NK activity has been described in various dermatological diseases including cancer (Reinhold et al., 1988). Similarly Azizi et al. (1987) suggested that basal cell carcinoma may arise through perturbations in structure or activity of epidermal Langerhan cells.

Nitrosamine

± ETHANOL

0 1 month 5 10 15 20 months

Figure 2. Animal Model of Immune Response Associated With Alcohol-Related Cancers. Rats are treated with a nitrosamine starting at time 0 (NMB$_Z$A at a dose of 2-5mg/kg 3 times a week for 3 weeks). Ethanol is administered one week later and continued until experiment terminated at 5, 10, 15 and 20 months.

Determinations

1. Incidence of preneoplastic lesions, persistent nodules and tumors.
2. Immunological assays. Samples from peripheral blood, peritoneal and lung lavage, lymphoid organs (spleen, liver and thymus*) and target tissue(s) analyzed for numbers and functions of T-lymphocytes and their subpopulations, monocytes/macrophages and natural killer cells.
3. Incidence of preneoplastic lesions, persistent nodules and tumors correlated with immune response.

*Thymus will be analyzed only at 5 month time-point because at later times it gets atrophied especially with chronic ethanol ingestion.

Based on the above observations, we suggest an animal model presented in Figure 2 to determine the effect of ethanol-induced immunosuppression on development of cancers. Such a system would use an organ specific carcinogen to initiate carcinogenesis. Since nitrosamines could induce tumors at sites relevant to alcohol use, these compounds could be usefully employed. A low dose of nitrosamine should be used that induces tumors in about 25-30% of animals in order that contribution of ethanol to the carcinogen-induced tumors could be determined. Dose finding studies described by Mufti et al. (1989c) show that both the dose and duration of treatment with the carcinogen are important for initiation of carcinogenesis. The model animal would receive ethanol administered as a tumor promoter after treatment with the carcinogen has been completed. Use of nutritionally balanced isocaloric liquid diet would be preferable. Our data indicates that a nutritionally balanced defined diet provides a better feeding regimen compared to regular chow diet since, apparently, ingredients in chow diet may act to increase tumor incidence. However, a liquid diet could be easily contaminated and serve equally well to nourish bacteria, fungi and other organisms. Cleanliness in preparation of diet and its feeding is, therefore, of utmost importance which should be combined with frequent sterilization or autoclaving of diet bottles and feeding tubes. For long term feeding, we also suggest a lowering of ethanol content to 5-6% for rats with a corresponding increase in dextrin maltose. This would ensure adequate health and body weight of animals for long term studies; a recommendation that is consistent with the suggestions of Rao et al (1987). Ethanol administration would then continue until the termination of experiment. Preliminary studies described above also indicate that in addition to persistent nodules and tumors, ethanol may effect incidence of preneoplastic lesions. Therefore, the study would determine the effect of increasing durations of ethanol consumption on immune resistance and the response of different immunity parameters would then be correlated with the incidence of preneoplastic lesions, persistent nodules and tumors. The course of immune response may have significant implications for the development of carcinogenesis, in determining the length of latency period or in an increased incidence of tumors and/or severity of malignancy.

Acknowledgments. Work described in this paper was partially supported by a grant (No. 03438) from the National Institute of Environmental Health Sciences and consultations by R.R. Watson from grant AA08037.

REFERENCES

American Institute of Nutrition (1977). Report of the American Institute of Nutrition Ad Hoc Committee on standards for nutritional studies. J Nutr 107:1340-1348.

Azizi E, Bucana C, Goldberg L, Kripke ML (1987). Perturbation of epidermal Langerhan cells in basal cell carcinomas. Am J Dermatopathol 9:465-473.

Burnett FM (1971). Immunological surveillance in neoplasia. Transplant Rev 7:3-25.

Doll R, Peto R (1981). The causes of cancer: quantitative estimates of avoidable risks of cancer in the United States today. J Natl Cancer Inst 66:1191-1308.

Gatti RA, Good RA (1971). Occurrence of malignancy in immune-deficiency diseases. Cancer 28:89-98.

Hakulinen T, Lehtimaki L, Lehtonen M, Teppo L (1974). Cancer morbidity among two male cohorts with increased alcohol consumption in Finland. J Natl Cancer Inst 52:1711-1714.

Kersey JH, Spector BD, Good RA (1973). Primary immunodeficiency diseases and cancer: the immunodeficiency-cancer registry. Int J Cancer 12:333-347.

Klein G (1976). Tumor immunology: a general appraisal. In Symington T, Carter RL (eds): "Scientific Foundation of Oncology," London: W Heinemann, pp 497-504.

Jensen OM (1979). Cancer morbidity and causes of death among Danish brewery workers. Int J Cancer 23:454-463.

Johnson RD, Williams R (1986). Immune responses in alcoholic liver disease. Alcohol Clin Exp Res 10:471-1479.

Lieber CS, DeCarli LM (1982). The feeding of alcohol in liquid diets: two decades of applications and 1982 update. Alcohol Clin Exp Res 6:523-531.

MacGregor RR (1986). Alcohol and immune defense. J Am Med Assoc 256:1474-1479.

Monson RR, Lyons JL (1975). Proportional mortality among alcoholics. Cancer 36:1077-1079.

Mufti SI, Prabhala R, Moriguchi S, Sipes IG, Watson RR (1988). Functional and numerical alterations induced by ethanol in the cellular immune system. Immunopharmacology 15:85-94.
Mufti SI, Darban HR, Watson RR (1989a). Alcohol, cancer, and immunomodulation. CRC Critical Rev Hematol Oncol, in press.
Mufti SI, Garewal HS, Watson RR (1989b). Role of environment, drugs of abuse, and nutritional factors in the etiology and prevention of cancers of oral cavity and esophagus. In Watson RR (ed): "Focus on Biochemistry and Physiology of Substance Abuse," Boca Raton FL: CRC Press, in press.
Mufti SI, Becker G, Sipes IG (1989c). Effect of chronic dietary ethanol consumption on the initiation and promotion of chemically-induced esophageal carcinogenesis in experimental rats. Carcinogenesis 10:303-309.
National Research Council (1982). Diet, Nutrition and Cancer. The Committee on Diet, Nutrition and Cancer, Assembly of Life Sciences, National Academy Press, Washington, DC.
Penn I, Starzl TE (1972). Malignant tumors arising de novo in immunodeficiency transplant recipients. Transplantation 14:407-417.
Phillips JC, Lake BG, Gangolli SD, Grasso P, Lloyd AG (1977). Effects of pyrazole and 3-amino-a,2,4-triazole on the metabolism and toxicity of dimethylnitrosamine in the rat. J Natl Cancer Inst 58:629-633.
Rao GA, Riley DE, Larkin EC (1987). Dietary carbohydrate stimulates alcohol diet ingestion, promotes growth and prevents fatty liver in rats. Nutr Res 7:81-87.
Reinhold U, Bauer R (1988). Eine Klinisch-immunologische Analyseuber deto Stellenwert naturlicher. Killerzellen bei dermato logischen Krankheiten. 39:129-135.
Rothman K, Garfinkel L, Keller AZ, Muir CS, Schottenfeld D (1980). The proportional of cancer attributable to alcohol consumption. Prev Med 9:174-179.
Tuyns AJ (1979). Epidemiology of alcohol and cancer. Cancer Res 39:2840-2843.
Van Rensburg SJ (1981). Advances in experimental cancer of the esophagus. S Afr Cancer Bull 25:66-76.

Van Rensburg SJ, Hall JM, Bruyn DuB (1985). Effect of various dietary staples on esophageal carcinogenesis induced in rats by subcutaneously administered N-nitrosomethylbenzylamine. J Natl Cancer Inst 75:561-566.

Watson RR (1984). Alcohol and immune functions. In Watson RR (ed): "Nutrition, Disease Resistance, and Immune Function," New York: M. Dekker, pp. 313-329.

Watson RR (1988). "Diagnosis of Alcohol Abuse," Boca Raton FL: CRC Press, in press.

Zetterman RK, Sorrell MF (1981). Immunologic aspects of alcoholic liver disease. Gastroenterology 81:616-624.

Alcohol, Immunomodulation, and AIDS, pages 373–382
© 1990 Alan R. Liss, Inc.

CHRONIC ALCOHOL CONSUMPTION PREVENTS THE SEPSIS-INDUCED INCREASES IN GLUCONEOGENESIS AND METABOLIC CLEARANCE RATE

Charles H. Lang, Patricia E. Molina,
Gregory J. Bagby and John J. Spitzer
Department of Physiology, Louisiana State University Medical Center, New Orleans, LA 70112

INTRODUCTION

An increased susceptibility to infections is one of the many complications of chronic alcohol abuse (Adams and Jordan, 1984; Louria, 1963). The mechanisms that predispose alcoholics to infection are not fully understood, but are undoubtedly due in part to the various metabolic alterations produced by the oxidation of ethanol. Previous studies have indicated that the shift in the hepatic redox potential to a more reduced state alters a number of NAD-dependent metabolic pathways (Lieber, 1982). One of the important effects of ethanol on hepatic carbohydrate metabolism is a shift in intracellular lactate flux away from gluconeogenesis and towards lactate release. Under conditions were the body's glycogen reserves are limited (i.e. prolonged fasting or malnutrition), the inhibition of de novo glucose synthesis may produce a marked hypoglycemia (Krebs et al, 1969). Similarly, ethanol may be expected to severely alter glucose homeostasis in any condition that has an increased reliance upon gluconeogenesis to meet peripheral demands for glucose.

Among the characteristic effects of sepsis in man and experimental animals are the increased rates of glucose appearance (Ra), glucose disappearance (Rd) and metabolic clearance (MCR). We previously demonstrated that the sepsis-induced increase in glucose Ra is predominantly due to an enhanced rate of gluconeogenesis (Lang et al, 1984). This increased glucose production during sepsis appears necessary to support the elevated energy demands of tissues rich in macrophages, such as the liver, spleen, lungs and skin (Meszaros et al, 1988). Since the optimal functioning of these tissues is dependent on a constant supply of glucose (Filkins and Kober, 1980), any condition or agent that interferes with glucose homeostasis is likely to impair the function of the reticulo-endothelial system and may increase morbidity and mortality.

Since alcoholics are predisposed to various types of infections, the purpose of our study was to determine whether chronic alcohol ingestion would prevent the sepsis-induced changes in carbohydrate metabolism. A significant attenuation of the characteristic changes in glucose flux induced by sepsis, could be a causal factor in eliciting the increased sensitivity to infection in these patients. In our present study in vivo glucose metabolism was studied in rats chronically fed ethanol, and in pair-fed control animals, with and without the induction of gram-negative sepsis.

MODEL OF CHRONIC ALCOHOLISM

Animals were maintained on a nutritionally adequate liquid diet (Sustacal, Mead Johnson) as the sole source of calories and fluid. This diet provided 36% of the total calories as ethanol, and was appropriately diluted with water to provide a final concentration of 1 calorie/ml. Pair-fed control animals received Sustacal in which the ethanol was isocalorically replaced with dextrin. Animals were maintained on this diet for a period of 5 weeks. Table 1 illustrates that over the 5 wk period alcoholic and nonalcoholic rats had similar caloric consumptions and weight gains. The daily alcohol consumption by the experimental animals was 16 $\pm$ 1 g ETOH/kg. These data are consistent with results obtained previously by other investigators using different types of liquid diets containing alcohol (Lieber and DeCarli, 1982). Animals maintained on this long term ethanol diet will be refered to as "chronic alcoholic."

Table 1. Food Consumption and Weight Gain of Rats Maintained on the Liquid Diet

	Alcoholic	Nonalcoholic
Initial Weight, g	220 ± 2	214 ± 2
Weight Gain, g/day	2.8 ± .2	3.2 ± .1
Diet Consumption, ml/day	85 ± 3	80 ± 1
Total Caloric Consumption cal/kg/day	265 ± 10	247 ± 3
Alcohol Intake, g/kg/day	16 ± 1	0

Values are means ± S.E.M. N = 24 for each group.

INDUCTION OF GRAM-NEGATIVE SEPSIS

After 5 weeks on the liquid diet, hypermetabolic sepsis was induced as described previously by our laboratory (Lang et al, 1984). Briefly, under anesthesia a small catheter (PE 50) was inserted down a subcutaneous tunnel on the dorsal surface of the animal for the subsequent injection of live Escherichia coli. Animals were administered E. coli (2-7 x 10^{10} CFUs/ml; E11775 ATCC) at 1200 and 1700 h on the first day, and at 0700 h on the second day. Time-matched control animals received an equal volume of saline. This regime has previously been shown to produce a hypermetabolic model of sepsis that is hemodynamically and metabolically stable.

When the subcutaneous catheter was implanted additional catheters were placed in the carotid artery and jugular vein using aseptic surgical techniques. Within 1 h of the final injection of bacteria, a tracer amount of [6-^{3}H] glucose (10 uCi/h) was infused into the venous catheter for the determination of in vivo glucose kinetics (Wolfe, 1984). The arterial catheter was used to collect blood for the determination of glucose and lactate concentrations, and glucose specific activity.

Because rats do not typically eat or drink for at least 24 h after surgery, and in order to prevent alcohol withdrawal, an intraperitoneal (IP) injection of ethanol (4 g/kg, 20% v/v) was administered at 1800 h on the day of surgery to the chronic alcoholic rats. Nonalcoholic animals received an equal volume (7-8 ml) of saline.

ALTERATIONS IN GLUCOSE METABOLISM

Gram-negative sepsis induced characteristic changes in whole body glucose metabolism in nonalcoholic rats consuming the liquid diet that were similar to those previously reported in rats provided solid rodent chow (Lang et al, 1984). The nonalcoholic septic animals tended to have lower blood glucose values than their time-matched nonseptic controls, but this change was not statistically significant (Fig. 1). However, sepsis did increase glucose Ra by 53%, compared to nonalcoholic nonseptic animals (Fig. 2). Under these experimental conditions where fasting has essentially eliminated glucose absorption from the gut and hepatic glycogenolysis as contributors to glucose output, the [^{3}H]-glucose determined rate of glucose production provides a reliable estimate of the rate of hepatic gluconeogenesis (Wolfe, 1984). Because these animals are in a metabolic steady-state, the rate of glucose disappearance or utilization was also proportionally increased. Likewise, the MCR for glucose was elevated by 94% in septic nonalcoholic animals (Fig. 3). This enhanced rate of glucose clearance indicates that the tissues in these animals have an increased ability to remove glucose at the same prevailing plasma glucose

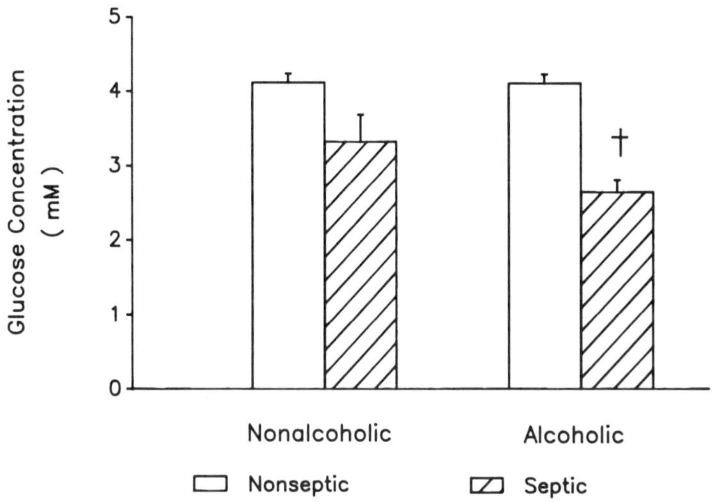

Figure 1. Plasma glucose concentration in alcoholic and nonalcoholic rats approximately 24 h after the induction of gram-negative sepsis. Values are means ± SEM. N = 7-15. †p<0.05 compared to time-matched nonseptic alcoholic animals.

concentration. The sepsis-induced increase in MCR does not appear to be associated with a corresponding increase in the plasma insulin concentration (Table 2). This septic insult was relatively mild, and while it did tend to increase the plasma lactate concentration this change was not statistically significant (Fig. 4).

The chronic consumption of ethanol by itself did not alter the plasma glucose concentration compared to nonalcoholic nonseptic rats (Fig. 1). However, alcohol feeding did reduce the rate of glucose production by 26%, without significantly altering the MCR. It is noteworthy that glucose Ra fell in these animals despite the nearly 7-fold increase in plasma glucagon levels (Table 2) which would be expected to maintain gluconeogenesis. Ethanol also produced a mild hyperlactacidemia, elevating plasma lactate levels by 260% (Fig. 4). The alcohol-induced increase in plasma lactate concentrations and the suppression of hepatic

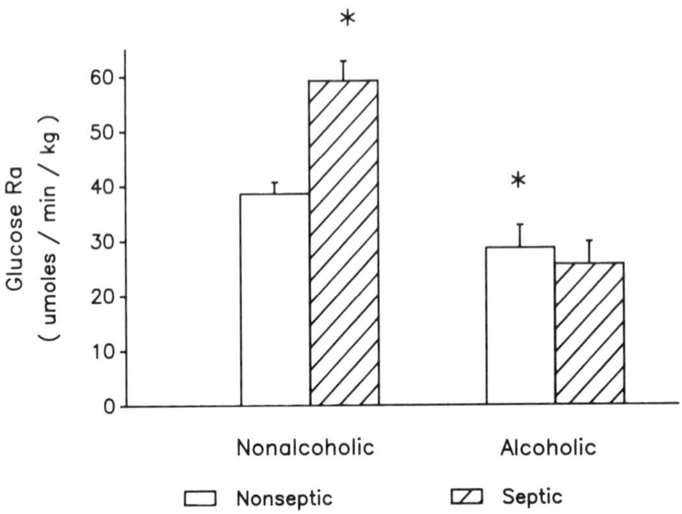

Figure 2. The rate of glucose appearance (Ra) in alcoholic and nonalcoholic rats approximately 24 h after the induction of sepsis. Values are means ± SEM. N = 7-15. *$p<0.05$ compared to time-matched nonseptic nonalcoholic animals.

glucose production have been reported previously in nonseptic subjects (Madison et al, 1967). These alterations have been attributed to the inhibition of lactate utilization that results from an increased cytosolic $NADH/NAD^+$ ratio in the liver following ethanol oxidation (Lieber, 1982).

Sepsis had a markedly different effect on carbohydrate metabolism in animals maintained on the alcohol-containing diet for 5 weeks, compared to pair-fed nonalcoholic animals. The blood glucose concentration was 36% lower in alcoholic animals that were septic versus the alcoholic nonseptic animals (Fig. 1). Furthermore, the characteristic sepsis-induced increases in glucose Ra and MCR that were observed in the nonalcoholic rats were absent in alcoholic animals (Figures 2 and 3). Sepsis did not produce an additional increase in plasma lactate

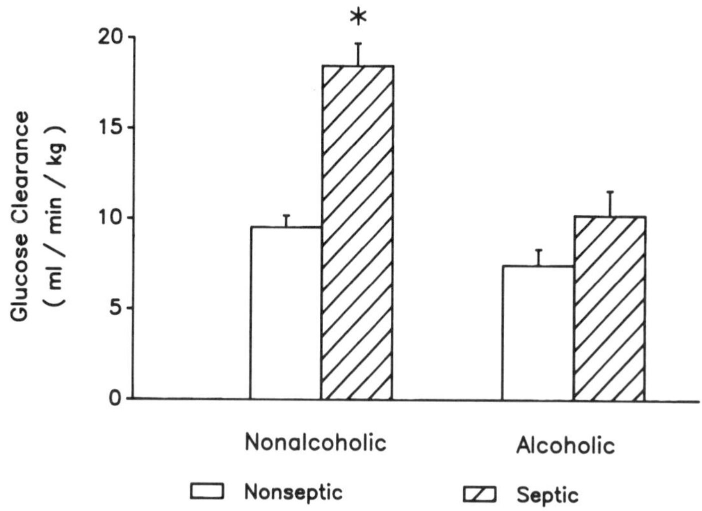

Figure 3. The glucose metabolic clearance rate (MCR) in alcoholic and nonalcoholic rats approximately 24 h after induction of sepsis. Values are means ± SEM. N = 7-15. *$p<0.05$ compared to time-matched nonseptic nonalcoholic animals.

concentration in alcoholic rats over that produced by alcohol alone (Fig. 4). The prevention of the sepsis-induced increase in glucose Ra by chronic alcohol is consistent with an impaired ability of the liver to utilize lactate as a gluconeogenic precursor, even at elevated prevailing lactate concentrations. These data are supported by our previous work in which a sustained infusion of ethanol decreased the rate of glucose recycling in endotoxic rats (unpublished data). These animals may also be resistant to the actions of glucagon, since the dramatic elevation in this glucoregulatory hormone in septic alcoholic rats (Table 2) would be expected to enhance hepatic glucose output. The attenuation of the sepsis-induced increase in MCR was not a result of a decrease in the plasma insulin concentration (Table 2), but might be due to the development of peripheral insulin resistance or the inhibition of insulin-like substances reported to be present in the circulation during sepsis (Filkins and Kober, 1980).

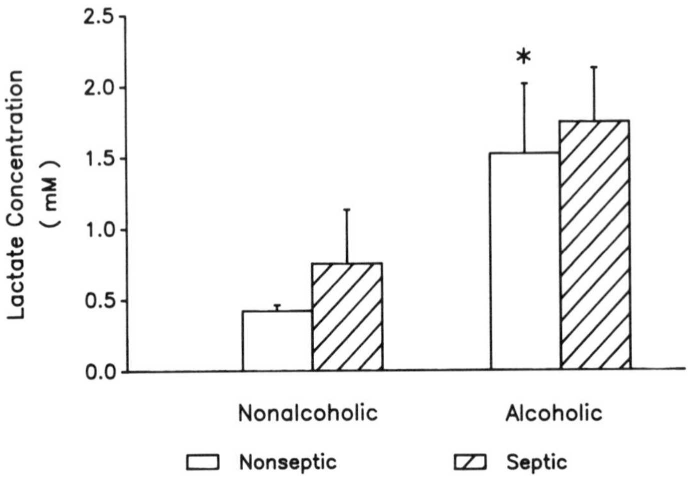

Figure 4. Plasma lactate concentration in alcoholic and nonalcoholic rats approximately 24 h after induction of sepsis. Values are means ± SEM. N = 7-15. *p<0.05 compared to time-matched nonseptic nonalcoholic animals.

The IP injection of ethanol lowered rectal temperature between 3-4°C in both septic and nonseptic animals. We have previously demonstrated that anesthesia-induced hypothermia of a more severe nature decreases glucose Ra (Lang et al, 1987) and, therefore, this alcohol-induced drop in body temperature may be partially responsible for the inhibition of gluconeogenesis seen in nonseptic alcoholic rats. However, in our previous work, hypothermic animals were still capable of increasing glucose output when challenged with epinephrine. This suggests that the inability of septic alcoholic animals to increase glucose production in the present study was an ethanol effect and was not due to the reduced body temperature.

Table 2. The Influence of Chronic Ethanol Feeding on the Sepsis-Induced Changes in Plasma Hormone Concentrations.

	Insulin, uU/ml	Glucagon, pg/ml
Non Alcoholic-Non Septic	22 ± 4	116 ± 5
Non Alcoholic-Septic	15 ± 4	655 ± 111
Alcoholic-Non Septic	38 ± 5	910 ± 288
Alcoholic-Septic	26 ± 4	1374 ± 255*

Values are means ± S.E. N = 4, 7, 5 and 8 for the four treatment groups, respectively. *$p<0.05$ compared to time-matched nonalcoholic-nonseptic animals.

CONCLUSIONS

It is well established that during the hypermetabolic phase of infection the peripheral tissues have an increased demand for metabolic substrates (Meszaros et al, 1988). Although mobilization of free fatty acids from lipid stores assumes increasing importance in meeting these energy needs, an adequate supply of glucose is also necessary for the normal functioning of various tissues. Macrophages are one such cell population whose function has been shown to be impaired by derrangements in glucose homeostasis (Filkins et al, 1980). Under nonalcoholic conditions, we have shown that sepsis increases the hepatic production of glucose to meet the increased demand by peripheral tissues. However, in alcoholic animals this enhanced rate of gluconeogenesis is absent. Therefore, alcohol may decrease the availability of glucose to immunological tissues, thereby compromising host defense against bacterial infection.

ACKNOWLEDGEMENTS

This work was supported by NIAAA Grant AA07287.

REFERENCES

Adams HG, Jordan C (1984). Infections in the alcoholic. Med Clin N Am 68:179-200.

Filkins JP, Kober PM (1980). Interrelations of RES endocytic and exocytic functions with glucose homeostasis in the pathogenesis of endotoxin shock. Adv Physiol Sci 26:171-180.

Krebs HA, Freedland RA. Hems R, Stubbs M (1969). Inhibition of hepatic gluconeogenesis by ethanol. Biochem J 112:117-124, 1969.

Lang CH, Bagby, GJ, Spitzer JJ (1984). Carbohydrate dynamics in the hypermetabolic septic rat. Metabolism 33:959-963.

Lang CH, Bagby GJ, Hargrove DM, Hyde PM, Spitzer JJ (1987). Alterations in glucose kinetics induced by pentobarbital anesthesia. Am J Physiol 253:E657-E663.

Lang CH, Bagby GJ, Spitzer JJ (1984). Carbohydrate dynamics in hypermetabolic septic rat. Metabolism 33:959-963.

Lieber CS, DeCarli LM (1982). The feeding of alcohol in liquid diets: Two decades of applications and 1982 update. Alcoholism: Clin Exper Res 6:523-531.

Lieber CS (1982). Metabolism of ethanol. Alcoholism: Clin Exper Res 22:1-42.

Lochner A, Wulff J, Madison LL (1967). Ethanol-induced hypoglycemia I. The acute effects of ethanol on hepatic glucose output and peripheral glucose utilization in fasted dogs. Metabolism 16:1-18.

Louria DB (1963). Susceptibility to infection during experimental alcohol intoxication. Trans Ass Am Physns 76:102.

Meszaros K, Lang CH, Bagby GJ, Spitzer JJ (1988). In vivo glucose utilization by individual tissues during nonlethal hypermetabolic sepsis. FASEB J 2:3083-3086.

Wolfe RR (1984). Tracers in metabolic research radioisotope and stable isotope/mass spectrometry methods. Alan R. Liss, Inc., New York.

Alcohol, Immunomodulation, and AIDS, pages 383–391
© 1990 Alan R. Liss, Inc.

ETHANOL AND SURVIVAL OF MYCOBACTERIUM AVIUM COMPLEX WITHIN MACROPHAGES

Luiz E. Bermudez, Lowell S. Young

Kuzell Institute for Arthritis and Infectious Diseases. Medical Research Institute of San Francisco at Pacific Presbyterian Medical Center, San Francisco, CA 94115

INTRODUCTION

Acute and chronic intoxication with ethanol has long been known to predispose to infection (Adams and Jordan, 1984). An extensive immunologic literature indicates that alcohol has profound effects on cell-mediated immune function (MacGregor, 1986). Chronic ethanol consumption is known to increase susceptibility to infectious diseases, and, in particular, classical tuberculosis and bacterial pneumonia (Bomalaski and Phair, 1982). Thus, decrease of neutrophil migration and adherence (Bryton, et al., 1970), decreased function of alveolar macrophages (Rimland, 1983), are all associated with intoxication with ethanol. There has been considerable speculation about the potential role of co-factors such as ethanol in predisposing patients with infection caused by the Human Immunodeficiency Virus-1 (HIV-1) to evolve into the full-blown AIDS syndrome with its characteristic opportunistic infections. Currently, approximately 60% of the patients with advanced stage of AIDS have evidence of M. avium complex infection (Young, 1988).

Our purpose in this study was to determine whether exposure to ethanol was associated with augmented intracellular survival of M. avium complex, and possible mechanisms involved in the survival.

MATERIAL AND METHODS

Bacteria: *Mycobacterium avium* complex (herein designated by MAC), strain 101, serotype 1 and strain 100, serotype 8, were obtained from patients with AIDS.

Macrophages: Human monocyte-derived macrophages were obtained and cultured in vitro as previously reported (Bermudez and Young, 1988). Mouse splenic macrophages were obtained from beige and C57 black mice as previously described (Bermudez et al, 1989). Kupffer cells were obtained and prepared as described by Bourgeois and Beaman.

Cytokines: Recombinant human and murine tumor necrosis factor (TNF) and granulocyte macrophage colony stimulating factor (GM-CSF) were provided by Genentech, Inc., South San Francisco and Immunex, Seattle, respectively.

Animals: C57 black mice, 6 week old females from Jackson Laboratories.

RESULTS

To determine whether exposure to ethanol was associated with increased intracellular survival of MAC, human macrophages were infected with strains 100 and 101 (ratio 100:1 of bacteria : cell). Monolayers were washed after 4 hours, and macrophages were lysed to quantitate the number of infecting organisms. Ethanol at 100 mg/dl was then added to the monolayers for 71 hours. Macrophages were lysed at 4 days to quantitate viable intracellular bacteria. As shown in Figure 1, MAC grows significantly faster in macrophages exposed to ethanol, in a dose-response manner.

As this finding could represent a non-specific impairment in the capacity of macrophages to inhibit growth of intracellular pathogens, we repeated the same experiment described above, using Listeria monocytogenes. Figure 2 shows that intracellular growth of L. monocytogenes was similar for cells exposed or not exposed to different concentrations of ethanol.

The continued presence of ethanol may be critical for other effects on phagocytic cells. To determine whether human macrophages and murine Kupffer cells under exposure to ethanol could be activated to kill MAC, we treated monolayers with TNF (10^3u/ml) and GM-CSF (10^2u/ml), two cytokines previously shown to stimulate the mycobactericidal activity in macrophages. Figures 3 and 4 show that both human macrophages and murine Kupffer cells have diminished response to stimulation with recombinant TNF and GM-CSF in presence of 100 mg/dl of ethanol ($p<0.02$ for all

INTRACELLULAR GROWTH OF M.AVIUM IN PRESENCE OF ETHANOL

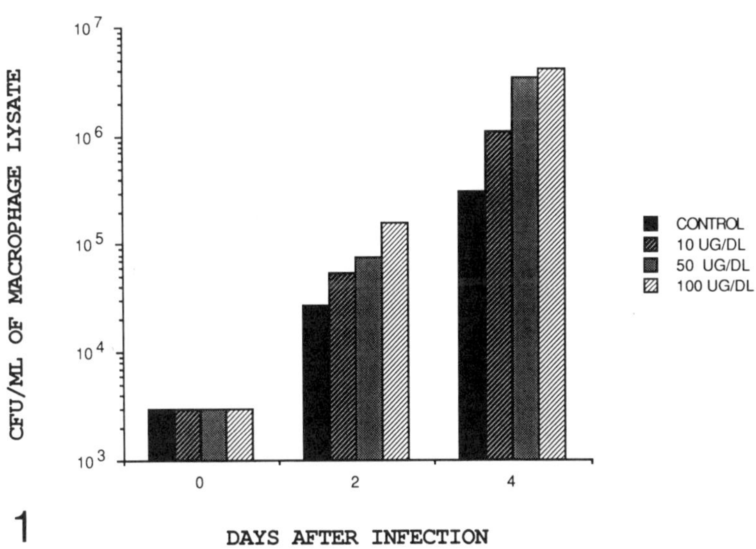

1

comparisons between ethanol-treated and control cells).

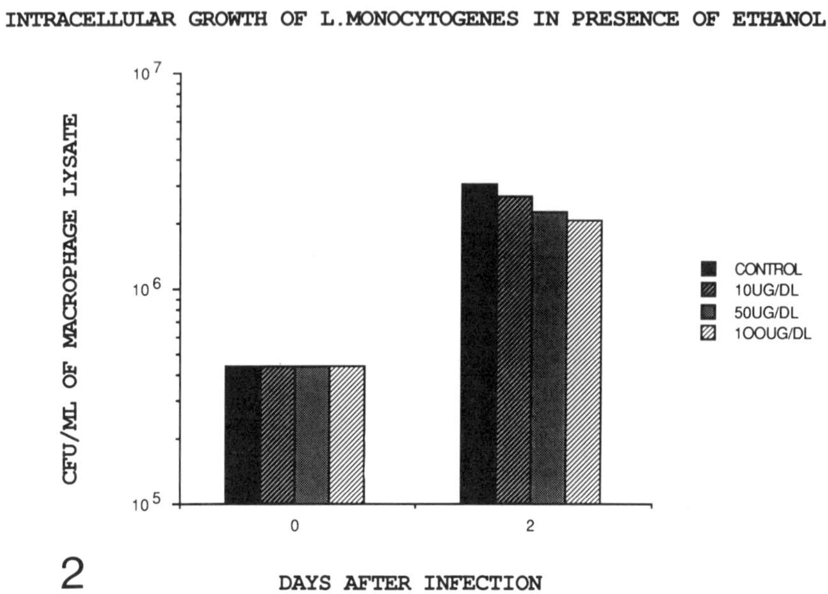

2

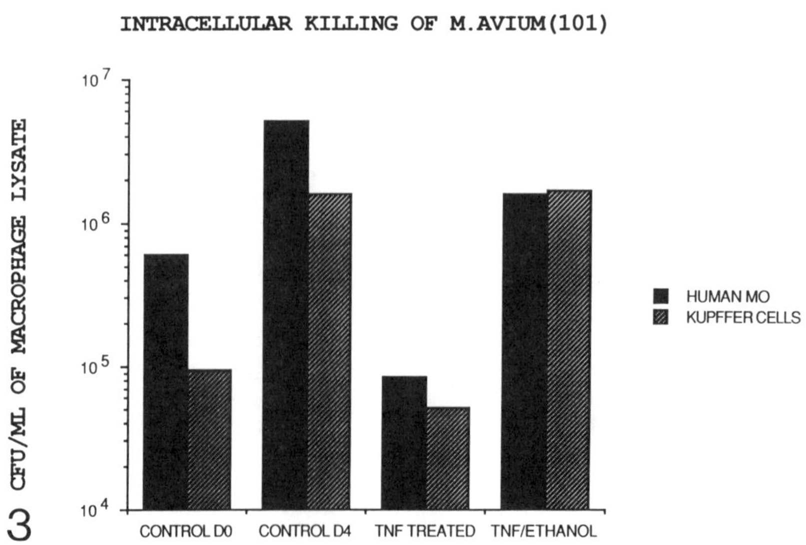

3

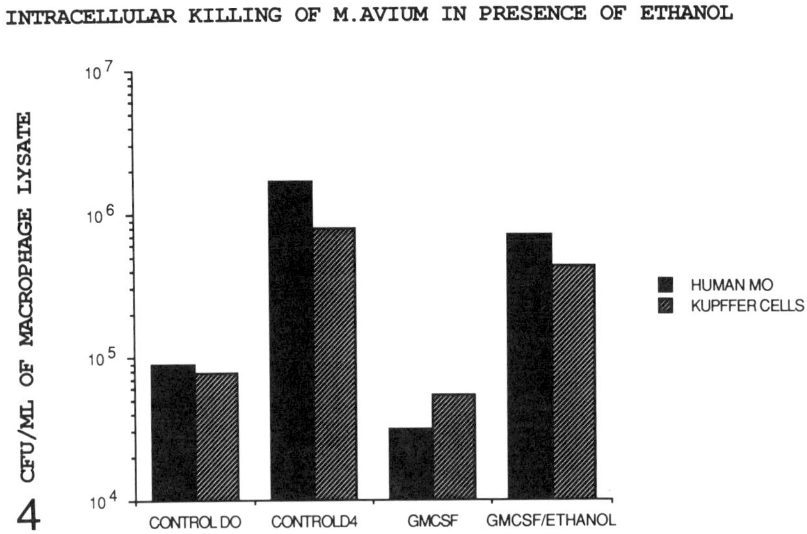

4

As ethanol could interfere with the production and release of cytokines by macrophages, which could be important autocrine factors in the defense against MAC, we treated human macrophages with lipopolysaccharide (LPS)(1ug/ml) in the presence or absence of different concentrations of ethanol (added 1 hour before LPS), and measured the concentrations of TNF and GM-CSF in the medium using the L929 assay for TNF (Bachwich et al, 1986), and an ELISA assay for GM-CSF (18 hours later). We observed that while low doses of ethanol were associated with decreased production and release of the tested cytokines, high concentrations of ethanol stimulate an increased release of TNF and GM-CSF. Since these results were not expected, we attempted repetitive stimulation of cultured human macrophages. We tested whether macrophages treated with ethanol and LPS (1 μg/ml) could respond to a second stimulus with LPS 18 hours later. We observed that in contrast to untreated cells, macrophages exposed to ethanol have an impaired response to the second stimulus, as measured by the release of TNF.

TABLE 1

PRODUCTION OF TNF AND GM-CSF (PROTEIN RELEASED) BY HUMAN MACROPHAGES

STIMULUS	TNF	GM-CSF
LPS	100±21 pg/ml	248±32 pg/ml
LPS + Ethanol (10 mg/dl)	60±15 pg/ml	98±8 pg/ml
LPS + Ethanol (50 mg/dl)	105±26 pg/ml	312±30 pg/ml
LPS + Ethanol (100 mg/dl)	204±20 pg/ml	350±41 pg/ml

Based on the results of 3 experiments.

TABLE 2

PRODUCTION OF TNF BY HUMAN MACROPHAGES

Stimulus	TNF First Stimulus	TNF Second Stimulus*
LPS	126±32 pg/ml	112±28 pg/ml
LPS + Ethanol (10 mg/dl)	74±17 pg/ml	62±12 pg/ml
LPS + Ethanol (50 mg/dl)	128±20 pg/ml	54±12 pg/ml
LPS + Ethanol (100 mg/dl)	190±31 pg/ml	59±19 PG/ml

Based on the results of 3 experiments.
*Treated with LPS 24 hours later.

Experiments were then carried out in C57 black mice in order to determine if continuous ingestion of ethanol could be associated with more progressive disseminated infection of MAC. Six week old females were given ethanol 15 mg/day for one week and then infected with the strain 101 (serotype 1) of MAC, IV (10^8 bacteria). Ethanol was continued for two more weeks (total of 3 weeks). Blood was obtained after 7 and 14 days, and, liver and spleen were harvested and homogenized after 14 days, for quantitation of the number of viable bacteria. As seen in Table 3, there were significantly greater numbers of MAC in blood, liver and spleen of animals receiving ethanol than in controls.

TABLE 3

DISSEMINATED INFECTION WITH M. AVIUM COMPLEX IN MICE

Groups	CFU/ml of Blood	CFU/g Liver	CFU/g Spleen
Control	$2.2 \pm 1.4 \times 10^4$	$1.8 \pm 0.5 \times 10^8$	$9.7 \pm 0.9 \times 10^7$
Ethanol intoxicated	$6.8 \pm 1.7 \times 10^4$ (+67.7%) ($p<0.05$)	$4.7 \pm 0.8 \times 10^8$ (+61.7%) ($p<0.05$)	$2.1 \pm 1.4 \times 10^8$ (+53.8%) ($p<0.05$)

Blood level of ethanol: 45-63 mg%

These results led us to study the function of splenic macrophages obtained from 57 black mice exposed to ethanol and then stimulated in vivo with TNF or GM-CSF. Ethanol and control groups were given TNF (25 ug/kg/day for 3 days) or GM-CSF (20 ug/kg/day for 3 days). The cells were harvested from mice, plated in vitro (10^5 cells/well), infected with MAC (100:1 cell) and the intracellular number of viable bacteria was determined after 3 days. While macrophages from animals not receiving ethanol had a 58±12% growth in the number of intracellular organisms, cells obtained from ethanol-intoxicated mice showed a 94±6% increase in the number of intracellular MAC. Macrophages from mice treated with TNF and GM-CSF killed 61±7% and 66±4% of the bacterial inoculum, respectively, compared with 21±7% and 29±6% killing observed with macrophages obtained from TNF and GM-CSF-treated animals which received ethanol as well ($p = 0.04$ for TNF and GM-CSF groups).

DISCUSSION

This investigation may provide insight into the effects of ethanol on macrophages during MAC infection. Ethanol is known to stimulate macrophages and neutrophils to produce superoxide (Hallengren and Forsgren, 1978). This effect is rapidly seen after exposure to ethanol and it is supposed to depend upon stimulation of protein Kinase C. Our studies show that human macrophages and murine Kupffer cells exposed to low concentrations of ethanol support a greater intracellular growth of MAC strains, a finding not observed in studies with L. monocytogenes. Interestingly, these macrophages also do not respond to activation with TNF and GM-CSF as normal cells do. Similarly, splenic macrophages obtained from mice intoxicated with ethanol have impaired capacity to respond in vivo to the stimulatio nwith TNF and GM-CSF. Ethanol also interferes with the production and release of TNF and GM-CSF by macrophages. Although human macrophages previously exposed to ethanol release greater concentrations of TNF and GM-CSF when they are stimulated by LPS, they do not respond to the second stimulus, suggesting blocking or exhaustion of intracellular pathways.

REFERENCES

Adams HG, Jordan C (1984). Infections in the alcoholic. Med Clin of N Am 68:179-200.

Bachwich PR, Lynch JP, Larrick J, Spengler M,Kunkel SL (1986). Tumor necrosis factor production by human sarcoid alveolar macrophages. Am J Pathol 125:421-425.

Bermudez LE, Kolonoski P, and Young LS (In press 1989). Natural killer cell activity and macrophage-dependent inhibition of growth or killing of Mycobacterium avium complex in a mouse model. J Leuk Biol.

Bermudez LE, Young LS (1988). Tumor necrosis factor alone or in combination with IL-2, but not IFNγ, is associated with macrophage killing of Mycobacterium avium complex. J Immun 140:3006-3013.

Bomalaski JS, Phair JP (1982). Alcohol, immunosuppression and the lung. Arch Intern Med 142:2073-2074.

Bourgeois L, Beaman BL (1974). Probable L-forms of Nocardia asteroides induced in cultured mouse peritoneal macrophages. Infect Immun 9:576-580.

Brayton RG, Stokes PE, Schwartz MS, Louna DB (1970). Effect of alcohol and various diseases on leukocyte mobilization, phagocytosis and intracellular bacterial killing. N Engl J Med 282:123-128.

Hallengren B, Forsgren A (1978). Effect of alcohol on chemotoxis, adherence and phagocytosis of human polymorphonuclear cells. Acta Med Scand 204:43-48.

MacGregor RR (1986). Alcohol and immune defense. JAMA 256:1474-1479.

Rimland D (1983). Mechanisms of ethanol-induced defects on alveolar macrophage function. Alcoholism 8:73-76.

Young LS (1988). Mycobacterium avium complex infection. J Infect Dis 157:863-867.

Alcohol, Immunomodulation, and AIDS, pages 393–401
© 1990 Alan R. Liss, Inc.

CLINICAL AND IMMUNOLOGIC SPECTRUM OF HIV INFECTION IN INFANTS AND CHILDREN AND DISEASE PATHOGENESIS

Savita Pahwa, Narendra Chirmule, Naoki Oyaizu

Division of Allergy/Immunology, Department of Pediatrics, North Shore University Hospital, Manhasset, NY 11030

The etiologic agent of acquired immunodeficiency syndrome (AIDS) is a lymphotropic retrovirus (1-3), termed the Human Immunodeficiency Virus or HIV. The major mode of acquisition of HIV infection in children is perinatal (4-8), from a HIV-infected mother. Intravenous drug abuse (IVDA) by the mother or by her sexual partner accounts for the HIV-infection in the mother in the majority of such cases.

A major problem in the field of pediatric HIV infection today is reliably diagnosing HIV infection in infants born to HIV positive women because of the difficulty in differentiating passively transferred maternal antibody from that synthesized by the infant de-novo. Such infants are classified as Class P-0 for "indeterminate HIV infection" which is indicative of an asymptomatic seropositive state in a child < 15 months of age who is the offspring of a HIV-infected women. Various assays that have been proposed to date for diagnosis of HIV infection in P-0 infants include serum HIV-specific IgM antibody (9), HIV antigen in serum (10), Western Blot profile differences between infant and maternal sera (11), and serial sample analysis for IgG subclass pattern changes in HIV antibodies in infant's serum (12). Individually, none of these assays have been entirely satisfactory. Actual evidence for the virus in the infant's blood would be the most desirable means of establishing the presence of HIV infection by virus culture; however this approach is labor intensive and not practical. More recently, the DNA amplification technique termed polymerase chain reactin (PCR) has been given much attention but still needs standardization (13,14). A major research interest of our laboratory is to develop an alternative assay for diagnosing HIV infection in asymptomatic infants. One assay we have persued is that of HIV antibody synthesis in vitro and is based on the premise that the infected infant would have memory B cells and activated B cells capable of secreting HIV antibody in-vitro. If the infant's peripheral blood lymphocytes are washed free of maternal antibody and cultured with appropriate stimuli, they would be expected to secrete newly synthesized HIV antibody in the event that the infant is infected. Initial data published by Amadori et al (15) and our own results (16) are promising, Table 1, and we are continuing to study this assay system.

Table 1: In-Vitro HIV-IgG Antibody Secretion

Study group	# tested	# positive
Healthy HIV negative controls	65	0
Seropositive Adults	18	18
Symptomatic children	25	24
Class "P-O" infants	36	11+

+5 infants have subsequently developed symptoms of HIV infection. Remaining 6 are still in P-O class.

At the present time, there are a number of puzzling issues pertaining to perinatal infection with HIV. Only about one third of women infected with HIV actually transmit the virus to their offspring. Among the cases born with HIV infection, there is no reliable clinical or laboratory marker which will predict the clinical outcome. Onset of clinical symptoms and diagnosis of HIV infection may be delayed until varying periods post birth, lasting from few months to several years (17,18). Table 2 lists the age of diagnosis of HIV infection in a cohort of children with perinatal infection that has been followed at our institution.

Table 2: Perinatal HIV Infection: Age at presentation

	<1 yr	1-4 yr	>4 yr
Male	17	9	2
Female	12	7	6
Total:	29	16	8

It is conceivable, and has been speculated that factors such as maternal state of health might influence rate of transmission and/or clinical outcome of an infant who gets infected perinatally. It also seems reasonable to speculate that the time in gestation when perinatal infection occurs would most likely influence time of onset of clinical disease. From the point of view of alcohol research, the influence of maternal alcohol intake on any of the above parameters merits serious investigation. It is not known for example, whether ethanol might facilitate or inhibit the passage of virus across the placenta or if it would result in earlier onset and/or increased severity of clinical disease in the offspring.

A clinical staging system for children with HIV infection has been developed by the CDC for diagnostic and surveillance purposes which is descriptive in nature and breaks down the symptoms of symptomatic cases into subclasses (8), Table 3. According to the current CDC classification system, children may be classified as symptomatic (Class P-2), asymptomatic (Class P-1) or indeterminate (Class P-0), which was discussed above. Table 4 indicates that the percentage of cases which fall into sublcasses under class P-2 for symptomatic children in our patient population.

Table 3: CDC Classification of pediatric HIV infection

Class P-0	=	Indeterminate infection
Class P-1	=	Asymptomatic infection
Class P-2	=	Symptomatic infection

Table 4: Clinical Features of 34 Children in P-2 Class

Clinical Classification	n	%
CLASS:		
P-2 A: NON SPECIFIC FINDINGS	30/34	(88%)
Lymphadenopathy	25/34	(73%)
Hepatomegaly	22/34	(64%)
Splenomegaly	17/34	(50%)
Failure to thrive	19/34	(55%)
Diarrhea	20/34	(58%)
Parotitis	4/34	(11%)
P-2 B: NEUROLOGIC DISEASE	17/34	(50%)
P-2 C: LYMPHOID INTERSTITIAL PNEUMONITIS	5/34	(14%)
P-2 D: SECONDARY INFECTION	30/34	(88%)
D-1: Opportunistic infections	16/34	(47%)
D-2: Bacterial infections	9/34	(26%)
D-3: Other infections	29/34	(84%)
P-2 E: SECONDARY MALIGNANCIES	1/34	(3%)
E-1: Malignancies	1/34	(2%)
E-1: Other Malignancies	0/34	(0%)
P-2 F: MISCELLANEOUS CONDITIONS	20/34	(58%)

This classification system does not attempt to and was not designed to grade the severity of disease or corelate clinical symptomology with immunologic status in more than a cursory mannor. In adults with HIV infection, in addition to the CDC designed clinical classification, a number of classification systems that attempt to indicate severity of disease based on clinical and/or immunlogic status have been designed (10). The corelation with falling CD4 positive T cells and disease progression has been well established in CD4 cells usually heralds an adverse course. However, definite studies are still ongoing with a number of immunologic markers.

Immunologic dysfunction in children with HIV infection has been discussed only briefly in the literature, but it is clear that some features are different in comparison to adults. A summary of cross sectional studies of immunologic parameters in our patient cohort is shown in Table 5.

Table 5: Class P-2 - Immunologic status at presentation in 34 children

Immunologic Abnormality	n	%
Hypergammaglobulinemia (<2 SD for age)	31	(91%)
Hypogammaglobulinemia (<2 SD for age)	3	(8%)
CD4 lymphopenia (<400/cu mm)	14	(41%)
Reversal of CD4/CD8 ratio (<1.0)	29	(85%)
Depressed lymphoproliferative responses (<2 SD below control)	28	(79%)

It should be noted that hypogammaglobulinemia may occur in children secondarily to HIV infection, which does not occur in adults. Even children who have profound hypergammaglobulinemia, often fail to mount specific responses upon immunization or upon exposure to infectious organisms (21). This defect of B cell function (22) makes children with HIV infection especially vulnerable to bacterial pathogens, in addition to the opportunistic infections which are a hallmark of AIDS, and forms the basis for treatment with intravenous immunoglobulin which is being given in some institutions.

Our laboratory has been investigating the pathogenesis of immune dysfunction in HIV infection, using a model system of normal T and B lymphocytes or cloned antigen specific T cells and HIV proteins (23-26). Briefly, thus far we have demonstrated that HIV whole virus extract or gp160 can induce polyclonal immunoglobulin secretion in a T dependent manner. The virus extract and gp 120 are however immunosuppressive for T cell activation that occurs as a consequence of T3/Ti receptor mediated signalling (Fig. 1).

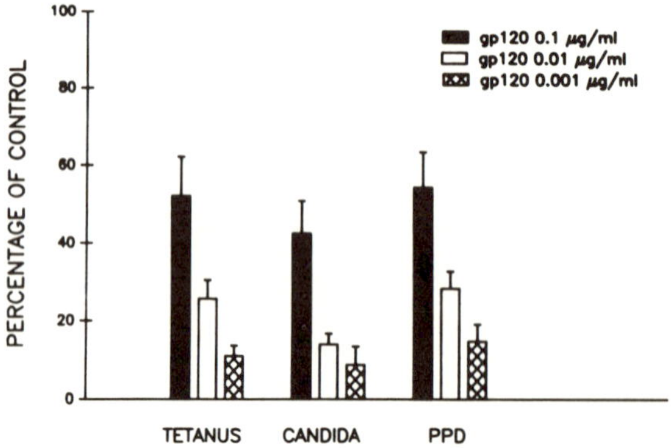

Fig. 1. Inhibition of antigen-specific lymphoproliferation by gp120. Lymphoproliferative responses were performed as described in the Methods section. Results denote mean ± SEM, n=5. Reprinted from Chirmule et al (25), with permission of Raven Press, Ltd.

Gp120 however does not influence activation signals delivered via CD2 and CD28 receptors or those elucited by a combination of phorbolester plus calcium ionophore (unpublished observations). The latter findings imply that the CD4 molecule (to which gp120 binds) must play a pivotal role in the antigen-specific T cell activation process. The influence of virus proteins on second messengers and on activation of genes regulating lymphocyte proliferation (eg. IL-2 and IL-2R) are currently under study. The additional secondary influences of ethanol on T cell activation and on T cell/gp120 interaction merit investigation. The observation that gp120 can so profoundly influence T cell function suggests that if such a mechanism is operative in vivo, it would explain the occurance of T cell immunedeficiency that precedes CD4 cell depletion (27).

REFERENCES

1. Gallo RC, Salandocin SZ, Popovic M, et al. Frequent detection and isolatin of cytopathic retroviruses (HTLV-III) from patients with AIDS and at risk for AIDS. Science 224:500-502, 1984.

2. Border S, and Gallo RC. A pathogenic retrovirus (HTLV-III) linked to AIDS. N Engl J Med. 511:1292-1297, 1984

3. Seligman M, Chess JL, Fahey AS, et al. AIDS - An immunologic reevaluation. N Engl J Med. 311:1286-1292, 1984.

4. Thomas PA, Jaffe HW, Spira TJ, Reiss R, Guerrero IC, and Auerbach D. Unexplained immunodeficinecy in children. A surveillance report. J Am Med Assoc. 252:639-644, 1984.

5. Oleske J, Minnefor A, Cooper R, et al. Immune deficiency syndrome in children. J Am Med Assoc. 249:2345-2349, 1983.

6. Scott GB, Buck BE, Leterman JG, Bloom FL and Parks NP. Acquired immunodeficiency syndrome in infants. N Engl J Med. 310:76-81, 1984.

7. Rubinstein A. Acquired immunodeficiency syndrome in infants. Am J Dis Child. 137:825-827, 1983.

8. MMWR: Classification system for Human immunodeficiency virus (HIV) infection in children under 13 years of age. 36:225-230, 1987

9. Gaetano C, Scano G, Carbonari M, et al: Delayed and defective anti-HIV IgM Response in infants . lancet 1:631, 1987

10. Wittek AE, Phelan MA, Wells MA et al. Detection of human immunodeficiency virus protein in plasma by enzyme immuno assay. Association of antigenemia with symptomatic disease and T-helper cell depletion. Ann Int Med 107:286-292, 1987.

11. Johnson JP, Nair P. Early diagnosis of HIV infection in the neonate. N Eng J Med. 316:273-274, 1987

12. Pyun KH, Ochs HD, Dufford MTW, and Wedgwood RJ. Perinatal infection with human immunodeficiency virus - specific antibody responses by the neonate. N Eng J Med. 316:272-273, 1987.

13. Kwok S, Mack DH, Mallis KB et at; Identification of human immunodeficiency virus sequences by using in vitro enzymatic amplification an oligomer cleavage detection. J Virol. Vol. 61: 1690-1694, 1987.

14. Ou CY, Kwok S, Mitchel SW et al; DNA amplification for direct detection of HIV-1 in DNA of peripheral blood mono-nuclear cells. Science 239:295-297, 1988.

15. Amadori A, DeRossi A, Giaquinto C. In-vitro production of HIV-specific antibody in children at risk of AIDS. Lancet i 852-854, 1988.

16. Lim W, Chirmule N, Slade HB, et al. In vitro synthesis of HIV antibody in infancy. Ped Research 23:356A, 1988 (abstract)

17. Pahwa S, Kaplan M, Fikrig S, Pahwa R, Sarangadharan Mg, Popovic M and Gallo RC. Spectrum of human T-cell lymphotropic virus type-III infection in children. J Am Med Assoc. 225:2299-2305, 1986.

18. Auger I, Thomas P, DeGruttola V, et al. Incubation periods for paediatric AIDS patients. Nature 336:373-377, 1988

19. Redfield RR, Wright DC, Tramont EC. The Walter Reed staging classficiation for HTLV-III/LAV infection. N Eng J Med 314:131-132, 1986

20. Polk BF, Fox R, Brookmeyer R, et al. Predictors of the acquired immunodeficiency syndrome developing in a cohort of seropositive homosexual men. N Eng J Med. 316:61-66, 1987

21. Bernstien JL, Ochs HD, Wedgwood RJ, et al. Defective humoral immunity in pediatric acquired immunodeficiency syndrome. J Pediatr. 107:352-357, 1985.

22. Pahwa S, Fikrig S, Menez R, et al. Pediatric acquired immunodeficiency syndrome: Demonstration of B lymphocyte defects in-vitro. Diagnostic Immunology. 4:24-30, 1986.

23. Pahwa S, Pahwa R, Saxinger C et al. Influence of HTLV-III/LAV virus on function of human lymphocytes: Evidence for immunsuppressive effects and polyclonal B-cell activation by banded viral preparations. Proc Natl Acad Sci. 82:8198-8202, 1985.

24. Pahwa S, Pahwa R, Good RC et al. Stimulatory and inhibitory influences of human T lymphotropic virus type-III on normal B lymphocytes. Proc Natl Acad Sci. 83:9124-9128, 1986.

25. Chirmule N, Kalayanaraman VS, Oyaizu N, Pahwa S. Inhibitory influenes of envelope glycoproteins of HIV-1 on normal lymphocyte responses. J AIDS 1:424-430, 1988.

26. Chirmule N, Saxinger C, Kalyanaraman VS, et al. Localization of B cell stimulatory activity of HIV-1 to the carboxyl terminus of gp41. Aids Research, (In press)

27. Lane HC, Depper J, Greene W et al. Qualitative analysis of immune function in patients with the acquired immunodeficiency syndrome. N Engl J Med. 313:79-84, 1985.

Alcohol, Immunomodulation, and AIDS, pages 403–412
© 1990 Alan R. Liss, Inc.

MALNUTRITION-INDUCED IMPAIRMENT OF RESISTANCE AGAINST EXPERIMENTAL PULMONARY TUBERCULOSIS

David N. McMurray, Rebecca A. Bartow and Carole Mintzer

Department of Medical Microbiology and Immunology, College of Medicine, Texas A&M University, College Station, TX 77843

INTRODUCTION

Primary malnutrition, alcoholism and AIDS are linked by the common themes of wasting, immune impairment and increased incidence of tuberculosis (Chaisson and Slutkin, 1989; Schieffelbein and Snider, 1988; Onwubalili and Scott, 1988). The importance of tuberculosis as a "malade signal" in these three seemingly disparate diseases suggests that each may be characterized by similar alterations in immune responses and antimicrobial resistance. To the extent that malnutrition, especially protein deprivation, is a co-factor in the pathogenesis of alcoholism and AIDS, the study of the impact of protein deficiency on resistance to tuberculosis may contribute to our understanding of altered host resistance in alcoholics and HIV-infected individuals.

A plethora of studies in humans and experimental animals has demonstrated clearly that the principal effects of malnutrition appear to be the loss of T lymphocyte functions, both effector and regulatory, and the subsequent impairment of resistance against infectious diseases like tuberculosis which require an intact cell-mediated immune response (Chandra, 1988; Keusch, et al., 1983). Thus, alterations in the proportions of T cells and T cell subsets, impairment of the response of T cells to antigens *in vivo* and *in vitro*, and reductions in the production of lymphokines and other immunoregulatory molecules have all been observed as sequelae of malnutrition (Chandra, 1979; Chandra, 1983; Hoffman-Goetz, 1988). The thymus and its hormones, which are critical to the development and maintenance of the T cell arm, are especially sensitive to nutritional insult (McMurray, 1984).

We have developed a model of moderate, chronic protein deficiency in the guinea pig in which to study the effects of malnutrition on resistance to tuberculosis. The model has been devised to mimic conditions under which humans acquire infection with mycobacteria (Smith and Harding; 1977). Thus, animals are exposed to a few virulent *Mycobacterium tuberculosis* by the respiratory route and the development of specific resistance is examined (McMurray, et al., 1986a).

METHODS

Outbred (Hartley) or inbred (Strain 2) guinea pigs were obtained commercially as weanlings (120-200 gr) and placed on purified, isocaloric diets containing either 30% ovalbumin (control - C) or 10% ovalbumin (low protein - LP) as the sole protein source (McMurray and Yetley, 1983). In some experiments animals were vaccinated with BCG vaccine or given a primary pulmonary infection with a low-virulence isolate of *M. tuberculosis*. About six weeks after initiation of experimental diets, animals were infected by the respiratory route with a few virulent *M. tuberculosis* H37Rv in a specially designed aerosol chamber (Wiegeshaus, et al., 1970). At intervals thereafter, guinea pigs from each treatment group were skin tested with tuberculin (PPD) and sacrificed. Viable lymphocyte populations were isolated from the blood, spleen and bronchotracheal lymph nodes draining the infected lung. Microtitre cultures were stimulated to proliferate by incubation with PPD (Cohen, et al., 1987). Total numbers of T cells were determined using E-rosette formation with rabbit erythrocytes (Stadecker, et al., 1973), and the proportions of T cells bearing Fc receptors for either IgG($T\gamma$) or IgM($T\mu$) were quantified with a modified double rosette assay (Bartow and McMurray, 1989). The degree of antimicrobial resistance was assessed by quantitative culture of viable *M. tuberculosis* from the lung and spleen (McMurray, et al., 1986a).

RESULTS

Chronic protein malnutrition interferes with the resistance normally afforded by BCG vaccination (Fig. 1). While BCG-vaccinated, normally nourished guinea pigs effectively controlled populations of viable mycobacteria in their tissues, protein-deprived counterparts demonstrated partial to complete loss of vaccine-induced resistance.

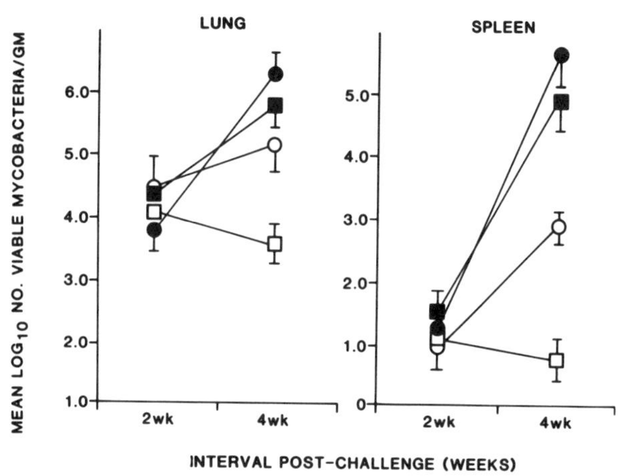

Fig. 1 - Viable mycobacteria recovered from LP (circles) and C (squares), BCG- vaccinated(open symbols) or non-vaccinated (closed symbols) guinea pigs; Mean $\pm$ SEM (4); (From McMurray, et al., 1986a).

In one set of experiments, BCG was replaced by a primary infection with a low-virulence (Lvsr) strain of *M. tuberculosis.* The animals were challenged several weeks later with a high-virulence (HV) strain to mimic the conditions under which debilitated individuals often develop exogenous re-infection tuberculosis (McMurray, et al., 1989a). The results (Fig. 2) indicate that reinfected, malnourished guinea pigs suffered more severe disease than their well-nourished counterparts. Control diet-fed animals were actually protected against exogenous reinfection, while protein-deprived animals were not protected.

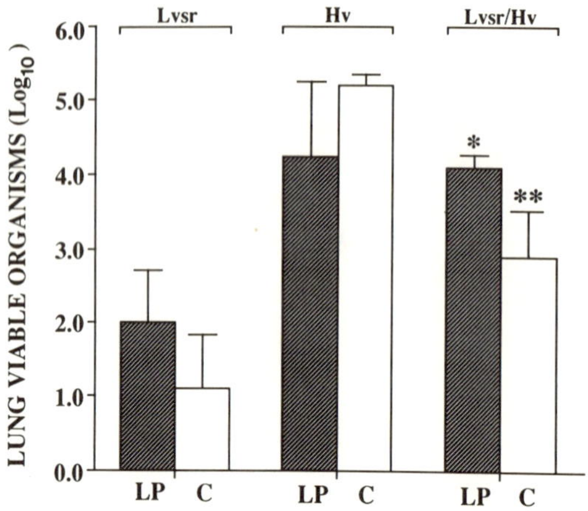

Fig. 2 - Viable mycobacteria recovered from LP and C guinea pigs infected with low-virulence (Lvsr) or high-virulence (Hv) isolates alone, or exogenously reinfected (Lvsr/Hv); Mean ± SEM (6-8); (From McMurray, et al.,1989a)

These observations suggested that specific immune responses against mycobacterial antigens were impaired in protein malnutrition. Evidence for such impairment was observed both *in vivo* and *in vitro* (Table 1). Tuberculin skin tests were dramatically reduced in size or absent in protein-deprived animals with tuberculosis, while PPD-induced proliferative responses of purified lymphocytes *in vitro* were markedly impaired. These diminished PPD-specific lymphocyte functions were even more remarkable given the extensive nature of the tuberculous disease in these animals.

Loss of PPD-induced immune responses in protein malnutrition could result from loss of T cells or their products, or alterations in the balance of regulatory cells which led to suppression of immunity. To test these hypotheses, the proportions of total T cells, $T\gamma$ and $T\mu$ subsets were determined. Figure 3 illustrates the temporal reduction of total E-rosette-forming T cells in the blood of protein-deprived guinea pigs 2 weeks post-challenge.

Table 1

Effect of diet on tuberculin skin reactions and PPD-induced proliferation of peripheral blood cells from guinea pigs infected with virulent *M. tuberculosis* H37Rv.

Diet	Skin test Diameter(mm)*	Stimulation Index**
Low Protein	4.2±2.3(6)	1.6±0.6(6)
Control	15.3±2.1(8)	11.8±3.8(8)

*Measured 24 hr after intradermal injection of 100 TU PPD. Mean ± SEM (number of animals)

**Ratio of counts per minute in PPD-stimulated (25μg/ml) over unstimulated lymphocytes after 4 days in culture ($2x10^6$ cells/ml).

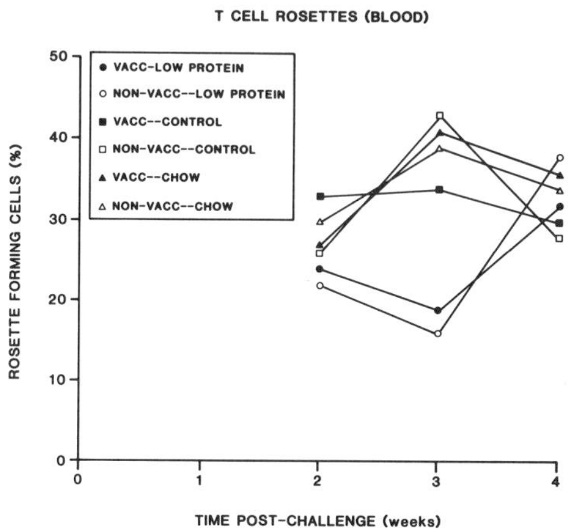

Fig. 3 - Proportion of the E-rosette-forming T lymphocytes in the blood of guinea pigs infected with virulent M. tuberculosis; Mean ± SEM of 4-5 animals.

Likewise, malnutrition was accompanied by changes in the proportions of FcR$^+$ T cells which were consistent with increases in the levels of putative suppressor (Tγ) cells and decreases in the levels of putative helper (Tμ) cells in the lymph nodes of tuberculous LP guinea pigs (Fig. 4)(McMurray, et al; 1989b).

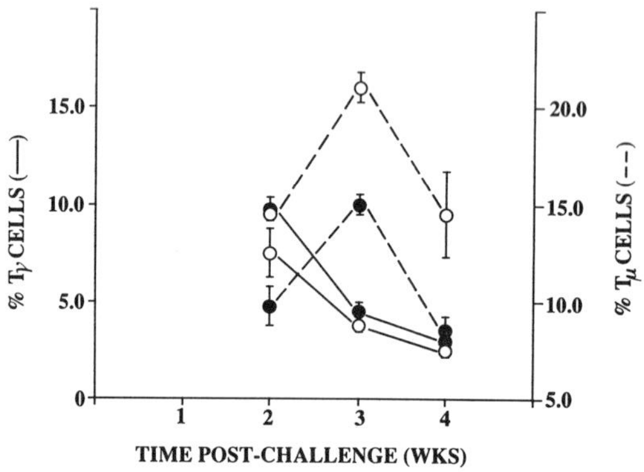

Fig. 4 - Levels of T_γ (———) and T_μ (-----) cells in the lymph nodes of LP (closed circles) and C (open circles) guinea pigs infected with M. tuberculosis; Mean ± SEM of 4 animals (From McMurray, et al., 1989b).

Finally, suppressed vaccine-induced protection and PPD-specific T lymphocyte functions appear to recover completely and rapidly following return of malnourished guinea pigs to a normal diet (McMurray, et al., 1986b). Thus, when BCG-vaccinated guinea pigs which had consumed the LP diet for six weeks were switched to an adequate diet at the time of virulent pulmonary challenge, they responded three weeks later by controlling mycobacterial loads in the tissues as though they had never been malnourished at all (Table 2). Their PPD reactions were actually greater than those of control animals. This dramatic return of normal immune function and disease resistance did not require any additional antigenic stimulus other than that which had been provided by BCG vaccine during the period of nutritional deprivation.

Table 2

Mean $\log_{10}$ number of viable *M. tuberculosis* H37Rv recovered from the spleen.*

	Control diet NV	Low protein VACC	Control VACC	Renourished VACC
Week 1	-0-	-0-	-0-	-0-
Week 2	3.84±0.32	-0-	0.82+0.60	-0-
Week 3	4.73±0.24	2.92±0.48	1.44+0.38	0.85+0.62
Week 4	6.00±0.18	3.22±0.81	1.08+0.74	0.78+0.70

*Mean±SEM of 4 animals per treatment per interval; Means underscored by a common line are not significantly different (Duncan's new multiple range test; $p>0.05$). (Reprinted from McMurray, et al., 1986b)

DISCUSSION

Alcoholism and AIDS are diseases which are accompanied by marked decline in nutritional status. The incidence of pulmonary tuberculosis in alcoholics and HIV-infected individuals is much higher than that observed in the general population (Chaisson and Slutkin, 1989; Schieffelbein and Snider, 1988). While alcoholism and AIDS each may be associated with unique mechanisms of immunodeficiency, they share a common cause of immune dysfunction, i.e. malnutrition.

Our results, taken together, suggest that chronic, moderate protein deficiency results in reversible impairment of antigen-specific T lymphocyte functions and loss of protection normally afforded by previous vaccination or self-limiting primary infection in guinea pigs infected with virulent *M. tuberculosis* (McMurray, et al., 1985; McMurray, et al., 1986a; McMurray, et al. 1989a). Thus, underlying protein malnutrition could contribute to the increased incidence of tuberculosis in alcoholics and AIDS patients quite apart from additional impairment of resistance to infection which accompanies those diseases. The data support the hypothesis that alterations in anti-tuberculous immunity are the result of imbalances in regulatory T cell subsets leading to active suppression of PPD-specific lymphocyte responses (McMurray, et al., 1989b). It is particularly interesting to note that protein-deprived guinea pigs with pulmonary tuberculosis have increased levels of circulating antibodies which bind PPD, in spite of tuberculin anergy (Mintzer, et al., 1986). Immune complexes containing IgG could interact with Tγ cells to induce suppression. This same immune paradox, increased antibody levels accompanying loss of cell-mediated immunity, is also seen in HIV-infected individuals (Chaisson and Slutkin, 1989).

Immune suppression in protein malnutrition is rapidly and completely relieved (See Table 2) when an adequate diet is given, implying that vaccination of malnourished individuals is capable of stimulating protective populations of antigen-reactive T cells, even though these cells cannot exert their beneficial effects until the nutritional deficits are corrected (McMurray, et al., 1986b). This suggests that nutritional support to correct metabolic imbalances in alcoholics and HIV-infected individuals might result in recall and appropriate expression of T cell reactivities which are being actively suppressed due to malnutrition.

REFERENCES

Bartow RA, McMurray DN (1989). Vaccination with *Mycobacterium bovis* BCG affects the distribution of Fc receptor-bearing T lymphocytes in experimental pulmonary tuberculosis. Infect. Immun. 57: (in press).

Chaisson R, Slutkin G (1989). Tuberculosis and human immunodeficiency virus infection. J Infect Dis 159:96-100.

Chandra RK (1979). T and B lymphocyte subpopulations and leukocyte terminal deoxynucleotidyl transferase in protein-energy malnutrition. Acta Paediatr Scand 68:841.

Chandra RK (1983). Numerical and functional deficiency in T helper cells in protein energy malnutrition. Clin Exp Immunol 51:126-132.

Chandra RK (1988). Nutrition and Immunology. Alan R. Liss, Inc., New York.

Cohen MK, Bartow RA, Mintzer CL, McMurray DN (1987). Effects of diet and genetics on *Mycobacterium bovis* BCG vaccine efficacy in inbred guinea pigs. Infect Immun 55:314-319.

Hoffman-Goetz L (1988). Lymphokines and monokines in protein-energy malnutrition In: Chandra RK, ed., Nutrition and Immunology; Alan R. Liss, Inc., New York, pp. 9-23.

Keusch GT, Wilson CS, Waksal SD (1983). Nutrition, host defenses and the lymphoid system. In Advances in Host Defense Mechanisms. vol. 2., Gallin JI, Fauci AS, eds. Raven Press, New York, p. 275-359.

McMurray DN, Yetley EA (1983). Response to *Mycobacterium bovis* BCG vaccination in protein- and zinc-deficient guinea pigs. Infect Immun 39:755-761.

McMurray DN (1984). Cell-mediated immunity in nutritional deficiency. Prog Food Nutr Sci 8:193-228.

McMurray DN, Carlomagno MA, Mintzer CL, Tetzlaff CL (1985). *Mycobacterium bovis* BCG vaccine fails to protect protein-deficient guinea pigs against respiratory challenge with virulent *Mycobacterium tuberculosis*. Infect Immun 50:555-559.

McMurray DN, Kimball MS, Tetzlaff CL, Mintzer CL (1986a). Effects of protein deprivation and BCG vaccination on alveolar macrophage function in pulmonary tuberculosis. Am Rev Resp Dis 133:1081-1085.

McMurray DN, Mintzer CL, Tetzlaff CL, Carlomagno MA (1986b). The influence of dietary protein on the protective effect of BCG in guinea pigs. Tubercle 67:31-39.

McMurray DN, Bartow RA, Mintzer CL (1989a). Impact of protein malnutrition on exogenous reinfection with *Mycobacterium tuberculosis*. Infect Immun 57:1746-1749.

McMurray DN, Bartow RA, Mintzer CL (1989b). Protein malnutrition alters the distribution of $Fc\gamma R^{+}(T\gamma)$ and $Fc\mu R^{+}(T\mu)$ T lymphocytes in experimental pulmonary tuberculosis. Infect Immun (submitted).

Mintzer CL, Carlomagno MA, McMurray DN (1986). Effect of dietary protein and zinc on anti-mycobacterial antibody responses in guinea pigs. Nutr Res 6:167-179.

Onwubalili JK, Scott GM (1988). Immune status in tuberculosis and response to treatment. Tubercle 69:81-94.

Schieffelbein CW, Snider DE (1988). Tuberculosis control among homeless populations. Arch Intern Med 148:1843-1846.
Smith DW, Harding GE(1977). Animal model of human disease. Pulmonary tuberculosis. Am J Pathol 84:273-276.
Stadecker M, Bishop G, Wortis H (1973). Rosette formation by guinea pig thymocytes and thymus-derived lymphocytes with rabbit red blood cells. J Immunol 111:1834-1837.
Wiegeshaus EH, McMurray DN, Grover AA, Harding GE, Smith DW (1970). Host-parasite relationships in experimental airborne tuberculosis. III. Relevance of microbial enumeration to acquired resistance in guinea pigs. Am Rev Resp Dis 102:422-429.

Alcohol, Immunomodulation, and AIDS, pages 413–418
© 1990 Alan R. Liss, Inc.

EFFECTS OF MORPHINE, COCAINE, AND HEROIN ON NUTRITION

Ronald Ross Watson, Ph.D., and Mary E. Mohs, Ph.D., R.D.
Department of Family and Community Medicine
University of Arizona, Tucson, Arizona 85724

Cofactors are clearly involved in aspects of HIV (Human Immunodeficiency Virus) infection, and development of AIDS (Watson, 1989). If they cause significant effects on nutrition, they may indirectly alter host defenses and ultimately development of AIDS after HIV infection. The nutritional effects of some addictive drugs of abuse can produce adverse immune effects. Nicotine (tobacco), marijuana, morphine, heroin, cocaine, and alcohol all impact on nutritional status and can cause alterations in food, water, and salt intake, weight maintenance, and the metabolism and status of specific nutrients. A more detailed review has recently been written which assisted in preparing this mini-review (Mohs and Watson, 1989).

MORPHINE

Morphine use in animals affects a variety of food consumption patterns as well as changes in the physiological utilization of nutrients and metabolic processes. The intake of food, water, and salt in experimental animals is affected, as is glucose metabolism, pancreatic function, digestion, thermic response, cholesterol levels, and calcium status (Celeste, 1984). Morphine injection produced uneven nutrient increases in food deprived rats, disproportionately increasing fatty foods intake compared to foods high in protein or carbohydrates (Vaswani, 1986). One hypothesis is that morphine depresses salt taste, reducing the aversiveness of high salt to appear palatable (Celeste, 1984). Concomitant use of naloxone, a narcotic antagonist, counteracted morphine's action by depressing the animals' preference for high levels of salt (Celeste, 1984).

Morphine has induced sustained hyperglycemia when injected intraventricularly in animals (Roane and Porter, 1986). In vitro studies showed that insulin and glucagon release were stimulated both by low and high doses of morphine (Giuigliano, 1984). Insulin, cortisol, glucagon, and epinephrine were also significantly increased above basal levels by the highest dose of morphine infusion only. Thus, at medium and high doses, morphine initiated a complex catabolic response (Radosevich et al., 1984). The low dose of (2mg/h) morphine lowered epinephrine basal levels. Morphine had a hypoglycemic effect due mainly to inhibition of the hepatic rate of appearance, which was independent of detectable changes in insulin, glucagon, cortisol, and epinephrine. The relationship of morphine-dependence and diabetes was studied in mice and rats. Diabetic animals showed reduced development of physical dependence on morphine (Shook and Dewery, 1986). Spontaneously diabetic mice were significantly less physically dependent upon morphine after a 9-day exposure to increasing doses of morphine-admixed food than controls, despite significantly greater morphine accumulation in their brains. Similarly, streptozotocin-diabetic rats showed significantly fewer behavioral signs of withdrawal after the infusion ended than non-diabetic rats with equal morphine brain levels following six days of intraperitoneal infusion of morphine.

These food intake changes need to be studied in humans. The changes in animals are not significant enough to cause severe malnutrition and hence immunosuppression. However, morphine does severely suppress immune functions and disease resistance (Yahya and Watson, 1987).

HEROIN

Heroin has limited documented nutritional effects, but does change insulin responses. Macaque monkeys given chronic intravenous self-administration of heroin hydrochloride in an ascending series of doses showed no statistically significant changes in food self-administration over 20 days regardless of how heroin self-administration changed (Mello et al., 1985).

Heroin addicts have shown flat glucose tolerance curves with an exaggerated and delayed insulin response following oral glucose loading (Reed and Hodse, 1973). They also showed significantly increased levels of glycosylated hemoglobin A_1, a useful index of the previous 3 to 4 weeks' glycemic control and they have a markedly reduced acute insulin response to i.v. glucose with low Kg values (Giuigliano, 1984). Clearly heroin use modified glucose use or subsequent further metabolism. The severe adverse effects of heroin on kidney function and glucose metabolism are of concern for human users. However, these changes are moderate compared to those seen in undernourished children which produce malnutrition.

COCAINE

Cocaine causes weight loss, food deprivation, and eating disorders. The type of cocaine administered, method of administration, dose level given, and dietary protein adequacy are important determinants of cocaine's effects on weight in rats (Burczynski et al., 1986). Self-administration of intravenous cocaine hydrochloride resulted in rats developing episodic drug intake patterns, losing up to 47% of body weight, and ceasing to groom themselves. The normal ability to accumulate body nitrogen in rats on low protein/high carbohydrate diets with low cocaine levels, suggested that cocaine helped spare amino acids by preferential utilization of fat under protein deprivation conditions. As seen in monkeys, food deprivation can lead to a dose-dependent increase in self-administration of cocaine (De La Garza and Johanson, 1987).

Cocaine abuse can lead to food deprivation or imbalance in humans. Young adult cocaine users ate significantly fewer complete/balanced meals per day, drank more alcoholic beverages per week, consumed more cups of coffee per day, and showed a nonsignificant increase in fatty food intake and decrease in low-fat food intake compared to non-users (Castro et al., 1987). Within the cocaine user group, moderate users ate fewer complete/balanced meals and perceived themselves as less healthy than light users did. It is also interesting that among cocaine abusers an elevated prevalence rate (32%) was seen for the eating disorders anorexia nervosa and bulimia (Mohs and Watson, 1989). Such changes could significantly reduce key nutrients such as to cause malnutritionally-mediated immunosuppression.

Table 1. Some Nutritional Effects of Selected Drugs of Abuse (Experimental Results)

	COCAINE	MORPHINE	HEROIN
HUMAN STUDIES	lower intake of complete/ balanced meals, higher alcohol and higher coffee intake, higher fatty food intake higher cocaine addiction seen in connection with eating disorders bulimia and anorexia nervosa		higher and delayed insulin response to IV glucose, Modified glucose use and higher and delayed insulin response
ANIMAL STUDIES	lower body weight, Normal food intake and Normal body weight with: 1. Low protein/high carbohydrate diet and 1mg/g cocaine or 2. High protein diet and 2/mg/g cocaine (rats) higher self-administeration of cocaine with food deprivation	lower fluid, lower salt intake (mice) lower fluid intake lower food intake (combined with naloxone) higher intake of fatty foods, higher food intake, higher insulin and higher glucagon release higher plasma glucose, higher gastric acid higher cholesterol, levels lower calcium uptake in brain Diabetes: lower physical dependence on morphine	No significant changes in food intake No change in body weight

Modified from Mohs and Watson (1989).

NUTRITIONAL TREATMENT OF THE EFFECTS OF DRUG ABUSE

The ways in which cocaine, heroin, and use change human food preference and weight maintenance are summarized in Table 1. To the extent that cocaine, or the other drugs of abuse modify nutritional state or food intake, dietary changes may be used help compensate for those changes.

ACKNOWLEDGMENTS. Supported in part by grants R01 DA 04827, and P50 AA08037 for the Specialized Alcohol Center. Appreciation is expressed to Mary Mohs whose assistance in preparation of a more detailed review (Mohs and Watson, 1989), and an oral presentation at the conference which made this mini-review possible.

REFERENCES

Burczynski, FJ, Boni, RL, Erickson, J, and Vitti, TG (1986). Effect of Erythroxylum Coca, cocaine and ecogonine methyl ester as dietary supplements on energy metabolism in the rat. J Ethnopharmacol 16:153-166.

Castro, FG, Newcomb, MD, and Cadish, K (1987). Lifestyle differences between young adult cocaine users and their nonuser peers. J Drug Educ 17:89-111.

Celeste, CK, Bryant, HU, Zabik, JE, and Yim, GKW (1984). Stress, endogenous opioids and salt intake. Appetite 5:53-60.

De La Garza, R, and Johanson, CE (1987). The effects of food deprivation on the self-administration of psychoactive drugs. Drug Alc Depend 19:17-27.

Giuigliano, D (1984). Morphine, opioid peptides, and pancreatic islet function. Diabetes Care 7:92-98.

Hollister, LE (1971). Hunger and appetite after single doses of marijuana, alcohol, and dextroamphetamine. Clin. Pharmacol. Ther., 12:44-49.

Mello, NK, Bree, MP, Lukas, SE, and Mendelson, JH (1985). Buprenorphine effects on food-maintained responding in Macaque monkeys. Pharmacol Biochem Behav 23:1037-1044.

Mohs, M and Watson RR (1989). Nutritional effects of selected drugs of abuse. In: Focus on Biochemistry and Physiology of Substance Abuse. CRC Press, Vol. I, in press.

Radosevich, PM, Williams, PE, Lacy, DB, McRae, JR, Stainer, KE, Cherrington, AD, Lacy, WW, and Abumrad, NN (1984). J Clin Invest 74:1473-1480.

Reed, JL, and Ghodse, AH (1973). Oral glucose tolerance and hormonal response in heroin-dependent males. Br Med J 2:582-585.

Roane, DS, and Porter, JR (1986). Nociception and opioid-induced analgesia in lean (Fa/-) and obese (fa/fa) Zucker rats. Physiol Behav 38:211-218.

Vaswani, K, Tejwani, GA, and Mousa, S (1986). Stress induced differential intake of various diets and water by rats: The role of the opiate system. Life Sci 32:1983-1986.

Watson, RR (Editor) (1989). Drugs of Abuse Immune Functions, and Resistance to Disease CRC Press Inc., Boca Raton, FL pp. 1-300.

Watson, RR, and McMurray, DN (1979). The effects of Malnutrition on the secretory and cellular immune processes. CRC-Critical Review Food Science and Nutrition. 12:113-159.

Yahya, MD and Watson, RR (1987). Minireview. Immunomodulation by morphine and marijuana. Life Sci. 41:2503-2510.

Alcohol, Immunomodulation, and AIDS, pages 419–432
© 1990 Alan R. Liss, Inc.

VITAMIN AND TRACE METAL DISTURBANCES IN ALCOHOLISM: POTENTIAL EFFECTS ON THE IMMUNE SYSTEM

Nancy W. Alcock
Department of Preventive Medicine and Community Health, University of Texas Medical Branch, Galveston, Texas 77550-5520

INTRODUCTION

Detrimental effects of excessive consumption of alcohol cover a broad spectrum. Metabolism of alcohol requires a greater expenditure of energy than equivalent calories from food carbohydrate. Increase in oxygen consumption in both man and rats has been observed (Pirola and Lieber, 1976). These observations could explain the weight loss which resulted when normal individuals were fed 50% of calories as ethanol (Pirola and Lieber, 1972) compared with equivalent calories as food. In addition to increased metabolic demands associated with excessive alcohol intake, anorexia frequently coexists. Gastritis caused by alcohol may result in the loss of iron due to bleeding (Davenport, 1969) and hence loss of iron may result. Alcoholics have impaired absorption of folate, thiamine, vitamin B_{12}, fat, xylose and a number of minerals and trace metals which may be due to nutritional deficiencies rather than malabsorption. With the exception of vitamin B_{12}, absorption appears to return to normal after withdrawal of alcohol and substitution of a nutritious diet (Lindenbaum and Lieber, 1975). Well nourished alcoholics have decreased levels of intestinal lactase, and are lactose intolerant (Perlow et al, 1977). Chronic pancreatitis occurs in a fraction of alcoholics, and has been associated with both low intakes of protein, fat and carbohydrates (Mezey et al, 1988), and high intakes of protein and fat (Sarles, 1973). Pancreatitis occurs at an earlier time in women than men exposed to the same intake of alcohol (Mezey et al, 1988). Malnutrition in the alcoholic is further accentuated by the direct effect of alcohol on the liver, and by impaired utilization of nutrients due to liver damage (Bunout et al, 1983). The economic impact of diversion of funds to satisfy the alcohol demands of the individual further compromises the chances of a healthy diet.

Many of the nutritional disturbances observed in experimental animals or humans consuming excessive amounts of alcohol also have been shown to have an effect on the immune system. Chandra (1986) cites malnutrition as the most common cause of acquired immune dysfunction throughout the world. Beisel et al (1981) reported on the effects of single nutrients on immunological functions. The extent of these is summarized in Figure 1.

Fig 1. Effects of Single-Nutrients on Immunological Functions

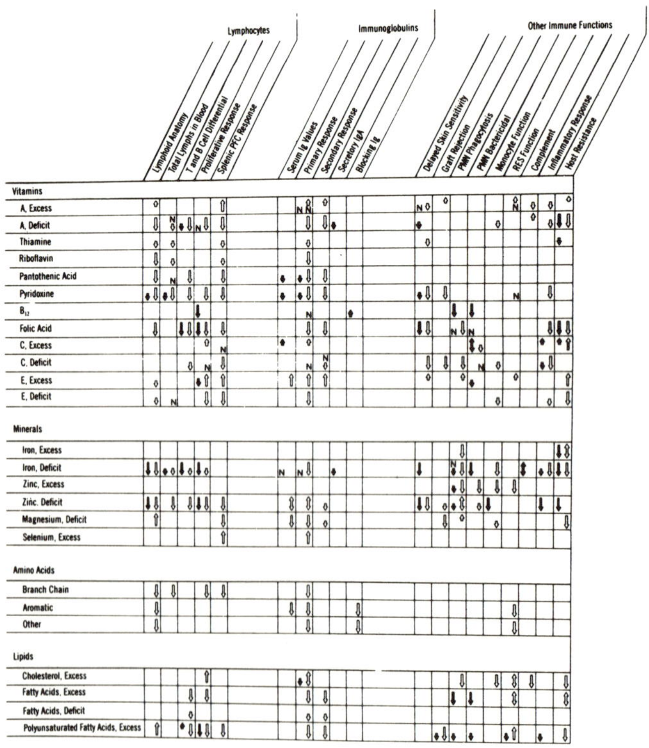

Any reported change in immune function (top) associated with nutritional variable (left) indicated by direction and length of arrows. Solid arrows indicate human studies; open arrows, animal findings; N, normal findings; PMN, polymorphonuclear leukocyte; PFC, plaque-forming colonies; RES, reticuloendothelial system.

From Beisel et al (1981). Reprinted by permission JAMA (1981) 245:53-58.

Patients with acquired immunodeficiency syndrome (AIDS) have low levels of serum zinc (Fabris et al, 1988), selenium (Dworkin et al, 1986), may be folate or vitamin B_{12} deficient, (Herbert et al, 1988), have demonstrable malabsorption of fat and carbohydrate (Gillin et al, 1985), and frequently lose excessive amounts of nutrients due to diarrhea. The relationship, if any, between the development of impaired immune function in individuals with AIDS and their nutritional status, including alcohol intake, requires elucidation, and any contribution of alcohol to the process documented. The pertinent literature involving relationships between alcohol intake, vitamins and trace metals and various parameters of the immune system is reviewed here.

ALCOHOL AND VITAMINS

Vitamin A is stored in the liver mainly as retinyl esters, which, on hydrolysis are linked to retinol binding protein for transport to most organs of the body. Predominent among its many functions retinol is involved in cell differentiation and in maintenance of corneal integrity. Liver vitamin A in autopsy specimens in man was found to be progressively decreased in persistent hepatitis, fatty liver, alcoholic hepatitis, and cirrhosis (Leo and Lieber, 1982). Baboons fed an adequate liquid diet containing 50% of total calories as ethanol produced a 59% decrease in liver vitamin A in 4 months compared with that of pair-fed controls fed isocaloric diet. The level decreased 95% in a 24-84 month period (Sato and Lieber, 1981). Fibrosis and cirrhosis developed during the latter period. Similar results were obtained in rats (Leo and Lieber, 1983). Serum vitamin A and the transport protein, retinol binding protein, were unaffected by the alcohol consumption in rats. A 5-fold increase in vitamin A intake did not restore the liver vitamin A. When vitamin A was removed from the diet, endogenous liver vitamin A was depleted 2.5 times faster in the alcohol consuming rats than in the control group. Increased catabolism of vitamin A in the liver and increased mobilization was evident since higher levels in the kidneys and testes of the rats was found.

Chronic alcoholism is frequently accompanied by a decreased intake of folate, diminished intestinal absorption (Halsted et al, 1967), and impairment of transport, tissue uptake, retention, and excretory mechanisms for this vitamin

(Lane et al, 1976). The effect of alcohol on folate bioavailability, and on the development of megaloblastic anemia (Blocker and Thenen, 1987) was assessed in monkeys . Decreased hemoglobin and red blood cell count occurred earlier in the alcohol group than in controls. Plasma, red blood cell and liver folate levels decreased. The increased excretion of formiminoglutamic acid in urine was approximately 2.5 times greater in the alcohol group than in the controls. Tritiated folic acid studies in the monkeys showed a decrease in folic acid in the urine of the alcohol group. Increased fecal excretion of the labelled folic acid could be explained by a postulated malabsorption of enterohepatically circulated folate in the alcohol group. The involvement of folate in DNA synthesis and in erythropoeisis requires adequate supplies and utilization of this vitamin. Although vitamin B12 absorption is impaired in chronic alcoholism (Lindenbaum and Lieber, 1975), resulting anemia is not a frequent occurrence in these individuals.

Results of experimental models to study the effect of alcohol on thiamin metabolism and thiamin status are conflicting. A review of the data by Shaw and Lieber (1988) indicates that no changes in brain and liver thiamin pyrophosphate resulted from chronic alcohol feeding with a formula diet. Measurement of bioavailability of thiamin in another study showed a decrease in blood and liver. In another study the cofactor thiamin pyrophosphate failed to enhance the activity of transketolase in blood, although the activity was lower than in controls. However, the Wernicke-Korsakoff Syndrome in which the brain is deficient in thiamin resulting in confusion, and even coma, occurs in some alcoholics. Furthermore, there is evidence that alcohol interferes with the active absorption of thiamin from the gastrointestinal tract (Hoyumpa, 1983; Tomasulo et al, 1968).

Pyridoxal phosphate, the active form of vitamin B_6, was decreased in the liver of rats fed a diet in which alcohol provided 36% of the caloric intake, whether the diet had adequate vitamin B_6, or was deficient in this vitamin (Veitch et al 1975). In vitro studies using perfused livers or isolated hepatocytes suggested that in vitamin B_6-deficient animals a decrease in pyridoxal phosphate from pyridoxine was dependent upon oxidation of alcohol. A deficiency of pyridoxal phosphate, the co-factor for many enzymes, may have an effect on the metabolism of carbohydrates, amino acids and lipids. Within 3 weeks of deprivation of the vitamin transaminases in blood may lose activity, and skin lesions and encephalographic changes occur.

Ascorbic acid content in the liver and in leukocytes from alcoholics was found to be low in more than 50% of the subjects with liver damage studied by Beattie and Sherlock (1976).

ALCOHOL AND TRACE METALS

Iron absorption may be increased due to excessive intake from beer and wine, or to increased solubility of ferric ion due to the action of alcohol on gastric acid secretion. If gastritis and bleeding occurs, iron will be lost via the gastrointestinal tract. Iron stores in the liver were increased in autopsy specimens from alcoholics even with early cirrhosis (Volini et al, 1968), and hence consideration of iron supplementation in alcoholics needs careful evaluation.

Disturbances in zinc metabolism in the alcoholic have been reviewed by McClain and Su (1983). Zinc intake is usually low, absorption from the gut decreased or clearance from the plasma increased (Sullivan et al, 1979), plasma zinc is low in those subjects with cirrhosis, and the urinary excretion is increased whether liver damage exists or not (Sullivan and Langford, 1965). Consequences of the ensuing zinc deficiency in the chronic alcoholic include acrodermatitis (Weismann et al,1980), abnormal ability to adapt to the dark, which requires both zinc and vitamin A for correction (Morrison et al, 1978), and hypogonadism (McClain et al, 1979). Normal vision and spermatogenesis both require the conversion of retinol to retinal; decreased activity of the zinc containing dehydrogenase may explain the development of night blindness and of hypogonadism in some alcoholics.

A role for zinc deficiency in the fetal alcohol syndrome has been suggested since congenital defects, especially of brain malformation, are common to both. However, the fetal alcohol syndrome occurred in non-human primates (Fisher et al, 1988) and in rats (Leitch and Rosemond, 1981) fed alcohol with an adequate zinc intake.

Zinc insufficiency could be a contributing factor to the anorexia frequently present in alcoholics. In experimental studies, zinc deprivation in animals results in anorexia at an early stage. Voluntary alcohol intake in rats was consistently increased when a zinc free diet was fed (Collipp et al, 1984).

Changes in copper metabolism in relation to alcohol intake have not been investigated systematically. Increased serum copper levels in alcoholics were reported by Hartome et al (1977) irrespective of the degree of liver involvement, and increased liver copper levels in cirrhosis were also reported (Volini et al, 1968).

Serum selenium was found to be decreased in all of 16 alcoholics with cirrhosis (Sullivan et al, 1971) and in alcoholics with and without advanced liver disease (Dworkin et al, 1985). Excretion of selenium in the urine in alcoholic patients was also increased (Rissanen et al, 1987). In view of the decreased levels of both selenium and vitamin E produced by alcohol (Bjorneboe et al, 1987), and the role of the selenium containing glutathione peroxidase and vitamin E in lipid peroxidation, cell membrane protection against oxidative products may be compromised.

Increased excretion of magnesium in the urine after alcohol ingestion is well documented (Rissanan et al, 1987; McCollister et al, 1963). Retention of magnesium from diet alone during the first 10 days after alcohol withdrawal (Jones et al, 1969) represents approximately 25% of the total exchangeable magnesium in a 70 Kg man, as calculated from the data of Barnes (1969).

RELEVANCE TO IMMUNE FUNCTION

Acrodermatitis enteropathica, an inherited autosomal recessive trait, is a syndrome in which moderate to severe zinc deficiency results, due to impairment of intestinal zinc abosrption (Moynahan and Barnes, 1973). The immunological abnormalities demonstrated in this disease in humans include impaired cutaneous delayed hypersensitivity responses and reduced lymphocyte proliferation *in vitro*. Polymorphonuclear chemotaxis is impaired. The proportion of T^{4+} helper cells is significantly reduced (Figure 2) and helper cell activity for B-cell function is decreased (Figure 3). Activity of the zinc requiring thymic hormone thymulin is decreased, and suppressor T-cell functions are decreased (Chandra, 1985).

The administration of daily supplements of zinc corrects the abnormalities cited.

Fig. 2

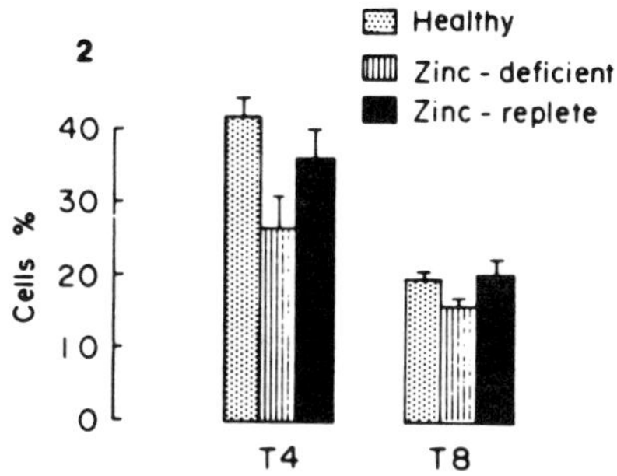

T-lymphocyte subsets enumerated by using monoclonal antibodies and immunofluorescence.

Fig. 3

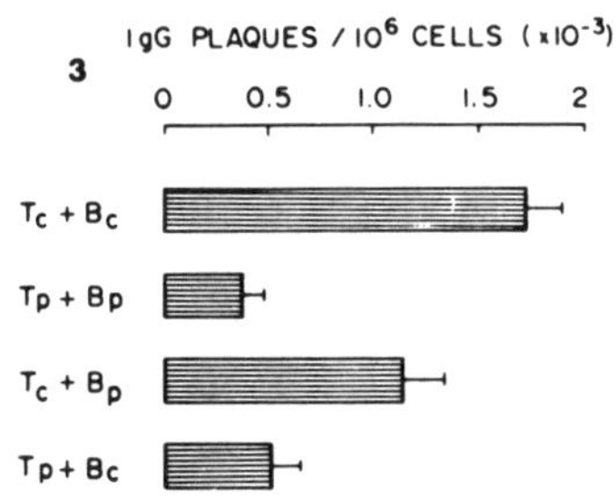

Results of coculture experiments using T cells and B cells from zinc-deficient patients (p) or zinc-replete controls (c). The number of pokeweed mitogen-induced IgG producing cells was counted by the reverse hemolytic plaque technique.

Reprinted by permission J Am Coll Nutr (1985) 4:5-16.

In experimental animals marginal intakes of zinc caused thymic atrophy (Fraker et al, 1986), lymphopenia and alterations in the proportions of the various subsets of lymphocytes and mononuclear phagocytes. Antibody mediated responses to both T-cell dependent and T-cell independent antigens were significantly reduced. Natural killer cell activity and delayed cutaneous hypersensitivity reactions were also depressed. Exposure in mice to suboptimal levels of zinc _in utero_ caused immunodeficiency in the offspring and this could be transferred to subsequent generations.

The thymic nonapeptide hormone thymulin is one of the numerous enzymes for which zinc is a co-factor (Dardenne et al, 1982). This hormone has been shown _in vitro_ to induce differentiation of normal human marrow T cell precursors into cells with T lymphocyte characteristics (Incefy et al, 1980).

Fabris et al (1988) reported low levels of zinc in the serum of patients with lymphadenopathy syndrome, and even lower levels in patients with acquired immunodeficiency syndrome, while virus-uninfected drug users had normal serum zinc levels. Thymulin activity in the patients with low serum zinc levels was depressed in the same proportion as the zinc. Activity of the hormone was restored to normal in the presence of added zinc to the assay medium where serum zinc was low, but was unaltered in the groups where serum zinc was normal.

Iron deficiency is rarely unaccompanied by other nutritional deficiencies, and therefore its effect on the immune system is difficult to define. Chandra has reviewed the relevant observations (Chandra 1985). Impairment of cell mediated immunity has been reported in patients with iron-deficiency anemia and both cell mediated and humoral immunity were affected in iron-deficient children. Polymorphonuclear neutrophils showed reduced bactericidal capacity in iron deficiency. The importance of adequate levels of transferrin in serum of patients receiving iron supplementation was discussed by Weinberg (1977). Bioavailability of iron to bacteria in the presence of low levels of transferrin, conceivably increase the susceptibility to infection.

Experimental copper deficiency in mice showed that the number of anti-body producing cells was reduced compared to those in pair-fed controls (Prohaska and Lukasewyez, 1981). Copper deficiency has also been associated with increased susceptibility to infection in these animals. Vyas and Chandra (1983) found decreased thymic factor activity in copper deficient mice.

A role for selenium in immunecompetence has been suggested by demonstration of suppressed antibody response (Chandra, 1983) in selenium deficient animals. However the suppression could be reversed by administration of vitamin E. The secondary antibody response to T-cell antigens was impaired in selenium deficiency (Mulhern et al, 1985).

Although normally present in biological tissues in higher concentrations than the trace metals discussed above, magnesium deficiency has been associated with impairment of immune function in experimental animals. Serum protein levels and IgG levels were markedly reduced in magnesium deficient rats (Alcock and Shils, 1974) and IgG, IgA and M levels in the serum of mice which were magnesium deficient were significantly decreased (Elin, 1975). The number of plaque-forming cells in the spleen of mice was also decreased. Thymic hyperplasia (Alcock et al, 1973), and thymic lymphosarcoma have been studied extensively in magnesium deficiency in the rat (Bois et al, 1969).

Observed effect on immune function associated with a deficiency of individual vitamins is indicated in Figure 1. Immunological competence in deficiencies of vitamin A (Watson, 1984), pyridoxine (Chandra and Puri, 1985), folate (Gross and Newberne, 1980), and vitamin C (Beisel, 1982), may be further impaired with excessive alcohol consumption.

AIDS AND NUTRITION

While disturbances in the single nutrients zinc, selenium, iron, folate and vitamin B_{12} have frequently been reported in symptomatic AIDS patients, the influence of protein-energy-malnutrition, together with the severe diarrhea frequently present, contribute to the severe wasting in the terminally ill patient. Co-ordinated studies of various parameters of immunological function and nutritional status, including alcohol intake, are required to monitor the initiation and progression of the various changes. A recent report (Shoemaker et al, 1988) showed marked alterations in the concentration of cellular cations, including calcium, magnesium and zinc, in lymphocytes from symptomatic AIDS patients. Virus infected cells in culture show similar abnormalities. The role of metabolites of vitamin D in mediating biological responses at the cellular level was recently reviewed (Minghetti and Norman, 1989) and emphasizes the central role these have in cell proliferation processes. Observations at the cellular level may be necessary to better assess nutritional status.

REFERENCES

Alcock NW, Shils ME, Lieberman PH, Erlandson RA (1973). Thymic changes in the magnesium depleted rat. Cancer Res 33:2196-2204.

Alcock NW, Shils ME (1974). Serum immunoglobulin G in the magnesium-depleted rat. Proc Soc Exp Biol Med

145:855-858.
Barnes B (1969) Magnesium conservation: A study of surgical patients. Ann NY Acad Sci 162: 787-801.
Beisel WR (1982) Single nutrients and immunity. Am J Clin Nutr 35:417-468.
Beisel WR, Edelman R, Nauss K, Suskind RM (1981). Single-nutrient effects on immunological functions. Report of a workshop sponsored by the Department of Food and Nutrition and its Nutrition Advisory Group of the American Medical Association. JAMA 245:53-58.
Bjorneboe GA, Johnsen J, Bjorneboe A, Morland J, Drevon CA (1987). Effect of heavy alcohol consumption on some concentrations of fat-soluble vitamins and selenium. Alcohol-Alcohol Suppl 1:533-537.
Blocker DE, Thenen SW (1987). Intestinal absorption, liver uptake, and excretion of 3H-folic acid in folic acid deficient, alcohol-consuming non-human primates. Am J Clin Nutr 46:503-510.
Bois P, Sandborn EB, Messier PE (1969). A study of thymic lymphosarcoma developing in magnesium-deficient rats. Cancer Res 29:763-775.
Bunout D, Gattas V, Iturriaga H, Perez C, Pereda T, Ugarte G (1983). Nutritional status of alcoholic patients: its possible relationship to alcoholic liver damage. Am J Clin Nutr 38:469-473.
Chandra RK (1983). Nutrition and immune responses. Canad J Physiol Pharmacol 61:290-294.
Chandra RJ (1985). Trace element regulation of immunity and infection. J Am Coll Nut 4:5-16.
Chandra RK (1986). Nutritional regulation of immunity and infection: from epidemiology to phenomenology to clinical practice. J Ped Gastroenterology and Nutrition 5:844-852.
Chandra RK, Puri S (1985). Vitamin B-6 modulation of immune response and infection. In Reynolds RD, Leklem JE (eds) Vitamin B-6: its role in health and disease, New York: Alan R Liss, pp 163-175.
Collipp PJ, Kris VK, Castro-Magana M, Shih A, Chen SY, Antoszyk N, Baltzell J, Noll J, Trusty C (1984). The effects of dietary zinc deficiency on voluntary alcohol drinking in rats. Alcoholism:Clin Exp Res 8:556-559.
Dardenne M, Pleau JM, Narbarra B, Lefrancier P, Derren M, Choay Bach JF (1982). Contribution of zinc and other metals to the biological activity of the serum thymic factor. Proc Natl Acad Sci 79:5370-5373.

Davenport HW (1969). Gastric mucosal hemorrhage in dogs. Effect of of acid, aspirin and alcohol. Gastroenterology 56:439-446.

Dworkin BM, Rosenthal WS, Wormser GP, Weiss L (1986). Selenium deficiency in the acquired immunodeficiency syndrome. J Parent Ent Nutr 10:405-407.

Dworkin B, Rosenthal WS, Jankowski RH, Gordon GG, Haldea D (1985). Low blood selenium levels in alcoholics with and without advanced liver disease. Correlations with clinical and nutritional status. Dig Dis Sci 30:838-844.

Elin RJ (1975). The effect of magnesium deficiency in mice on serum immunoglobulin concentrations and antibody plaque-forming cells. Proc Soc Exp Biol Med 148:620-624.

Fabris N, Mocchagiani E, Galli M, Irato L, Lazzarin A, Moroni M (1988). AIDS, zinc deficiency and thymic hormone failure. JAMA 259:839-840.

Fisher SE, Alcock NW, Amirian J, Altshuler HL (1988). Neonatal and maternal hair zinc levels in a nonhuman primate model of the fetal alcohol syndrome. Alcoholism:Clin Exp Res 12:417-421.

Fraker PJ, Gershwin ME, Good RA, Prasad A (1986). Interrelationships between zinc and immune function. Fed Proc 45:1474-1479.

Gillin JS, Shike M, Alcock NW, Urmacher C, Krown S, Kurtz RC, C, Winawer SJ (1985). Malabsorption and mucosal of the small intestine in the acquired immunodeficiency syndrome. Ann Intern Med 102:619-622.

Gross RL, Newberne PM (1980). Role of nutrition in immunological function. Physiol Rev 60:188-302.

Halsted CH, Griggs RC, Harris JW (1967). The effect of alcoholism on the absorption of folic acid (3H-PGA) evaluated by plasma levels and urine excretion. J Lab Clin Med 69:116-131.

Herbert V, Gulle V, Stopler T, Shevchuk O, Tsougranis M, Javali S . Clinically unsuspected negative vitamin B-12 balance in patients. Clin Res 36:796A.

Herbert V, Jacobson J, Colman N, Shevchuk O, Javali S, Tsougranis M, Castellar L, Stopler T (1989). Negative folate balance in AIDS. FASEB J 3:A1278.

Hoyumpa Jr. AM (1983). Alcohol and thiamine metabolism. Alcoholism:Clin Exp Res 7:11-14.

Hartoma TR, Sontaniemi Ea, Pelkonen O, Ahlqvist J (1977). Serum zinc and serum copper and indices of drug metabolism. Eur J Clin Pharmacol 12:147-151.

Hurley LS (1979). The fetal alcohol syndrome: possible implication of nutrition deficiencies. In Li TK, Schenken S, L (eds): "Alcohol and Nutrition" Research monograph 2, US Dept HEW pp36-....
Incefy GS, Mertelsmann R, Yata K, Dardenne M, Bach JF, Good RA (1980). Induction of differentiation in human marrow T cell precursors by the synthetic serum thymic factor FTS. Clin Exp Immun 40:396-406.
Jones JE, Shane SR, Jacobs WH, Flink EB (1969). Magnesium balance studies in chronic alcoholism. Ann NY Acad Sci 162:934-946.
Lane F, Goff P, McGuffin R, Eichner ER, Hillman RS (1976). Folic acid metabolism in normal, folate deficient and alcoholic man. Br J Haematol 34:489-500.
Leo MA, Lieber CS (1982). Hepatic vitamin A depletion in alcoholic liver injury in man. New Eng J Med 37:597-601.
Leo MA, Lieber CS (1983). Interaction of ethanol with vitamin A. Alcoholosm:Clin Exp Res 7:15-21.
Lindenbaum J, Lieber CS (1975). Effects of chronic alcohol administration intestinal absorption in man in the absence of nutritional deficiency. Ann NY Acad Sci 252:228-234.
McClain CJ, Van Thiel DD, Parker S, Badzin LK, Gilbert H (1979). Alterations in zinc, vitamin A, retinol binding protein in chronic alcoholics: A possible mechanism for night blindness and hypogonadism. Alcoholism:Clin Exp Res 3:135-141.
McCollister RJ, Flink EB, Lewis MD (1963). Urine excretion of magnesium in man following ingestion of ethanol. Am J Clin Nutr 12:415-420.
Mezey E, Kolman CJ, Diehl AM, Mitchell MC, Herlong HF (1988).Alcohol and dietary intake in the development of chronic pancreatitis and liver disease in alcoholism. Am J Clin Nut 48:148-151.
Morrison SA, Russell RM, Carney EA, Oaks EV (1978). Zinc deficiency: a cause of abnormal dark adaptation in cirrhosis. Am J Clin Nutr 31:276-281.
Moynahan EJ, Barnes PM (1973). Zinc deficiency and a synthetic diet for lactose tolerance. Lancet 1:676-677.
Mulhern SA, Taylor GL, Magruder LE, et al (1985). Nutr Res 5:201-205.
Minghetti PP, Norman AW (1989). 1,25(OH)2-Vitamin D3 receptors: gene regulation and genetic circuitry. FASEB J 2:3043-3053.

Pirola RC, Lieber CS (1972).The energy cost of the metabolism of drugs, including alcohol. Pharmacology 7:185-196.

Pirola RC, Lieber CS (1976). Hypothesis: energy wastage in alcoholism and drug abuse. Possible role of hepatic microsomal enzymes. Am J Clin Nutr 19:90-97.

Prohaska JR, Lukasewyez OA (1981). Copper deficiency suppresses the immune response of mice. Science 213:559-561.

Rissanen A, Sarlio-Lahteenkorua S, Alfthan G, Gref C-G, Keso L, Salaspuro M (1987). Am J Clin Nutr 45:456-461.

Sarles H (1973). An international survey on nutrition and pancreatitis. Digestion 9:389-403.

Sato M, Lieber CS (1981). Hepatic vitamin A depletion in alcoholic liver injury in man. New Eng J Med 37:597-601.

Shaw S, Lieber CS (1988). Nutrition and diet in alcoholism. In Shils ME, Young VR (eds) "Modern Nutrition in Health and Disease" 7th Edition, Philadelphia: Lea and Febiger, pp1423-1449.

Shoemaker JD, Millard MC, Johnson PB (1988). Zinc in human immunodeficiency virus infection. JAMA 260:1881-1882.

Sullivan JF, Jetton MM, Burch RE (1979). A zinc tolerance test. J Lab Clin Med 93:485-492.

Sullivan JF, Lankford HG (1965). Zinc metabolism and chronic alcoholism. Am J Clin Nutr 17:57-63.

Sullivan JF, Williams RV, Burch RE (1979).The metabolism of zinc and selenium in cirrhotic patients during 6 weeks of zinc digestion. Alcoholism:Clin Exp Res 3:235-239.

Tomasulo PA, Kater RMH, Iber FL (1968) Impairment of thiamin absorption in alcoholism. Am J Clin Nutr 21:1341-1344.

Veitch RL, Lumeng L, Li TK (1975). Vitamin B-6 metabolism in chronic alcohol abuse. The effect of ethanol oxidation on hepatic pyridoxal-5-phosphate metabolism. J Clin Invest 55:1036-1032.

Volini F, Huergo J, Kent G (1968). Trace metal studies in liver disease using atomic absorption spectrophotometry. In Sunderman FW, Sunderman FW Jr., Green WH (eds) "Laboratory Diagnosis of Liver Disease". St. Louis, WH Green.

Vyas D, Chandra RK (1983). Thymic factor activity, lymphocyte stimulation response and antibody producing cells in copper deficiency. Nutr Res 3:343-349.

Watson RR (ed) (1984). Nutrition, disease resistance, and immune function. New York:Marcel Dekker, pp 325-343.

Weinberg E (1977). Infection and iron metabolism. Am J Clin Nutr 30:1485-1490.

Weismann K, Hoyer H, Christensen E (1980). Acquired zinc deficiency in alcoholic liver cirrhosis. Report of 2 cases. Acta Dermatol 60:447-449.

Alcohol, Immunomodulation, and AIDS, pages 433–444
© 1990 Alan R. Liss, Inc.

ETHANOL INDUCED MALNUTRITION, A POTENTIAL CAUSE OF IMMUNOSUPPRESSION DURING AIDS

Mary E. Mohs, Ph.D, R.D., and Ronald R. Watson, Ph.D.
Director, NIAAA funded specialized Alcohol Research Center
Department of Family and Community Medicine
University of Arizona
Tucson, Arizona 85724

INTRODUCTION

Alcohol affects every stage in nutrient metabolism including nutrient intake, digestion, absorption, activation, storage, utilization, degradation and excretion (Leonard et al., 1987). Reductions in micro and macro nutrient intakes can be related to significant immunosuppression (Beisel, 1982, Watson and McMurray, 1979). Such suppression during progression from HIV infection to AIDS may accelerate the process by reducing host defenses and permitting greater bacterial stimulation of T cells as targets for retroviral infection (Leonard-Green and Watson, 1989). The effects of alcohol intake on nutritional status are dependent upon the frequency and amount of alcohol intake, the pattern of intake, the duration of alcohol use, the user's socioeconomic status, the presence or absence of disease, the use of medications, dietary intake and nutrient adequacy, and nutritional status (Mohs et al., 1988).

Alcohol often leads to a decrease in food intake and is substituted for more nutritious foods. Alcohol can decrease absorption of nutrients through physiological alterations in the absorptive surface of the gastrointestinal tract. Alcohol increases the utilization of nutrients secondary to the metabolism of alcohol. The activation of nutrients to their metabolically active forms is decreased with alcohol use due to organ damage.

Alcohol is transported throughout the body system giving it the potential to affect most organs and tissues. Alcohol effects the gastrointestinal tract by alterations in stomach acid secretion and delayed gastric emptying. Alterations in the mucosa of the small intestine leads to alterations in the production of enzymes, decreased absorptive capacity, malabsorption, and altered transport of nutrients. Alcohol also negatively affects pancreatic function with the potential for maldigestion of foods and altered glucose tolerance (Leonard et al., 1987).

The liver is the primary site for many important functions such as the metabolism, activation, and storage of many nutrients. The liver is also the site of alcohol metabolism. If hepatic damage occurs this can profoundly affect nutritional status. Adequate nutritional status does not protect against the hepatotoxic effect of alcohol. Injury to body systems due to alcohol intake imposes increased demand for many nutrients for repair which depletes body stores increasing the requirement for these nutrients.

Ethanol consumption affects nutrition through a number of mechanisms. A number of nutrients function as catalysts, co-enzymes, and/or metalloenzyme co-factors in the metabolism of alcohol. Chronic alcohol use leads to the increased utilization or turnover of B vitamins, biotin, niacin, pantothenic acid, magnesium, and zincs. The repair of damaged tissues increases the utilization of antioxidants such as vitamin C. Increased collagen synthesis increases the requirement for vitamin C. Increased cell reproduction and protein synthesis that accompany tissue repair increases the utilization and therefore need for vitamin B_6, vitamin B_{12}, and folic acid. Alcohol intake can lead to inflammation of the stomach, small intestine and pancreas resulting in inhibition of the absorption of vitamins. Alcohol and its metabolites can alter the ability of the liver to change vitamins like vitamins B_1 and B_6 to their active metabolites or to store them (Ryle and Thomas, 1984). The elimination of alcohol breakdown products increases the excretion of some vitamin and minerals (Leonard et al., 1987).

EFFECTS OF SINGLE NUTRIENTS ON IMMUNOCOMPETENCE AND OF ALCOHOL ON SINGLE NUTRIENTS

Inadequacies of single or multiple nutrients can affect immunocompetence. It is difficult to prove cause and effect relationships between single nutrients and alterations in immune function because deficiencies of multiple nutrients often occur together, the deficiency of one nutrient can affect the utilization of another, and often an infectious process or toxin occurring concomitantly can itself impart a direct impact on immune function (Leonard et al., 1987).

Vitamin A

Retinoids and carotenoids play a number of roles in immune competence. Vitamin A deficiency has been associated with an increased incidence in a variety of cancers and to an increased susceptibility to infection (Leonard-Green and Watson, 1989). Animals with a vitamin A deficiency have decreased thymic weights, depressed levels of lymphocytes and plasma cells. Vitamin A deficiency may decrease antigen binding due to alterations in surface membrane glycoproteins (Cunningham-Rundles, 1985). Beta carotene, a precursor to vitamin A (retinol) stimulates immune cells when present in adequate quantities. In addition, carotenoids function as antioxidants. The effects of low serum levels of beta carotene on the immune system is unknown (Beisel, 1982), but it is low in alcohol abuses as is vitamin A (Aoki et al., 1987).

Chronic alcohol use increases the catabolism of retinol leading to a depletion of existing hepatic vitamin A stores. In addition, there is a decrease of hepatic storage of vitamin A (Grummar and Erdman, 1983). Vitamin A (retinol) is converted to its storage form, retinal, in the liver by alcohol dehydrogenase. Alcohol competes for this enzyme in its metabolic pathway potentially depleting available enzyme altering liver storage of retinol. Zinc deficiency, common in alcoholics, can perpetuate the shortage of enzyme through its role as a co-factor in dehydrogenase. A study looking at the serum and hepatic level of vitamin A in patients with various stages of alcoholic liver disease found hepatic levels of vitamin A were depleted at all stages of alcoholic liver disease even when levels of serum vitamin A, retinol binding protein and prealbumin are unaltered (Leo and Leiber, 1983).

A study looking at the relationship between smoking and/or alcohol habits and serum carotene levels in healthy individuals found a lower serum B-carotene level in current smokers and regular alcohol users. Dietary intake of carotene did not differ between groups. Alcohol had a greater negative effect on serum carotene levels than smoking. The combination of smoking and alcohol use had the greatest negative effect (Aoki et al., 1987).

Supplementation of non-toxic doses of retinoids and of the carotenoids showed that each stimulated immunocompetence. Retinoids and carotenoids have different effects on immune function (Watson and Rybski, 1988). Retinoids play a role in the differentiation of immune cells increasing mitogenesis of lymphocytes and the phagocytosis and activation of monocytes/macrophages. Retinoids stimulate cellular immune functions of increasing T-lymphocyte proliferation, increased numbers of mature T-helper lymphocytes, increased response of T-lymphocytes to certain mitogens, and enhanced growth of granulocyte/macrophage precursor cells (Watson and Rybski, 1988). The carotenoids activate lymphocytes and monocytes and potentially enhances the immunosurveillance of natural killer cells (Abril et al., 1989). Beta-carotene increases the percent of total T-cells, T-helper cells, natural killer cells, and can lead to increased production of interferon by T-lymphocytes (Prabhala et al., 1989; Watson and Rybski, 1988). In addition beta-carotene inhibits damage by free radicals. Canthaxanthin increases the percent of T-helper cells and increases the activation of monocytes. Thus, changes in the adequacy of retinoids and carotenoids could play key roles in alcohol associated immunosuppression. However, while the association is suggested, studies to test for this relationship has not been studied in alcohol abusing animals or people.

Vitamin D

The hormonal form of vitamin D, calcitriol, has antineoplastic properties. Morphological and biochemical changes that occur in human monocytes treated with calcitriol. Vitamin D deficiency can occur in alcoholics as indicated by decreased serum levels, depressed bone mass and low calcium levels. Vitamin D is converted to its active hormonal form by the liver. Alcohol related liver damage may be the mechanism by which vitamin D deficiency occurs in alcoholics. Low calcium levels common in chronic alcohol use may in part be due to vitamin D inadequacy leading to negative effects on calcium absorption and mobilization (Mohs et al., 1988). A study of calcium status and regulating factors of hospitalized male alcoholics found significantly decreased circulating levels of 25-hydroxyvitamin D3 and 1,25-dihydroxy vitamin D3 as compared to controls. There was no difference in the dietary intake of vitamin D between groups. Sun exposure was higher in the alcoholic group. Low levels of circulating vitamin D metabolites in alcoholics may be due to a decrease in hepatic or renal enzymes or hormones necessary for conversion to vitamin D3 metabolites. In chickens ethanol inhibits the activity of the renal enzyme responsible for vitamin D3 conversion. In rats ethanol intake results in decreased muscle and adipose tissue stores of vitamin D3. This depletion of stores may limit the level of available substrate for hepatic conversion (Bjorne-Boe et al., 1988). The effects, if any, on reduced calcium such as seen in alcohol abusers on cellular immunity is not known (Mohs and Watson, 1990).

Vitamin E

High levels of vitamin E stimulate T-helper lymphocytes, antibody response, delayed cutaneous hypersensitivity reactions, the reticuloendothelial system, host resistance, phagocytosis, mitogen responsiveness increased T-helper cell activity and enhanced humoral immune response. Animal studies have correlated a decreased serum vitamin E level with alcohol use. The decreased serum levels of vitamin E and selenium may affect the integrity of cell structure and function as indicated by an increase in lipid peroxidation and enhance free radical activity (Bjorne-Boe et al., 1988b). It is less clear that these decreases are low enough to affect immune functions to suppress them, as the usual diet has a large excess of vitamin E. Serum selenium concentration was also decreased in alcoholics as compared to controls. Severe selenium and vitamin E malnutrition is unlikely, so their potential deficiencies significant enough to cause immunosuppression is small.

Vitamin B_1 and B_2

Very little is known of what role vitamin B_1 and B_2 plays in immunocompetence. However, vitamin B_1 deficiency can occur with chronic alcohol use due to decreased intake, absorption, and metabolism, increased catabolism, decreased activation and hepatic storage. Alcohol significantly impairs thiamin absorption primarily by decreasing the rate of active thiamin absorption which occurs at low intakes. Both human and rat studies have shown that folate deficiency can lead to a significant reduction in vitamin B_1 absorption and perpetuate the deficiency (Mohs and Watson, 1989). Vitamin B_2 deficiency is common in chronic alcohol use. One study found 23% of patients with alcohol-related illness had vitamin B_2 deficiency (Baines, 1978).

Vitamin B_6

Vitamin B_6 deficiency leads to thymic epithelial tissue dysfunction, decreased thymic factor activity, decreased humoral immune response to T-dependent and independent antigens, depressed cell mediated immune response, delayed cutaneous hypersensitivity, depressed antibody response to vaccines, and depressed proliferation responses. A study on mice found that those fed higher levels of vitamin B_6 had greater immunological response to antigen than those fed lower levels (Gridley et al., 1988).

Alcohol and acetaldehyde can lead to vitamin B_6 deficiency through decreased intake, malabsorption, increased catabolism, decreased activation and increased excretion. Vitamin B_6 deficiency is estimated to occur in 80-100% of alcoholics with liver disease and plasma co-factor levels of vitamin B_6 are depressed in 57% of alcoholics with no hepatic or hematologic signs.

Vitamin B_{12}

Vitamin B_{12} deficiency alters immunocompetence with a decreased antigen responsiveness of T- and B-lymphocytes and depressed phagocytic function (Cunningham-Rundles, 1985). Vitamin B_{12} deficiency may occur with alcohol abuse due to decreased absorption resulting from alterations in the mucosal surface of the gastrointestinal tract and alterations in the production of intrinsic factor. It is difficult to identify vitamin B_{12} deficiency because the maintenance of serum levels may hide tissue depletion. Significantly low levels of liver vitamin B_{12} with high serum levels of vitamin B_{12} was found in alcoholic patients.

Folate

Folate deficiency resulting in megaloblastic anemia and alterations in DNA synthesis leads to a decreased cell mediated immunity and proliferative responses. Folate deficiency related to alcohol consumption is associated with an increased urinary excretion of folate, decreased intake, impaired absorption, and alteration of folate storage and release (Weir et al., 1985). Alcoholic cirrhosis results in a decrease in hepatic ability to bind and retain folate. In addition, alcohol may block a specific folate metabolic pathway or it may inhibit the function of a specific co-enzyme form of folate. A study of alcoholic megaloblastic patients who were post treatment for megaloblastic anemia were given a challenge of a low-folate diet and the equivalent of 1 pint of whiskey per day. They exhibited a drop in serum folate levels in 4 days and megaloblastic bone marrow 2 to 3 weeks post challenge. A study on rats found alcohol produces a depression of serum and liver folate. Thus, alcohol induced severe folate inadequacy and immunosuppression may be associated.

Vitamin C

Vitamin C deficiency leads to a reduced delayed cutaneous hypersensitivity delayed mitogenic responsiveness, a decreased phagocytic cell function, T-cell lymphopenia and decreased macrophage mobilization and aggregation (Leonard-Green and Watson, 1989). Vitamin C deficiency is common in chronic alcohol users. Vitamin C may increase the oxidation and, therefore, clearance of alcohol, leading to increased vitamin C utilization and depletion. One study of patients with alcohol related illnesses found 91 percent of these patients deficient in vitamin C. In animal studies of vitamin C deficient guinea pigs chronic alcohol intake lead to a decrease in the efficiency of the metabolism by the microsomal ethanol oxidizing system resulting in an increase in the plasma half-life of drugs. The vitamin C level of liver, kidney, and adrenal glands was lower in the alcohol treated groups than in controls. Chronic high alcohol intake leads to vitamin C inadequacy even with adequate vitamin C intake, and that vitamin C may have some role in alcohol metabolism. Substantial vitamin C deficiency is needed to cause immunosuppression; so the extent of correlation needs detailed study.

Iron

Iron deficiency results in reduced T-cell number, impaired lymphocytic mitogen response, decreased granulocytic bacteriocidal activity, inhibition of total and active E-rosette formation, suppression of cell mediated community, and alterations in the synthesis of granulocytes and macrophages (Sherman, 1986). Some of the immune function changes may be due to alterations in folate metabolism resulting from iron deficiency.

Alcohol intake increases iron absorption due to alcohol induced increase in gastric acid production. Elevated iron levels in chronic alcohol use may be due to alterations in liver function, enhanced iron absorption or due to folate deficiency. Iron deficiency can be seen in chronic alcohol may be related to blood loss. Anemia may also be seen secondary to alterations in bone marrow function induced by alcohol (Marietta et al., 1988).

Magnesium

Very little information is available related to what role magnesium has in immunocompetence (Beisel 1982; Leonard-Green and Watson, 1989). However, low serum magnesium levels are common in chronic alcohol abusers. Urinary magnesium excretion can increase 2-3 times above that of normal controls. Plasma magnesium levels fall during alcohol withdrawal indicative of increased losses or utilization during this stress. Magnesium deficiency may exert a role in the effect alcohol has on vitamin B_1 metabolism and, therefore, status (Mohs and Watson, 1989). Chronic alcohol intake decreases magnesium levels in various body organs. Magnesium is an essential co-factor in thiamin metabolism, so magnesium deficiency can perpetuate a thiamin deficiency and affect the efficacy of thiamin supplementation.

Zinc

Zinc plays a very important role in immunocompetence and exerts crucial regulatory effects on specific immune functions. Zinc deficiency leads to depression of cell-mediated immunity with decreased T-cells and B-cells in lymphoid tissue, decreased T-helper cell number and activity, an inverted ratio of T-helper to T-suppressor cells, a depressed reactivity of T-lymphocytes to tumor cells, a delayed cutaneous hypersensitivity, decreased synthesis of lymphokine and cytotoxic T-cells, reduced T-helper cell dependent antibody responses, decreased natural killer cell activity, a depression of thymic hormone levels, and a depression of IgM (Mohs and Watson, 1989; Beisel, 1982; Leonard-Green and Watson, 1989). Alterations in T-cell subpopulations and natural killer cell activity is associated with chronic, mild zinc deficiency of the type that may be found in chronic alcohol use.

Zinc deficiency is common with chronic alcohol use. Zinc deficiency may occur with chronic alcohol use due to inadequate dietary intake, altered absorption and increased urinary excretion. One study found that 90% of alcoholics with or without liver disease had inadequate dietary zinc intake. In animals ethanol intake decreased zinc absorption. In humans there is an increase in urinary zinc excretion in alcoholics with or without liver disease. Individuals with severe liver disease lost the most zinc through urinary excretion. Plasma zinc levels can be decreased to 60% of normal in chronic alcohol users. Zinc deficiency can affect vitamin A status due to alterations in vitamin A metabolism manifesting with impaired visual function. Zinc plays a role in the storage and mobilization of vitamin A. Zinc is a part of a metalloenzyme that is responsible for alcohol metabolism. In animals zinc deficiency impairs alcohol metabolism. This slows the elimination of alcohol from the body resulting in increased levels of alcohol in the blood and tissues for a longer duration of time. If this similarly occurs in humans chronic alcohol use such as in alcoholism, leading to or occurring with zinc deficiency, places a high load on body systems that must metabolize alcohol and exposes the body to higher levels of alcohol for a longer duration leading to liver disease and further malnutrition.

Research related to the interrelationships between alcohol, malnutrition, and immunocompetence has been conducted. Both alcohol intake and malnutrition can adversely affect immunocompetence and alcohol intake can affect nutritional status (Mohs and Watson, 1989).

EFFECTS OF ALCOHOL INTAKE ON IMMUNOCOMPETENCE

Moderate as well as severe protein-calorie malnutrition in non-alcohol users results in immunosuppression: lymphopenia, decreased T-helper cells as compared to T-suppressor cells, decreased natural killer and cytotoxic cell activity, depression of cell mediated immunity, and decreased humoral immunity (Watson and McMurray, 1979).

Chronic alcohol users have a number of similar alterations in immunocompetence including a depression of serum bacteriocidal activity, alterations of immunoglobin production, leukopenia, defects in chemotaxis, decreased antigen trapping and processing, and decreased T-cell mitogenesis. Alcohol abuse also decreases cellular immune surveillance. In animals alcohol use produces thymic and splenic atrophy, alterations in circulating lymphocytes, and in cellular and humoral immunity (Marietta et al., 1988). Resistance to infection and susceptibility to liver damage may be related to alterations in antibody synthesis, the direct effects of alcohol use, or nutritional deficiencies of one or more nutrients that can occur with alcohol use (Watson and Darban, 1988). Much research related to alcohol and cellular immune function has been conducted on alcoholic hepatitis patients. They have a reduced skin test reactivity to common antigens, reduced numbers of circulating T-lymphocytes and normal levels of B-lymphocytes. Effects of moderate or chronic alcohol use without severe organ damage can't be extrapolated from this. In animals without liver damage alcohol intake induces rapid cellular immune function changes. Unfortunately, the nutritional status of patients in the above studies, and the extent of nutritional stresses were generally not measured to be able to correlate them to immunosuppression associated with alcohol use (Darban and Watson, 1988).

One study looked at cellular immune function in four groups of individuals: previous alcohol abusers, current alcohol abusers, those with alcoholic cirrhosis or pancreatitis, and a control group of life long abstainers. In current and previous alcohol abusers T-cell number remained within normal levels with a non-statistically significant decrease in T-lymphocyte mitogenesis. In the alcoholic cirrhosis and pancreatitis group, levels of T-helper and suppressor cells were increased significantly (Watson, et al., 1985).

Acknowledgments. Supported by grants DA04827 and also AA08037 which sustains the NIAAA specialized Alcohol Research Center at The University of Arizona. Appreciation to T. Leonard-Green, and M. Mohs who helped draft longer reviews which facilitated this paper is recognized. In addition the oral presentation of much of this material by M. Mohs at the conference is appreciated.

REFERENCES

Abril, ER, Rybski, JA, Scuderi, P and Watson, RR (1989). Beta-carotene stimulates human monocyte secretion of a novel tumoricidal cytokine. J. Leuk. Biol. 45:255-261.

Aoki, K, Ito, Y, Sasaki, R, Ohtani, M, Hamajima, N and Asano, A. (1987) Smoking, alcohol drinking, and serum carotenoids levels. Jpn J Cancer Res 78:1049-1056.

Baines, M. (1978) Detection and incidence of B and C vitamin deficiency in alcohol-related illness. Ann Clin Biochem 15:307-312.

Beisel, WR. (1982) Single nutrients and immunity. Am J Clin Nutr 35:417-418.

Bjorne-Boe, G, Bjorne-Boe, A, Johnson, J, Skylv, N, Oftebro, H, Gautvik, K, Hoiseth, A, Morland, J and Drevon C. (1988) Calcium status and calcium-regulating hormones in alcoholics. Alcoholism 12:229-231.

Bjorne-Boe, GA, Johnsen, J, Bjorne-Boe, A, Bache-Wiig, J, Morland, J and Drevon, CA. (1988) Diminished serum concentration of vitamin E in alcoholics. Ann Nutr Metab 32:56-61.

Cunningham-Rundles, S. (1985) Effects of nutritional status on immunological functions. Am J Clin Nutr 35:1202-1215.

Gridley, D, Shultz, T and Stickney D. (1988) In vivo and in vitro stimulation of cell-mediated immunity by vitamin B_6. Nutrition Research 8:201-207.

Grummer, M and Erdman, J. (1983) Effect of chronic alcohol consumption and moderate fat diet on vitamin A status in rats fed either vitamin A or beta carotene. J Nutr 113:350-64.

Leonard, TK, Mohs, ME, and Watson, RR. The cardiovascular effects of alcohol. (1987) In: Nutrition and Heart Disease Volume I. CRC Press, Inc., Boca Raton, Florida, Ed. RR Watson, pp. 19-47.

Leonard-Green, TK and Watson, RR. The AIDS-immunocompetence-nutrition-infection cycle. (1989) In Press: CRC Press Inc., Boca Raton, Florida.

Marietta, CA, Jerrells, TR, Meagher, RC, Karanian, JW, Weight, F, Eckhardt, MJ. (1988) Effects of long-term alcohol inhalation on the immune and hematopoietic systems of the rat. Alcoholism 12:211-222.

Mohs, ME, Leonard, TK and Watson, RR. (1988) Interrelationships among alcohol abuse, obesity, and Type II diabetes mellitus: Focus on Native Americans. Wld Rev Nutr Diet 55:93-172.

Mohs, ME and Watson, RR. (1989) Changes in the nutrients associated with alcohol abuse. In press: Diagnosis of Alcohol Abuse, CRC Press, Inc.

Prabhala, RH, Maxey, V, Hicks, MJ and Watson, RR (1989). Enhancement of the expression of activation markers on human peripheral blood mononuclear cells by in vitro culture with retinoids and carotenoids. J. Leuk. Biol. 45:249-254 (1989).

Ryle, PR and Thomas, AD. (1984) Nutrition and vitamins in alcoholism. In: Clinical Biochemistry of Alcoholism. Ed. Rosalki, SB. New York:Churchill Livington, 188-224.

Sherman, AR. (1986) Alterations in immunity related to nutritional status. Nutrition Today 7-13.

Watson, RR and Darban, H (1988). Alcohol and immunosuppression. Clinical Immunol. Newsletter 9:129-131.

Watson, RR, and Rybski, J (1988). Immunological response modification by vitamin A and other retinoids. Nutrition and Immunology, ed. (R.K. Chandra) 87-99, A.R. Liss, New York.

Watson, RR, Jackson, JC, Hartmann, B, Sampliner, R, Mobley, D and Eskelson C. (1985) Cellular immune functions, endorphins, and alcohol consumption in males. Alcoholism: Clin Exp Res 9:248-254.

Watson, RR and McMurray, DN (1979). The effects of malnutrition on the secretory and cellular immune processes. CRC-Critical Rev. Food Science Nutr. 12:113-159.

Weir, DG, McGing, PG and Scott, JM. (1985) Folate metabolism, the enterohepatic circulation and alcohol. Biochem Pharmacol 34:1-7.

Index

Acetaldehyde (ACHO)
  and cell-mediated cytotoxicity, 145, 148-151
  immune response to, 333-339
  and Kupffer cell function, 256, 257, 259, 261
  and mitogenesis, 158-161
  and natural killer activity, 165-171
  and T-lymphocytes, 157-158, 295
Acetaldehyde/protein adducts, 333-339
Acetate, effect of on T-cells, 295
Acetic acid, effect of on mitogenesis, 159
Acetyl-CoA, and ethanol metabolism, 114
Acquired immunodeficiency syndrome. *See* AIDS/HIV infection
Acrodermatitis enteropathica, 424
ACTH (corticotropin), ethanol effect on, 314, 316, 317
Adducts, acetaldehyde/protein, as immunogens, 333-339
Adolescents, alcohol use and sexual risk-taking in, 11-18
Adrenals, ethanol effect on, 317
AIDS/HIV infection
  and alcohol use or abuse, 33, 35, 69-71, 94, 161, 211, 218, 221, 229, 231, 267, 383
    in adolescents, 15
    CNS effects of, 57-64
    in homosexuals, 32, 284, 351
    incidence in, 69-70
    and modulation of CD4(+) cells, 267-270
    prevention approaches, 44
  and auditory brainstem response, 60-64
  and azidothymidine (AZT)
    in animal model, 296
    reduced effectiveness of, 232-237
  beta-carotene supplements in, 293
  and cancer risk, 285
  central nervous system effect of, 57-58, 60-61
  cofactors in, 94-95, 123, 284, 351, 413
  and drug abuse, 69-71, 94-95, 231, 308, 413
  in heterosexuals, 21-22
  and immune dysfunction, 70, 123
    pathogenesis of, 397-398
  incidence of, 284
  and Kaposi's sarcoma, 93, 96-99
  lymphocytes' role in, 161, 229
  malnutrition as co-factor in, 403, 410
  M. avium infection in, 383
  mechanism of infection, 351-352
  murine model of, 287-290
  and nitrate inhalants, 93, 97-99
  nutritional disturbances in, 427
    vitamin/trace metal deficiencies, 421, 426
  pediatric HIV infection
    classification of, 395-396
    diagnosis of, 393-394
    immunological abnormalities in, 397
    prediction of outcome, 394-395

research, methodological issues in, 1-8, 95
transfusion-related, 96
tuberculosis in, 409
tumor necrosis factor level in, 217
zinc deficiency in, 421
see also ARC (AIDS-related complex); HIV (human immunodeficiency virus); Risk-taking behavior
Albumin, reduced clearance of, 341
Alcohol
and auditory brainstem response, 58-60
in HIV infected patients, 61-64
as cofactor in HIV infection, 69-71, 94, 161, 211, 218, 221, 229
interactive effects of alcohol and HIV, 57-64
and modulation of CD4(+) cells, 267-270
correlation of use of with drug use, 105, 107, 108, 231
effect of on immune function, 57, 70-71, 104-107, 123-131, 135, 142, 145, 155, 211-212, 221, 229, 231, 255, 313, 351-352
and nutritional status, 181-188
and receptor modulation, 305-310
role of gastric tissue in, 75-77
fetal exposure to
and immune function, 178, 191-199
and placental transport of IgG, 201-208
and gastric emptying, 242, 252-253
metabolism of, 419, 433
role of zinc in, 441
in methadone treatment group, 109
and nutrient metabolism, 413, 433-434
as part of diet, 87, 89-90, 203-205, 314-317, 419
prenatal exposure to
and IgG transport, 201-208
immune effects of, 178, 191-199
from paternal consumption, 47-54
route of administration of, and varied effects, 314
suppression of tumor necrosis factor by, 211-218
see also Acetaldehyde; Alcoholism; Drinking behavior; Ethanol
Alcohol dehydrogenase (ADH), and ethanol metabolism, 239, 252
Alcoholics/alcoholism
acetaldehyde adduct antigens in, 333, 339
animal model of, 374-375
anorexia in, 419, 423
and carcinogenesis, 283-285
and cellular immunity, 295-296
costs of, 283
diagnosis of, 30-32
and drug abuse, 27, 107-109, 305-309
HIV infection in, 69-70
effect of on interferon system, 123-131
hepatitis B virus in, 67-68
incidence of, 69
and HIV infection, 69-70, 94, 123
hormonal alterations in, 314
immune alterations in , 321-322
incidence of, 321
liver damage in, 161, 255, 263, 342, 346, 419-420
NK cell activities of lymphocytes in, 225-226
nutritional disturbances in, 419-421, 433-435
protein malnutrition, 403, 410
trace metal deficiencies, 423-424, 439-441
vitamin deficiencies, 421-423, 435-439
pancreatitis in, 419
RES depression in, 341
and susceptibility to infection, 135, 142, 255, 341, 373-374, 383
tuberculosis in, 383, 409
see also Drinking behavior
Aldehyde/protein adducts, 335-339
Alveolar macrophages (AM)
and ethanol, 364, 365, 383
after bacterial challenge, 215
effect on superoxide in, 135-143
role of, 211
Anemia
iron-deficiency, 426, 439
megaloblastic, 422, 438, 439
Animal research
of AIDS transmission, 95
murine model of AIDS, 287-290
of opiate immunosuppression, 103-104
see also Mouse; Rat
Anorexia, in alcoholics, 419
and zinc deficiency, 423-424
Anorexia nervosa, 415
Antibodies
to aldehyde/protein adducts, 333-339
crossreactivity of, 337

cellular translocation of, and ethanol exposure, 202
Antibody-dependent cell-mediated cytotoxicity (ADCC)
acetaldehyde effect on, 145, 148
ethanol inhibition of, 145-147, 149-151
recovery of by calcium ionophore, 149-150
Antigen(s)
competitive inhibition studies, 336-337
HLA, 323-325, 327, 330
major histocompatibility complex (MHC), 325
p24 antigen, 268-270, 353
Antigen presenting cell (APC), 323
Arachidonic acid (AA)
and platelet aggregation, 118, 121
and T cell proliferation, 318
ARC (AIDS-related complex), 284
immunostimulation in, 293
Ascorbic acid (vitamin C), deficiency of in alcoholism, 419, 422
Aspirin, and ethanol inhibition of platelet-activating factor, 119, 121
Auditory brainstem response (ABR)
alcohol effect on, 59, 60
and brain temperature, 59-60
HIV effect on, 60-61
and interaction of alcohol and HIV, 61-64
as test of CNS function, 58
Avidin-biotin peroxidase complex (ABC) method, 326
Azidothymidine (AZT), 296
effect of alcohol intake on, 232-237

Bacterial clearance, ethanol inhibition of, 136
B cells
dysfunction of, 104
and HIV antibody, 394
in liver disease, 321, 329
in murine model for AIDS, 288, 289
suppression of proliferative responses in, 224, 229
in zinc deficiency, 440
BCG vaccine, 404, 405
Beta-carotene, 286, 297
ethanol effect on tissue levels of, 80
immune response enhanced by, 285, 293-294
and macrophage secretion of TCF, 85-88
monocyte response to, 79, 83-84, 88
production of, 82
see also Vitamin A
Blood alcohol concentration
and effect of sodium acetate, 239-253
and Kupffer cell function, 258-261
and testing of auditory brainstem response, 63
Blood flow, ethanol effect on, 343, 345, 346
Blood transfusions, and AIDS-related Kaposi's sarcoma, 96
Bovine serum albumin (BSA), aldehyde adducts on, 334-337
Brain temperature, and ABR latencies, 59-60
Bronchoalveolar lavage (BAL), and alcohol effect on tumor necrosis factor, 212-216
Bulimia, 415
Butanol, effect of on mitogenesis, 159
Butyraldehyde adducts, 335, 336

Calcitriol, 436-437; *see also* Vitamin D
Calcium
decreased levels in alcholics, 436
intracellular mobilization of, 136-142
reversal of ADCC inhibition by, 149-151
Cancer
in AIDS patients, 284-285
alcohol-related, 283-284, 287
animal models of, 294
and dietary supplementation, 286, 291-294
epidemiology of, 283-284
and immune response, 359-368
types of, 359
esophageal, 284, 287-290, 359-368
in immune deficiency, 366
and NK activity, 367
and retrovirus infection, 287-289, 296
Canthaxanthin, 285, 286, 291-294, 297
effects of supplementation, 436
Carbohydrate metabolism, alcohol effect on, 373, 378
Carbon tetrachloride, and liver damage, 256, 263
Carotenoids, and immune competence, 435-436; *see also* Beta-carotene; Canthaxanin; Vitamin A
Catabolic response, in morphine use, 414
Catecholamines
and immune responsiveness, 53
and lymphocyte activity, 273, 280
CD4 cells, 106, 108-109, 355

in alcoholic liver disease, 321, 322, 327, 330
and HIV infection, 267, 270, 308, 352, 397, 398
CD8 cells, 330, 352
ratio of to CD4 cells, 322, 327, 397
role of in resistance to HIV, 356
Cell-mediated cytotoxicity
antibody-dependent, 145-151
and Kupffer cells, 262-263
see also Cytotoxicity
Cell-mediated immunity
alcohol effect on, 70, 173, 285, 295-296, 313, 364-366, 383, 441-442
in liver disease, 321-330
prenatal alcohol exposure to, 51
in HIV infection, 410
in iron deficiency, 426
and resistance to tuberculosis infection, 403
retinoid effect on, 436
stimulation of, 293
Cell membranes, effect of drug abuse on, 309
Cellular physiology, ethanol effect on, 270
CEM cells, and alcohol effect on HIV infection, 267-270
Center for Disease Control (CDC), classification of HIV infection, 395-396
Central nervous system (CNS)
alcohol and HIV effects on, 57-58
and auditory brainstem response, 59-64
effect of on immunity, 53
Chemotaxis, reduction of following alcohol treatment, 75-77
Children, HIV infection in
classification of, 395-396
diagnosis of, 393-394
immunological abnormalities in, 397
prediction of outcome, 394-395
Cigarette smoking
and beta carotene, 293, 435
demographic characteristics of, 127
and interferon levels, 124-131
see also Tobacco
Cirrhosis
biopsy results, vs. hepatitis, 327, 328
and ethanol in diet, 421
and folate deficiency, 438
immunosuppression in, 155, 160-161, 295-296
incidence of, 321
see also Liver disease
Cocaine
and alcohol use, 105, 107, 108
and E-rosette formation, 307
nutritional effects of abuse of, 415, 416
Cognitive impairment, alcohol induced, 16
Colloidal carbon, ethanol effect on, 260, 262
Concanavalin A (Con A)
ethanol inhibition of, 140-143, 321-322
and lymphocyte proliferation, 316
morphine effect on, 274, 275
Condoms, use or nonuse of, 15, 24, 25, 39, 44
Contraceptive behavior, and alcohol use, 11, 15, 39-40, 43
Copper
in alcoholism and liver disease, 424
deficiency of, 426
Corticosteroids
and ethanol induced immunosuppression, 177
and morphine induced immunosuppression, 274, 277-279
Corticotropin (ACTH), ethanol effect on, 314, 316, 317
Corticotropin releasing factor (CRF), ethanol effect on, 314, 316, 317
Cutaneous hypersensitivity. *See* Hypersensitivity, delayed cutaneous
CV 3988, and ethanol, 114-115
Cytokines, 385
ethanol interference with release of, 387
and Kupffer cell function, 262, 263
Cytolytic activity, morphine effect on, 274, 276-279
Cytomegalovirus (CMV), and Kaposi's sarcoma, 96-97
Cytotoxicity, beta-carotene effect on, 80, 81, 83-90, 294; *see also* Cell-mediated cytotoxicity
Cytotoxic-T-lymphocytes (CTL)
and alcoholic liver disease, 322, 328, 329
ethanol inhibition of, 146-148
growth and differentation of, 323
target cell killing by, 324

De novo pathway, 114, 121
Diabetes, and morphine dependence, 414

Diet
alcohol as part of, 87, 89-90, 203-205, 314-317, 374-375, 419, 433
carotenoids as immunostimulants, 79-90, 285, 286, 291-294, 297
and drug abusers
altered preferences in, 413, 415, 416
nutritional treatment of, 417
effect of fasting on alcohol metabolism, 250-253
and hypermetabolic phase of infection, 375-381
and NK activity, 181-188
and tumor incidence, 364, 368
see also Malnutrition
DiGeorge syndrome, 194-196, 199
Disinhibition, alcohol induced, 16-17, 22, 41
DNA
folate involvement in synthesis of, 422
incorporation of AZT and thymidine into, 237
replicating, and carcinogenesis, 286-287
sperm, alcohol-induced changes in, 52-54
Drinking behavior
in adolescents, 11-18
anticipatory excuse drinking, 17
demographics of, 3, 127
disinhibition model of, 16-17, 22, 41
and drug abuse, 27, 107-109, 305-309
as excuse for unacceptable behavior, 41-42
in homosexual men, 27-33
methodological issues, 1, 3, 11
and sexual activity, 36-39
and sexual risk-taking, 1, 11-18, 21-25, 39-44, 70, 267
See also Alcohol; Alcoholism
Drug abuse
in adolescents, 11
and alcohol use, 27, 107-109, 305-309
in HIV infection, 69-70
as cofactor in AIDS, 93-95, 103-104
difficulty in study of, 94-95
effects of on nutrition, 413-417
and hepatitis infection, 69, 71
and immune function, 103-107, 305-310
laboratory tests for, 95
of nitrate inhalants, and Kaposi's sarcoma, 93, 97-99
polydrug abuse, interactive effects of, 307
questionaires for, 95
see also Alcohol use and abuse

Ear-canal temperature, alcohol effect on, 60, 63
Effector/target cell ratios, morphine effect on, 276, 277
Endocrine hormones, and immune function, 313-314
Endocytosis, receptor-mediated, 202, 208
Endotoxins
beneficial vs. toxic effects of, 342
and liver disease, 342-343, 346-347
Epithelial tissues, effect of alcohol exposure on, 204-208
Epitope specificity, of acetaldehyde adduct antibodies, 333-339
E-rosette formation
alcohol effect on, 307
in prenatal exposure, 160
cocaine effect on, 307
iron deficiency effect on, 439
and malnutrition in mycobacteria infection, 406, 407
opiate effect on, 306
Esophagus, cancer of
and alcohol consumption, 284, 359
experimentally induced, 287-290, 360-368
Ethanol (ETOH)
acetaldehyde's role in toxicity of, 145
and cell-mediated cytotoxicity, 145-147, 149-151
and cellular immunity, 285, 295-296
circulatory response to, 343, 346
and immune function, 285
and carcinogenesis, 285-287, 292-294, 359-368
HPA axis hormones in, 313-318
mechanisms of suppression, 173-179
and intracellular calcium levels, 138
and Kupffer cell role in liver injury, 255-263, 342-343, 346-347
and LAK cell generation, 223
liver microscopy following acute ingestion of, 341-347
and lymphocytes
and mitogenesis, 155-161
proliferative response of to HIV peptides, 227-228
metabolism of, 252-253
and gastric emptying, 242, 245

by Kupffer cells, 255
and oxydized nucleotides, 239
modulation of platelet-activating factor by, 113-121
and natural killer activity, 165-171, 222-223
response to in target cells, 232-237
and signal transduction, 135-143
and survival of *M. avium* after exposure to, 383-390
see also Alcohol
Exocytosis, 202, 208

Fasting, and alcohol metabolism, 250-253
Fatty foods, drug-abusers preference for, 413, 415, 416
Fetal alcohol exposure
immune effects of, 178, 191-199
from paternal consumption, 47-54
and placental transport of IgG, 201-208
and zinc deficiency, 423
Folate, alcohol-induced deficiency of, 419, 421-422, 438

Gastritis, in alcoholics, 419
Gastrointestinal tissue
acetate effect on alcohol level in, 242, 243, 245, 248, 253
alcohol effects in, 433
and immune function, 75-77
Glucocorticoids
ethanol effect on, 317, 318
and immunosuppression, 274, 277-279, 314
Gluconeogenesis, sepsis-induced increases in, 373-374, 376-377
ethanol prevention of, 373, 378-381
Glucose appearance, increased rates of, 373, 376-380
Glucose metabolism, in heroin users, 414-415
Golgi elements, hypertrophy of, 204, 205
Gp120, and T cell function, 397-398
Gp160, 397
Granular endoplasmic reticulum, alcohol effect on, 204, 205
Granulocyte macrophage colony stimulating factor (GM-CSF), 384, 389-391
Guinea pigs, experimental tuberculosis in, 403-410
Hemophiliacs, 284
CMV infection in, 97
Hepatitis, alcohol-induced
biopsy results, vs. cirrhosis, 327, 328
immune function in, 332, 441-442
incidence of, 321
and Kupffer cell function, 263
see also Liver disease
Hepatitis B virus
and drug abuse, 69, 71
incidence of in alcoholics, 67-69
Heroin, 103
and alcohol use, 105, 107, 108
immunological effects of, 305-306
metabolic effects of, 414-415
Heterosexuals
and AIDS
CMV infection in, 97
and intravenous drug use, 69-70, 103, 305
contraceptive use in, 40
sexual risk-taking by, 21-25, 69-70
HIV (human immunodeficiency virus), 123
alcohol modification of, 211
and hepatitis B virus, 68
research pertaining to, 231, 397-398
survival of in macrophages, 142-143
transmission of, 68
see also AIDS/HIV infection
HIV-1
and CD4 cells, 308
and immune dysfunction, 104
HIV antibody, 394
HIV peptides, lymphocyte proliferative responses to, 227-229
HL-60 cells, biochemical changes in after ethanol treatment, 231-237
HLA antigens, 323-325
in alcoholic liver, 325, 327, 330
HLA-DR5 phenotype, 96
Homeostasis, PAF synthesis in, 114
Homosexual men
alcohol use or abuse in, 1, 27-33
vs. that of heterosexuals, 28
and risk of AIDS, 32, 284, 351
and unsafe sexual behavior, 39-40, 42
Kaposi's sarcoma in, 96
nitrate inhalant use in, 97
HTLVI/II infection, and immune dysfunction, 104
HuIFN-Ĩ, 125, 128-129
HuIFN-Ì, 125, 129
Human immunodeficiency virus. *See* HIV
Hypergammaglobulinemia, 397
Hyperglycemia, morphine-induced, 413-414
Hypermetabolism, sepsis-induced, 376-377
Hypersensitivity, delayed cutaneous
in dietary deficiencies, 425, 439, 440

in prenatal alcohol exposure, 198
Hypogammaglobulinemia, 397
Hypogonadism, in alcoholics, 423
Hypothalamic-pituitary-adrenal axis
and ethanol effect on immune function, 313-318
and opiate receptors, 273
Hypothalamus, ethanol effect on ACTH and CRF, 314, 316
Hypothermia, and alcohol, 59, 380

Imipramine, and reversal of effect of prenatal alcohol exposure, 50-51
Immobility response, in alcohol-sired rats, 49-50
Immune function
and alcohol-induced organ damage, 333
alcohol interference with, 142, 161, 165, 284-285, 351
and carcinogenesis, 294-295, 359, 366-367
in chronic alcohol use, 123-131, 145, 155, 255, 441-442
in drug users, 105-109
due to fetal exposure, 178, 191-199
in hepatitis, 322
and HPA axis hormones, 313-318
and malnutrition, 181-182, 419-420
mechanisms of suppression, 173-179, 322-323
alveolar macrophage in, 135, 211
assays of, 290
and cigarette smoking, 126-131
CNS influcence on, 53
and dietary supplementation, 285, 286, 291-294, 297, 410, 436, 438
and drug use, 103-109, 305-310, 414, 415
and E-rosetting, 306-307
in HIV infection, 70, 123, 397-398
and IgG transport, 201-202
interferons in, 123-124
morphine effect on, 273-280
and nutritional disturbances, 420, 424-427, 434-441
and retrovirus, 285, 292-294
and stress reactivity, 53
T-cells in regulation of, 308, 309
see also Cell-mediated immunity; Infections; Interferons; Surveillance system
Immunoglobulin G (IgG)
alcohol effect on placental transport of, 201-208
and T cell function in malnutrition, 404, 410
Immunoglobulin M (IgM), 404
and retroviral infection, 296
Immunomodulators, effect on tumor cell cytotoxic activity, 79-80, 82, 88-90; *see also* Interferons
Immunostimulants, carotenoids as, 79-90, 285, 286, 291-294, 297
Infants, HIV infection in, 393-394
Infections
hypermetabolism in, 373-377
alcohol effect on, 377-381
susceptibility to
alcohol-induced, 135, 142, 255, 341, 373-374, 383
and gastric-derived immunosuppressors, 77
morphine effect on, 89
and prenatal alcohol consumption, 50-51
secondary, 211-212 , 216
See also Immune function
Inflammation, PAF synthesis in, 114
Insulin, in heroin and morphine users, 414-415
Intercellular-adhesion molecule (ICAM), 324, 330
Interferons
in alcoholics and cigarette smokers, 123-131
alpha (HuIFN-α), 125, 128-129
effect of ethanol on cellular response to, 235, 237
gamma (HuIFN-γ) 125, 129
and meclomen, 131
morphine efect on, 89
and natural killer activity, 166-167, 170
Interleukin(s)
in alcoholic liver disease, 325, 330
and growth and differentiation of CTLs, 323
Interleukin-1 (IL-1), stimulated production of, 293-294
Interleukin-2 (IL-2)
and ethanol effect on immune function, 175, 177-179
in PMBC, 353, 354
Intrauterine growth (IUG) retardation, and fetal ethanol exposure, 195

Iron
alcohol-induced deficiency of, 423, 426, 439
in gastritis, 419
and immune function, 439

Kaposi, Moriz, 95
Kaposi's sarcoma (KS)
AIDS-related, 96-99, 284, 285
classical, 95, 96
and drug abuse, 94
and nitrate inhalant abuse, 93, 97-99
Kennedy-Wise pathway, 114
Klebsiella pneumonia, 212-215
Kupffer cells
and alcoholic liver disease, 341-342
effect of ethanol on, 255-262, 391
phagocytic function, 343-347
recovery of, 263

Laboratory tests, for drug abuse, 95
Lactate, plasma, 378
chronic alcohol effect on, 379, 380
Large granular lymphocytes (LGL), and natural killer activity, 167, 171, 222
Leukocytes, typing of, 308
Leukoplakia, oral, 293
Leukotriene B_4 (LTB-4), 263
Leukotrienes, and T cell proliferation, 318
Lipopolysaccharide (LPS), 216, 387, 390
Listeria monocytogenes, 385, 390
Liver, 434
alcohol effect on
blood flow changes, 346
vitamin deficiencies, 421-423
biopsies of, 325-328
in vivo microscopy of, 341-347
Liver disease
and alcohol use, 161, 255, 263, 342, 346
cell-mediated immunity in, 321-330
and endotoxins, 342
impaired mitogen response in, 155, 160, 295-296
NK cells in, 108, 181
and nutritional deficiencies, 421-424, 435, 436
pathogenesis of, 322-323
role for Kupffer cells in, 255-264, 341-342
see also Cirrhosis; Hepatitis
Locomotor activity, effect of fetal alcohol exposure on, 49-50
LP-BM5 virus, 80, 287-289, 293
Lymphocyte activated killer (LAK) cells, 321
Lymphocyte blastogenesis, in study of immune system, 314
Lymphocyte function-associated (LFA) antigens, 324
Lymphocyte phenotypes, correlations with alcohol use, 106
Lymphocyte proliferative responses
alcohol effect on, 224, 229, 315-316
in children with HIV infections, 397
and HIV peptides, 227-228
influence of virus proteins on, 398
in mycobacterial infection, 406
Lymphocytes
alcohol effect on, 89, 155-162, 352, 366
carotenoid and retinoid effect on, 436
catecholamine effect on, 53
large granular (LGL), 222-223
mitogenesis of, 157, 160
morphine effect on, 89, 273-280
mouse, ethanol effect on, 145-147, 151
prenatal exposure, 191-199
NK activity of, 221-223, 225-226
subpopulations of, 156-158
susceptibility of to HIV infection, 267
see also T-cells
Lymphoid cells
canthaxanthin effect on, 291
vitamin A effect on, 292
Lymphokine activated killer (LAK) cell activity, alcohol effect on, 221-223, 229
Lymphokines, 403
Lysosomes, primary, 204, 205

Macrophage(s)
alcohol-induced defect of, 70-71, 135, 211, 262
and AIDS, 211
dietary stimulation of, 84-90, 293-294
and glucose homeostasis, 374, 381
PAF synthesis in cell line, 114-121
survival of *M. avium* in after ethanol exposure, 383-390
and vitamin C deficiency, 439
see also Alveolar macrophages (AM); Kupffer cells
Magnesium, deficiency of
alcohol-induced, 424, 440
immune function, 426-427
Major histocompatibility complex (MHC) antigens, 325, 339
Malnutrition/nutritional disturbances

in AIDS patients, 403, 410, 427
in alcoholism, 419-421, 433-435
trace metal deficiencies, 423-424, 439-441
vitamin deficiencies, 421-423, 435-439
in drug abuse, 413-416
treatment of effects of, 417
and immune function, 403, 424-427, 434-435, 441
effects of single nutrients on, 420
and impaired resistence to experimental tuberculosis, 403-410
and NK cell activity, 181-188
protein, and resistence to experimental tuberculosis, 403-410
Meclomen, 131
Metabolic clearance (MCR), sepsis-induced increase in, 373, 376
alcohol effect on, 377
Metabolism
of alcohol, 419, 433
effect of fasting on, 250-253
role of zinc in, 441
in infections, 376-377
role of liver in, 434
Metals, trace, deficiencies of, 423-424, 439-441
Methadone, and immune system, 103, 104, 108-109
Methanol, effect of on lymphocytes and mitogenesis, 158, 159
Methylbenzylnitrosamine (NMB_ZA), and ethanol effect on esophageal lesions, 287, 360-363, 367
Michigan Alcohol Screen Test (MAST), 124, 127
Microscopy, of liver in vivo after ethanol ingestion, 341-347
Mink cell focus (MCF) murine type C retrovirus, 288
Mitochondria, alcohol-induced changes in, 204, 205
Mitogenesis
impairment of by alcohol, 155-161, 175-176, 295-296
and risk of AIDS, 161
and vitamin C deficiency, 439
Monoclonal antibodies, 308
and aldehyde/protein adducts, 333, 339
Monocytes
beta-carotene stimulation of, 79, 83-84, 88
calcitriol-induced changes in, 436
as targets for HIV, 352
Mononuclear leukocytes
alcohol effect on, 224, 225
and HIV peptides, 227-228
Morphine
effect of on tumor cell cytotoxicity, 83-86, 89
and E-rosette formation, 306
immunosuppressive effects of, 80, 273-280
nutritional effects of, 413-414, 416
treatment of, 417
Mouse
alcohol effect on cell-mediated cytotoxicity in, 145-151
beta-carotene effect on cytotoxicity in, 79-90
canthaxanthin immunostimulation in, 285-293
prenatal exposure to ethanol in, 191-199
Murine L929S leukemia cells, 81, 83
Murine LP-BM5 retrovirus
beta-carotene stimulation of, 85-88
as model for AIDS, 287-289
Murine macrophages, 80
beta-carotene stimulation of, 84-85, 88
Mycobacteria, in macrophages, 142
Mycobacterium avium complex (MAC)
in AIDS patients, 383
ethanol effect on survival of, 384-390
Mycobacterium tuberculosis
experimentally induced infection with, 404-405
and protein malnutrition, 406-409

Naloxone
and E-rosette formation, 306
reversal of morphine-induced salt preference by, 413
Naltrexone, and lymphocyte proliferation, 275-279
Natural killer (NK) cells
alcohol effect on, 106, 130, 131, 221-223
acetaldehyde, 148, 165-171
ethanol, 146-147, 165-171, 295
in liver of alcoholics, 321, 322, 329
in lymphocytes of alcoholics, 225-226
and nutritional factors, 181-188, 293
various alcohols, 157, 158
and cigarette smoking, 130, 131

morphine effect on, 274-279
opioid effect on, 309
and resistance to cancer, 367
in zinc deficiency, 425, 440
Neural cell adhesion molecule (NCAM), 324
Neural crest, 194-195
Neutrophils
alcohol effect on, 71, 75-77, 383
in iron deficiency, 426
and superoxide production, 136, 142
Nicotine. *See* Tobacco
Night blindness, in alcoholics, 423
Nitrate inhalants, and Kaposi's sarcoma, 93, 97-99
Nitrosamines
and ethanol effect on esophageal lesions, 287, 360-363, 365, 367, 368
in tobacco, 365
Non-Hodgkin's lymphona, and drug abuse, 93, 94
Nucleotides, oxidized (NAD), in ethanol metabolism, 239, 253
Nutrition. *See* Diet; Malnutrition

Opiate receptors, stimulation of, 273, 279
Opiates, immunological effects of, 305-310; *see also* Heroin

Pancreatitis
in alcoholics, 419
immunosuppression in, 295-296
Parenchymal cell, alcohol-induced alterations in, 255, 261
PDP (tuberculin), 404
effect of diet on skin reaction, 407
and protein malnutrition, 406, 410
PDP-specific lymphocyte functions, 406, 408, 410
Peptides, HIV, lymphocyte proliferative responses to, 227-229
Periaqueductal gray, morphine effect on, 279
Peripheral blood mononuclear cells (PBMC), 157, 159, 227, 228
alcohol effect on HIV replication in, 352-356
Phagocytosis
by alveolar macrophages, 364-365
ethanol effect on, 117, 120, 364, 365, 385
dose-related variance in, 346-347
by Kupffer cells, 255-259, 261
and vitamin C deficiency, 439
Phorbol ester (PMA), 136
ethanol inhibition of, 140-143
Phytohemagglutinin (PHA), 104, 106, 107
ethanol effect on, 315
Pituitary, ethanol effect on ACTH in, 314, 316
Pituitary hormones, and morphine effect on lymphocytes, 280
Placental transport, of IgG
alcohol effect on, 201-208
in-vitro and *in-vivo* models of, 205
Plasma alcohol level (PAL)
effect of sodium acetate on, 243-247
effect of potassium butytrate on, 249
and ethanol metabolism, 250-253
Plasma membrane microviscosity, ethanol effect on, 257, 260, 261
Platelet-activating factor (PAF), ethanol modulation of, 113-121
Pneumonia, in AIDS patients, 211-212
Pokeweed mitogen (PWM), 104, 106, 107, 316
Poly-IC
as IFN inducer, 167, 170
influence of on NK activity, 165-166, 169, 170
Polymerase chain reaction (PCR), 394
Polymorphonuclear leukocytes (PMN), alcohol suppression of, 215-218
Potassium butyrate, and gastric emptying, 245, 249, 253
Pregnancy
alcohol use during
immune effects of, 178, 191-199
and placental transport of IgG, 201-208
and zinc deficiency, 423
and pediatric HIV infection, 393-395
Primates, nonhuman, absence of HIV related abnormalities in, 288
Propanol, effect of on lymphocytes and mitogenesis, 158, 159
Prostaglandin E_1 (PGE_1), 262
Prostaglandin E_2 (PGE_2), 262-263
Protein kinase C, 136, 137, 391
Protein malnutrition
in alcoholism and HIV infection, 403, 409-410
experimentally induced, 404-409
Pseudomonas aeruginosa, susceptibility to, and paternal alcohol consumption, 50-51

Pyridoxal phosphate (vitamin B_6), alcohol-induced deficiency, 422, 426

Randomized response technique (RRT)
  and sample size, 3-9
  unrelated question model, 2-3
  Warner model, 2
Rat
  alcohol-related cancers induced in, 359-368
  Kupffer cells' role in liver injury in, 255-263
  as model of chronic alcoholism, 374-375
  natural killer activity in, 165-171
  paternal alcohol exposure in, 47-52
  placental transport of IgG in, 201-208
  and sepsis-induced hypermetabolism, 375-381
  signal transduction in, 135-143
  suppression of tumor necrosis factor in, 212-216
Receptor function, ethanol effect on response to interferon, 237
Receptor modulation, alcohol and drug effect on, 305-310
Reticuloendothelial function
  ethanol effect on, 341
  and glucose homeostasis, 374
Retinoids, and immune competence, 435-436; *see also* Vitamin A
Retinyl palmitate, 80-81, 285, 286, 291-294, 297; *see also* Vitamin A
Retrovirus infection
  animal model of, 287-289
  and beta-carotene stimulation of cytotoxicity, 85-90
  ethanol effect on, 161
Risk-taking behavior
  and alcohol consumption, 39-44, 70, 267
    in adolescents, 11-18
  and drug abuse, 1, 94
  See also Sexual behavior, risky
RNA virus, and activation of HIV infection, 352
Rosettes. *See* E-rosette formation

Salt, intake of in morphine users, 413
Selenium
  in alcoholics, 424
  and immune function, 426
  and integrity of cell structures, 437
Sepsis. *See* Infections
Serotonin, and immune responsiveness, 53
Sexual behavior
  in adolescents, 11, 15, 36
  alcohol effect on, 21-25, 36-44, 70, 267
  and drug abuse, 1, 94
  risky, 39-44
    disinhibition model of, 16-17, 22, 41
    in heterosexuals, 21-25, 69-70
    in homosexual men, 39, 40
    methodological issues about, 1, 11, 21
Signal transduction, ethanol effect on, 135-143
Sinusoids, ethanol effect on blood flow in, 343, 345, 346
Smoking. *See* Cigarette smoking
Sodium acetate, and ethanol metabolism, 239-253
Soluble immune response suppressor (SIRS), alcohol depression of synthesis of, 354-355
Speedball, and alcohol use, 105, 107, 108
Sperm, alcohol effect on, 47, 48, 423
  and DNA alteration, 52-54
Spleen
  alcohol effect on, 295
    and dietary variations, 183-185, 188, 361, 365
    mechanism of action, 176, 177
    and NK activity, 165-171, 183-185
  morphine effect on, 274-279
  in retroviral infection, 85, 296
Squamous cell carcinomas, 284-285
Staphyloccus aureus, 212-215
Stress reactivity
  effect of paternal alcohol consumption on, 49-50
  and immune function, 53
Superoxide, ethanol effect on, 135-138, 140-142, 391
Surveillance system
  and cancer, 366
  and Kaposi's sarcoma, 285
Surveys
  and drug-abuse research, 95
  randomized response techniques of, 2-9
  sample sizes in, 3-9
Syncytium formation, as measure of HIV replication, 352, 353
2-5A Synthetase, and receptor function, 235-237

T-cells
activation of, 293
alcohol effect on, 155-161, 295, 307, 442
mechanism of effect, 318
beta-carotene effect on, 436
in drug abusers, 305-310
and E-rosetting, 306, 307
helper vs. suppressor cells, 441
and immunoresponsiveness, 308, 309, 352, 410
in malnutrition, 403-410
mechanism of impairment of, 175-179
in nutritional deficiencies, 439
and pathogenesis of immune dysfunction in HIV infection, 397-398
responsiveness of to alcoholic hyalin, 323
retroviral effect on, 288-292
suppression of proliferative responses in, 224, 229
and vitamin E levels, 437
in zinc deficiency states, 424, 425, 440
see also Cell-mediated immunity; Cytotoxic-T-lymphocytes
Temperature, alcohol effect on, 59-60, 380
Teratogens, alcohol effect on thymus, 191-199
Thiamin (vitamin B_1), alcohol-induced deficiency in, 422, 436
and magnesium, 440
Thymidine, effect of alcohol intake on, 233-237
Thymosin alpha-1 (TA-1), paternal alcohol effect on, 51, 52
Thymulin, and zinc deficiency, 425, 426
Thymus
CNS control over, 53
ethanol efect on, 176, 177, 315, 317, 365
prenatal exposure, 191-199
and malnutrition, 404
Tobacco
nitrosamines in, 294, 365
and nutritional status, 413
see also Cigarette smoking
Trace metals, deficiencies of, 423-424, 439-441
Transferrin, and iron supplementation, 426
Transplantation, and malignancy, 366
Tuberculin. *See* PDP (tuberculin)
Tuberculin skin reaction, effect of diet on, 407
Tuberculosis
in alcoholism, 383, 409
experimentally induced, 404-410
in HIV infection, 409
malnutrition and immune impairment in, 403, 410
Tumor cell line, morphine effect on, 276
Tumor cytotoxic factor (TCF), and beta-carotene, 83-90, 294
Tumor necrosis factor (TNF)
alcohol suppression of, 212-214, 216, 218, 346
and intracellular survival of *M. avium*, 384, 388-390
beta-carotene stimulation of, 79
in HIV infection, 217
release of from Kupffer cells, 342

Virus
gp120, and T cell function, 397, 398
gp160, 397
Vitamin A
in alcohol users, 421, 435
function of, 421
and immune function, 427, 435
as stimulant of, 88-89, 285, 286, 291-294, 297, 436
role of zinc in metabolism of, 441
in smokers, 435
supplementation of, 436
Vitamin B_1(thiamin), deficiency of in alcoholism, 422, 431, 437
and magnesium, 440
Vitamin B_2, deficiency of in alcoholism, 437
Vitamin B_6, deficiency of in alcoholism, 422, 431, 438
Vitamin B_{12}, deficiency of in alcoholism, 419, 438
Vitamin C (ascorbic acid), deficiency of in alcoholism, 422, 427, 431, 439
Vitamin D
and cellular proliferation, 427
deficiency in alcoholics, 436-437
Vitamin D_3, in alcoholics, 436-437
Vitamin E, 424, 437
and selenium deficiency, 426

Wernicke-Korsakoff syndrome, 422
Western Blot profile, 393

YAC target cells, 276
Yolk-sac epithelial tissues, effect of alcohol
exposure on, 204-208

Zinc
deficiency of, 424-426
alcohol-induced, 440-441
role of in immune function, 440
and vitamin A metabolism, 441
Zymosan, 116, 117, 120